Wrestling with Behavioral Genetics

Wrestling with Behavioral Genetics

Science, Ethics, and Public Conversation

Edited by

Erik Parens
Senior Research Scholar, The Hastings Center
Garrison, New York

Audrey R. Chapman
Director, Dialogue on Science, Ethics and Religion
American Association for the Advancement of Science
Washington, D.C.

and

Nancy Press
Professor, School of Nursing
Oregon Health and Sciences University
Portland, Oregon

The Johns Hopkins University Press
Baltimore

© 2006 The Johns Hopkins University Press
All rights reserved. Published 2006
Printed in the United States of America on acid-free paper
9 8 7 6 5 4 3 2 1

The Johns Hopkins University Press
2715 North Charles Street
Baltimore, Maryland 21218-4363
www.press.jhu.edu

Library of Congress Cataloging-in-Publication Data

Wrestling with behavioral genetics : science, ethics, and public
conversation / edited by Erik Parens, Audrey R. Chapman, and
Nancy Press.
        p. ; cm.
    Includes bibliographical references and index.
    ISBN 0-8018-8224-9 (hardcover : alk. paper)
    1. Behavior genetics—Popular works.
    [DNLM: 1. Genetics, Behavioral.   2. Genetics, Behavioral—
ethics. QH 457 W945 2005]   I. Parens, Erik, 1957–   II. Chapman, Audrey R.   III. Press, Nancy, 1947–
    QH457.W747 2005
    155.7—dc22   2005006475

A catalog record for this book is available from the British
Library.

With admiration and gratitude to our wise mentor,
V. Elving Anderson,
who did not always agree with us, but always helped us.

Contents

Contributors

Jonathan Beckwith, Ph.D., American Cancer Society Professor, Department of Microbiology and Molecular Genetics, Harvard Medical School, Boston, Massachusetts

Dan W. Brock, Ph.D., Professor of Medical Ethics, Harvard Medical School, Boston, Massachusetts

Celeste Condit, Ph.D., Research Professor, Department of Speech Communication, University of Georgia, Athens, Georgia

Troy Duster, Ph.D., Professor of Sociology and Director, Institute for the Study of Social Change, University of California at Berkeley, Berkeley, California

Harold Edgar, LL.B, Julius Silver Professor of Law, Science and Technology and Director of the Julius Silver Program in Law, Science, and Technology, Columbia Law School, New York, New York

Leonard Fleck, Ph.D., Professor of Philosophy, Center for Ethics and Humanities, Michigan State University, East Lansing, Michigan

Tina Harris, Ph.D., Assistant Professor, Department of Speech Communication, University of Georgia, Athens, Georgia

Steven E. Hyman, M.D., Ph.D., Professor of Neurobiology, Harvard University, Cambridge, Massachusetts

Gregory E. Kaebnick, Ph.D., Editor, *Hastings Center Report,* and Associate for Philosophical Studies, The Hastings Center, Garrison, New York

Roxanne Parrott, Ph.D., Professor of Communications Arts and Sciences, Pennsylvania State University, Hershey, Pennsylvania

Kenneth F. Schaffner, M.D., Ph.D., University Professor of History and Philosophy of Science, University of Pittsburgh

Eric Turkheimer, Ph.D., Professor, Department of Psychology, University of Virginia, Charlottesville, Virginia

Robert Wachbroit, Ph.D., Research Scholar, Institute for Philosophy and Public Policy, University of Maryland, College Park, Maryland

Rick Weiss, M.A., Staff Writer, *Washington Post,* Washington, D.C.

Acknowledgments

This book is one product of a large project undertaken by The Hastings Center and the American Association for the Advancement of Science (AAAS) and funded by the Ethical, Legal, and Social Implications (ELSI) division of the National Human Genome Research Institute. Two people who were involved from the beginning of the grant application process deserve special mention. Mark Frankel, director of the Scientific Freedom, Responsibility and Law Program (at AAAS), led our initiative to hold a public meeting about behavioral genetics in 2003 at AAAS; he also took the lead on shepherding Catherine Baker's primer on behavioral genetics (available at www.aaas.org/spp/bgenes/publications.shtml) through to publication. V. Elving Anderson, professor emeritus of genetics at the University of Minnesota, helped us at every step, from writing the grant application to planning the meetings. We could not have done this project without Elving's tireless, erudite, and wise advice. All of us who participated in this project owe Elving a great debt of gratitude.

The project steering committee, consisting of Mark, Elving, Catherine, and this volume's three editors, was part of a larger working group, which included Jonathan Beckwith (Harvard Medical School), Dan W. Brock (Harvard Medical School), Troy Duster (New York University and University of California–Berkeley), Harold Edgar (Columbia University School of Law), Lee Ehrman (State University of New York), Marcus Feldman (Stanford University), Leonard Fleck (Michigan State University), Irving Gottesman (University of Minnesota), Bruce Jennings (The Hastings Center), Gregory E. Kaebnick (The Hastings Center), Patricia King (Georgetown University Law Center), Yvette Miller (American Red Cross), Thomas H. Murray (The Hastings Center), Karen Porter (Brooklyn Law School), Kenneth F. Schaffner (George Washington University), Robert Wachbroit (University of Maryland), and Rick Weiss (*Washington Post*). This volume never would have come into being if it were not for the conscientious efforts of the entire working group.

When we did not have the expertise we needed within the working group, we sought and received the help of a distinguished roster of consultants, including Greg Carey (University of Colorado), Celeste Condit (University of Georgia), Carl Elliott (University of Minnesota), Elliot Gershon (University of Chicago), John Holmfeld (Science Policy Research), Steven E. Hyman (Harvard University), Kay Redfield Jamison (Johns Hopkins University), Toby Jayaratne (University of Michigan), Robert F. Krueger (University of Minnesota), Karen Lebacqz (Pacific School of Religion), John Loehlin (University of Texas), David Lubinski (Vanderbilt University), Jonathan Marks (University of North Carolina at Charlotte), Matt McGue (University of Minnesota), Sue Levi-Pearl (Tourette Syndrome Association), Jo C. Phelan (Columbia University), John Rice (Washington University), Janice Robinson (Grace Episcopal Church), Margo Smith (Depression and Related Affective Disorders Association), Eric Turkheimer (University of Virginia), and Irwin Waldman (Emory University).

We were joined at one of our working group meetings by members of the United Kingdom's Nuffield Council, which has explored similar questions: Tom Baldwin, Martin Bobrow, Tor Lezmore, Yvonne Melia, Paul Pharoah, Martin Richards, and Sandy Thomas. Not only did we benefit from their comments at our meeting, but we benefited from the superb report they published in 2002: *Genetics and Human Behaviour: The Ethical Context* (London: Nuffield Council on Bioethics).

Administering such a complicated grant isn't always easy. We are deeply grateful to Joy Boyer at the ELSI office for her always thoughtful and kind support of our work. We also want to thank Vicki Peyton at The Hastings Center, who has cheerfully and carefully helped us with the technical aspects of bringing this volume of essays together.

Finally, we want to thank Wendy Harris at the Johns Hopkins University Press, who, from the start of our research project, supported our effort to create this book. Without Wendy's care and patience, this volume would not now be in your hands.

Introduction

Nancy Press, Audrey R. Chapman, and Erik Parens

Hardly a month goes by without a media report that researchers have discovered the "gene for" some complex human behavior or trait. One month it's "intelligence," the next it's "language" or "dyslexia" or "novelty seeking" or "shyness" or "homosexuality." The array and conceptual span of these behaviors is so stunning that it can be difficult for a reader to comprehend the rubric—behavioral genetics—that is supposed to encompass all this scientific activity.

In addition, people who study behavioral genetics come from a wide variety of disciplinary backgrounds, including molecular genetics, psychology, and medicine. Though their disciplinary backgrounds differ, they share the aim of investigating how genes influence individual variation in human traits and patterns of behavior. As the field has developed, in addition to studying how genes help to explain why individuals appear and act differently, behavioral geneticists increasingly study how genes interact with environments to create such differences.

Because the methods and aims of behavioral genetics are so heterogeneous and complex, communicating about (and even within) the field can be difficult. It is not surprising that many of the field's more complex debates and findings never find their way into the larger public conversation. When findings from behavioral genetics do appear in the popular media, they are too often couched in the "gene for" language, which implies that a single gene has been isolated and can explain why some of us are risk takers, or can't read well, or are shy. Sometimes such "gene for" language is just shorthand for a complex idea that reporters lack the room to explain. And sometimes it's hype to help make some small step in the daily work of normal science sound dramatic. Unfortunately, overglamorizing the findings' significance , or underreporting their complexity, can allow even educated readers to imagine that there is no need to wrestle with the field of behavioral genetics.

In fact, of all the new lines of inquiry that have grown out of genetics, behavioral genetics may be the most germane to the day-to-day life of individuals and communities. Behavioral genetics raises questions about human behavior that concern us all: What is normal? How should we think about the great range of variation among individuals with respect to most complex traits? How should we understand the ways that humans, as opposed to other animals, react to, are shaped by, and, in turn, affect their environments? Are traits with strong genetic underpinnings really less malleable than those heavily shaped by the environment? The answers to these questions have the potential to influence how we think about free will, guilt and innocence, as well as equality and distributive justice.

Behavioral genetics is clearly anything but arcane. It concerns matters of great societal and individual importance, and it is a branch of science that has brought significant good. By helping us to understand, for example, that genes contribute to many of the most severe mental illnesses, behavioral genetics has provided relief to parents who no longer need to blame themselves for their children's illnesses. The field's important and ultimate ambition is to find better treatments, if not cures, for those same illnesses. Yet because behavioral genetics is so tightly linked with major areas of personal and social life, its findings—or at least pernicious interpretations of them—also have the power to do great harm by, for example, bolstering a belief that differences in educational attainment between groups are genetic, unalterable, and so need not be addressed through social measures.

Besides the complex mix of good and bad results that grows out of the science, the science itself is complex and thus poses a set of conceptual and mathematical challenges to nonscientists. To make things more complicated still, there is considerable internal contention within the field itself over core concepts and the potential limits to what can be learned using its methods. This makes it difficult for even the most educated layperson to know what methods and findings to trust, much less to understand what those findings mean for how we think about who we are.

For all these reasons, The Hastings Center and the American Association for the Advancement of Science (AAAS) sought to create tools to help members of the general public to understand and discuss behavioral genetic science and the implications of that science—tools that would make it easier to sift through media reports to separate the kernel of important finding from the chaff of sensationalist reporting.

With a generous grant from the Ethical, Legal, and Social Implications program at the National Human Genome Research Institute (RO1 HG001873), The Hastings Center and the AAAS brought together a group of scientists and humanists from various disciplines and launched a three-year multidisciplinary project to explore the methods, findings, and implications of behavioral genetics. (For a lengthy report on the project and a synopsis of its findings, see Erik Parens, "Genetic Differences and Human Identities: On Why Talking about Behavioral Genetics Is Important and Difficult," *Hastings Center Report Special Supplement* 34, no. 1 [2004], available at www.thehastingscenter.org.)

Most of the contributors to this volume were members of the project's working group, and the others served as consultants at one or more meetings. The chapters are intended to help readers to evaluate better what behavioral geneticists have and have not found, the benefits that may accrue from such research, the concerns it may raise, and the implications it may have for how we think about who we are. The chapters are also intended to help readers to discern and assess for themselves claims they hear and read about developments in behavioral genetics.

Conversations and Contributions

To better understand the structure and content of the volume, we believe it helps to have a sense of the conversations out of which it grew. Although the chapters appear separate and bounded, each emerged out of the interactions among project participants. Individual chapters were polished as one author's ideas rubbed up against the views of others in the group, sometimes long after the last project meeting ended. Even if that rubbing was in the end always valuable, it wasn't always easy.

What made our conversation so difficult? The working group was multidisciplinary, including the people who do the science for a living, people who think about the history and sociology and ethics of the science for a living, and people who do other things (like be a reporter or doctor or lawyer). Nobody assumed that molecular biologists or experimental psychologists would learn the finer points of law or philosophy, or that the lawyers or philosophers would learn the finer points of molecular biology. All we assumed was that everyone brought to the table a commitment to engage in an open and respectful conversation. Yet despite the considerable good will clearly manifested by all, our conversation was sometimes difficult. We set out to create tools for public conversation, but we underestimated how difficult it would be to conduct a fruitful conversation among ourselves.

One altogether surprising difficulty was that working group members came from different disciplinary backgrounds, with those from the humanities and social sciences occasionally intimidated by the languages of statistics and genetics, while those from behavioral genetics were at times impatient with the language and concerns of scholars in the humanities and social sciences. Behavioral genetics research has attracted considerable attention and controversy over the years, some of it more—or less—warranted. Many of the humanists and social scientists wanted to review these issues; others were interested in understanding the philosophical and ethical implications of the findings for the individual and society. After all, this is what they have been trained to do. Some of the geneticists, however, seemed to interpret the philosophical analysis or ethical concerns as implying criticism of the integrity of the field. Perhaps more particularly, they felt these conversations lacked an appreciation of the actual and potential contributions of behavioral genetics to scientific understanding and societal benefit. These difficulties were to be expected from a multidisciplinary endeavor.

Our working group conversation was also difficult because nobody comes to the table without feelings about what the facts *should* be. Nor can these feelings be divided neatly between scientists and humanists. During our meetings, it appeared, some from both sides of the disciplinary divide fervently wanted genetic differences to go a long way toward explaining behavioral differences, and some from both sides equally fervently wanted genetics to be of little use. If a given genetic finding might suggest that genetic differences can play an important role in explaining variation in intelligence, or novelty seeking, or sociality, then that finding seemed to gladden some people as it simultaneously depressed others.

Why such intense feelings? Because in some cases, no less seemed to be at stake than human identities and the proper organization of societies. To what extent are privileges people enjoy the consequence of natural gifts instead of luck and "gifts of nurture"? Does our current social order reflect the way things are "by nature" meant to be? Or does it reflect the contingent effects of power-seeking animals? Is it an inexorable fact of nature, or a contestable product of human choices? Ultimately, to what extent are current forms of inequality rooted in natural differences, and to what extent in human intentions? Few issues inspire as much feeling. Moreover, we eventually realized that some of us simply seemed to have an almost esthetic preference for the minimalist clarity of reductionist explanations, while others were drawn to the messy complexity of a holistic view.

But perhaps most surprising, and in some ways most difficult for the non-scientist editors of this volume, was the degree of disagreement about the facts of the matter that we found *among the scientists*. For example, molecular geneticist Jonathan Beckwith was critical of some foundational assumptions of early behavioral genetics, such as the equal environments assumption, which posits the similarity of the environments of children raised together, regardless of their degree of biological relationship, in contrast to the dissimilarity of environments of children raised apart, again regardless of their degree of biological relatedness; this assumption is a major pillar of the centrally important twin and adoption studies of early behavioral genetics. Some behavioral geneticists in the group disagreed among themselves about the magnitude of the influence of what is called the "nonshared" component of the environment; as readers will see in Eric Turkheimer's contribution to this volume, some behavioral geneticists are skeptical about the very possibility of modeling sufficiently complex gene-environment interactions.

While disputes within science are certainly the norm, not the exception, these disagreements seemed particularly important. It finally appeared to us that we were in what might be termed a "transformative" moment in behavioral genetics, in which an awareness of complexity at a variety of levels is causing a reexamination of many terms and assumptions, as well as some hard thinking about whether it will turn out to be true that identifying statistical correlations between genotypes and phenotypes will help us to *influence* or *predict* behavior.

Our original plan was to start with the science and, with that knowledge as a baseline, to move on to the social and philosophical issues raised by the science. However, as the editors of this volume looked back at the agendas for our five meetings, it became clear that the original, carefully constructed balance among behavioral genetics science, social and philosophical concerns, and issues surrounding public conversation became skewed as the humanists and social scientists felt a continuing need to have the contested and seemingly elusive nature of the "facts" of behavioral genetic science explicated. In response to that need, additional behavioral geneticists, with varying methods and points of view, were invited to participate in meetings. Inevitably, this took up more meeting time than had been anticipated. For example, while we initially expected to spend a considerable portion of time discussing the issue, "is it genetics or is it the environment?" we found that the issues that took more of our attention were: What *is* the environment? How is it measured? How does it interact with genes? And how is it that genes—those of small effect, those of large effect, those in interaction—work? What is the role of protein folding and structure? And what do all the failures to replicate initial gene findings mean for the future of the field?

The Historical Context of Public Concerns and Conversation about Behavioral Genetics

Two pieces of background may help orient readers as they approach this volume. Some readers likely will already be familiar with one or both. The first is a brief history of behavioral genetics in relation to its societal uses and abuses; this is a crucial baseline in understanding the concerns of the social critics of behavioral genetics. The second is some rudimentary facts about the science of behavioral genetics.

The history of behavioral genetics is inextricably bound up with that of statistics. Statistics as a discipline was born in the middle of the nineteenth century, when L.A.J. Quetelet introduced the bell-shaped curve to describe the variation in heights among French soldiers. Later in that century, investigators like Francis Galton began to try to understand how inherited differences could help to explain what seemed to be a naturally and predictably occurring range of phenotypic differences among humans (Kevles, 1985).

The recognition that human traits were distributed in a way that could be represented by the bell-shaped curve, just like animal and plant traits, was part of the larger effort, then gaining steam, to understand human beings as part of the natural world. Indeed, behavioral genetics can be understood as an expression of that same marvelous, radical, naturalistic desire that is most famously associated with Galton's cousin, Charles Darwin: the desire to understand human beings as part of the natural world, to give a natural scientific explanation for why human beings appear and behave as they do.

But almost from the beginning—and repeatedly—the marvelous, radical, naturalistic desire to integrate the study of humans into the study of the rest of nature, the desire to *explain* why human beings appear and behave differently, has converged with, or has been co-opted by, one of the ugliest and meanest of human desires—the desire to *justify* the status quo, to give a naturalistic account of why those who have, have, and why those who lack, lack. Efforts to explain human differences scientifically certainly do not logically entail efforts to justify hierarchical forms of social organization. Still, the history of how the sciences of human differences have been used is long and sordid (Paul, 1995).

In 1869, 10 years after Darwin published *The Origin of Species,* his cousin, Francis Galton, published *Hereditary Genius.* That book advanced the idea that intellect and character were "natural abilities" that could be bred into future generations. Galton envisioned a meritocracy in which intelligence and character, not money, would determine one's place in the social hierarchy—an inherently liberal idea with clear roots in Enlightenment philosophy.

Galton's view that intelligence was a unitary phenomenon soon led to the idea of testing to measure this trait and determine an individual's natural "intelligence." The first such "intelligence test" was created by the French psychologist Alfred Binet at the beginning of the twentieth century. Binet's original and innocent intention was to use such tests to identify children with cognitive disabilities so that they could receive the special attention they needed. But the American H. H. Goddard took Binet's tests and put them to less innocent uses. Goddard's research around the time of World War I convinced him that, among the newly arrived Jews, Hungarians, Italians, and Russians, a huge percentage were "feeble-minded"—or to use his technical term, "morons." Given his view that intelligence was a trait transmitted from generation to generation in the same simple pattern that color was transmitted in Mendel's pea plants, Goddard recommended that "the feeble-minded [should] be identified and kept from breeding" (Gould, 1996, 108).

The term that Galton originally used, *eugenics,* or "good birth," has become inextricably bound up with behavioral genetics and goes a long way toward explaining the contentious nature of the field in the public imagination even today. Eugenics became a prominent movement in the United States in the early part of the twentieth century, taking much of its language and purpose from animal breeders. County fairs became sites of "fitter family" contests, in which purportedly "fit" humans were displayed, like livestock, and given awards and prizes; breeding among these "fit" individuals was to be encouraged. Negative eugenics sought to discourage breeding among those considered to be of genetically inferior stock, including the so-called feeble-minded, criminal, and the mentally ill. Prominent scientists in the United States, such as Charles Davenport, director of the Eugenics Record Office at Cold Spring Harbor Laboratory, were proponents of measures to actually prevent reproduction among "unfit" individuals. By the late 1920s, 28 states had passed laws allowing for compulsory sterilization of those considered unfit.

In the wake of World War II, the recognition of the extent to which Nazi "science" had borrowed from U.S. eugenic theories led to an abrupt hiatus of a couple of decades in discussions about eugenics. In 1969, however, Arthur Jensen published a paper that insinuated that, on average, "whites" score better than "blacks" on IQ tests because of a natural or "genetic" difference between the "races" (Jensen, 1969). In 1994, Richard Herrnstein and Charles Murray revisited Jensen's claim. Their book, *The Bell Curve*, criticized environmental explanations for the black-white gap on various educational tests and marshaled evidence for the genetic influence on intelligence. Further, they warned against squandering scarce resources on social approaches to narrowing the gap. Like Jensen, they never explicitly say that blacks are genetically inferior to whites with respect to intelligence, but they imply that the difference is genetic. So though these authors profess merely to be explaining why blacks and whites score differently on IQ tests, it's easy to see how their work can all too easily be used to justify the fact that in this country whites enjoy more social power than blacks.

Contemporary behavioral geneticists often point out that some of their predecessors fell prey to deeply simplistic ideas, for example, that traits like "intelligence" or "mental deficiency" can be transmitted in "true Mendelian fashion"; they argue that past abuses are not likely to recur, as behavioral geneticists no longer give these theories credence. In this vein, it is important to note that much new behavioral genetics work is painting a more complex picture of gene-environment interactions, yielding insights into why, for example, some people may suffer more than others when exposed to environmental pathogens like child abuse and stress (Caspi et al., 2002, 2003). In addition, many behavioral geneticists, importantly including members of our working group, have spoken eloquently against behavioral genetics claims that could be used to justify a system of racial hierarchy.

Yet some of the social critics in our working group pointed out that none of this has stopped behavioral genetics from being used by some to make invidious comparisons that justify the status quo, and that whether or not these claims are being made by the most respected scientists in the field may be less important than the public attention they get. Thus, within our working group, those who were social critics of behavioral genetics did not differ from the enthusiasts in terms of decrying wrongs of the past, but rather in their belief about how difficult it would be to keep the "eugenic" and discriminatory genie in the bottle, as well as about the extent of the good that behavioral genetics could bring to society.

Behavioral Genetics Today

The first large class of behavioral genetic methodologies used today is sometimes labeled "classical" (or "traditional" or "quantitative" or "epidemiological"). Classical approaches to behavioral genetics employ twin, adoption, and family studies to determine how much influence genes have on a trait—in a particular population, in a particular environment, at a particular time—in comparison to the environment. As mentioned earlier, behavioral geneticists working in this vein take advantage of "the natural experiment" provided by identical twins (who are 100% genetically similar) and fraternal twins (who, on average, are only 50% similar). They make the crucial assumption that while the genetic component of these two types of twins differs, both kinds of twins experience equally similar environments. Conversely, they assume that the environments of identical twins reared apart are completely different, while their genotypes are the same. Using these and other assumptions, behavioral geneticists use straightforward equations to ascertain the magnitude of the genetic influence on the particular trait of interest. These classical approaches are explained at considerable length in chapter 1; for now, the important point is that, since the first twin study in 1924, researchers have found identical twins to be more similar than fraternal twins on a wide range of traits, from height to intelligence to schizophrenia (Plomin et al., 2001). That is, the classical approaches have gathered significant evidence to suggest that genetic differences go a long way in explaining why individuals appear and act differently.

If the classical methodologies aim to discover *whether* (and then *how much*) genetic differences help to explain why people appear and act differently, then the aim of the "molecular" methodologies is to discover *which* genes explain those differences. These molecular studies, which ultimately aim at helping to explain *how* genetic differences help to explain phenotypic differences, are where most of the action and enthusiasm is in behavioral genetics today. Molecular genetics is exciting to behavioral geneticists because it seems that it now will be possible to look, as it were, inside the "black box" of twin and adoption studies and discern precisely which genes lead to differences and similarities.

Yet, despite the methodological advances that the molecular geneticists have achieved, the actual results of molecular approaches to behavioral genetics have been very modest thus far. Few gene variants have been linked to behavioral traits and disorders, and many exciting, initial findings have not been replicated (Hamer, 2002). It is not clear whether this is mainly because the methodologies and technologies are not yet powerful enough, or mainly because the complex behaviors at issue result from stochastic, unpredictable processes that will always make them resistant to the methodologies of behavioral genetics. To the more optimistic behavioral geneticists, the science is new and the problems seem surmountable. They believe that technological and methodological advances will produce more replicable and useful results. As Michael Rutter put it, "the identification of multiple genes of small effect . . . will be quite difficult. Nevertheless, through the use of multiple research strategies, it is likely that delivery will come even if it takes longer than some expect" (Rutter, 2002, 4). To the more pessimistic behavioral geneticists, the fundamental problem is with the theory, which overestimates how much analysis beginning from genes can explain about the origins of complex human behaviors. As behavioral geneticist Eric Turkheimer has put the point, "no amount of physics would ever lead to an explanation of why some objects are carpets" (Turkheimer, 1998, 784). Understanding gravity, the strong and weak forces within the atoms that make up any given carpet, and so on, may in some sense be relevant to an ultimate understanding of what a carpet is. But to understand how a carpet works, to know what you need to do to repair it if it rips, how some carpets are different from others, and how carpets are different from desks, physics is of little help.

Did the working group's emphasis on the "science" mean that we ultimately saw no further philosophical or political or social problems associated with behavioral genetics? Certainly not. Most, if not all, members of the working group agreed that even if behavioral genetics will never explain as much of human behavior as was once promised—and feared—behavioral genetics will continue to have an influence on some concepts that bear directly on how we think about who we are.

A Few Basic Ethical and Social Issues

In the West there is a long tradition of dualist accounts of the self, beginning with Plato and extending to St. Augustine, Descartes, Kant, and even into the present. According to this tradition, body and mind (or "soul") are different substances, one, part of the physical or natural world, the other, part of a world beyond it, a "*meta*physical" world. If you think that freedom depends on the existence of an extra- or meta- or non-natural substance that "rules over" the substance that is your body, then behavioral genetics is just not relevant to your interpretation of freedom. Behavioral genetics does not say anything about extranatural or metaphysical phenomena. It cannot touch the idea of an extranatural mind or soul. The discussions in our project and as represented in this volume, however, proceed from the naturalistic premise that when we speak of body and mind, we are in both cases speaking about entities in the natural world. Even though we do not believe that natural science can give a full or adequate account of our experience, we assume that our experience emerges out of natural (as opposed to extranatural or metaphysical) processes. Insofar as behavioral genetics investigates the relationship between genes and human behaviors, however, the results of those investigations will be relevant to, and potentially have implications for, naturalistic understandings of what we call our choices—and what we call our freedom.

Gregory Kaebnick (chapter 10), in the tradition of Daniel Dennett and others, suggests that we can continue to talk about freedom of the will, as long as we do so in ways that are compatible with the understanding that all behavior is itself causally determined by other natural events. We can do so, according to the "compatibilist" view, if we adopt down-to-earth definitions of terms like *freedom of the will* so that they make no grand metaphysical claims but are instead merely descriptions of behaviors that have evolved in humans and that humans exhibit in some circumstances. In this view, to say that a person acts freely is merely to say that the person has the cognitive capacities to set goals, think about how to pursue them, and then act so as to pursue them, and that in deciding to act, the person was not unduly coerced or constrained. If the action was compelled by physical or social circumstances ("I was forced to do it," "I was tricked and did it unknowingly," "A drug administered to me deprived me of muscle control"), then it wasn't "freely taken." So we might even say that, whereas the dualist account of freedom is about what an agent does to the world, the compatibilist account of freedom is about whether the world is doing something to the agent.

But freedom is not the only self-concept that may be affected by behavioral genetics. As Robert Wachbroit discusses in chapter 11, our understanding of normality is also central to our self-conception. How we understand it affects our categorization of people and behaviors as okay and acceptable by virtue of their normality, or deficient by virtue of their abnormality. Persons considered to be abnormal run the risk of stigmatization. Nevertheless, because we have several different approaches to conceptualizing normality, it is difficult to anticipate how behavioral genetics will affect our understandings.

Most of the chapters in this volume, as most of the discussion in our working group, are thus skeptical about the idea that any time soon scientists will know enough about the genetic basis of complex behaviors to manipulate those traits. But what if researchers did discover enough to manipulate them? Specifically, what would a commitment to distributive justice require? According to philosopher Dan Brock, until recently, many political philosophers have argued that, while there is an obligation for societies to compensate for socially created disadvantages, there is no such obligation to compensate for disadvantages that are rooted in nature. Thus, if you believe that individuals are essentially stuck with their draw in the natural lottery, then you concentrate on responding to disadvantages that do not depend on biology; you spend your time concentrating on disadvantages that in general seem more amenable to social intervention. Leaving aside for the moment the mistake in thinking that natural differences are fixed, it seems possible at least to ask, *if*—and this is a gigantic *"if"*—it were feasible to genetically enhance human traits and capacities, would there be an obligation to use that power to equalize the opportunities of those whose opportunities are limited by a bad draw in the genetic lottery? Even more bluntly: if it is sometimes appropriate to respond to social inequalities with social responses such as affirmative action, then would it be appropriate—or even morally necessary—to respond to those same inequalities with genetic or medical means? Brock suggests that a fair equality of opportunity might require such efforts, while acknowledging that it is unlikely that there would be a political commitment to do so.

These philosophical questions about the effect of behavioral genetics on our understandings of freedom of choice and the conceptualization of the normal were centrally important to some working group members because of the effect they might have directly—or indirectly—on the law and the justice system. Indeed, Kenneth Schaffner frames his chapters on behavioral genetics science largely around a discussion with an imaginary "Judge Jean." Much of Schaffner's chapters aims to help Judge Jean avoid easily made but mistaken inferences about the relevance of behavioral genetics findings to judicial (and other sorts of administrative) decision making.

Harold Edgar considers ways that actual judges—many less informed than Judge Jean—might bring to bear their understanding of how genes act to influence temperament in considering sentencing for behaviors that were thought to have a strong genetic component. Like David Wasserman before him, Edgar argues that a belief in a strong genetic underpinning could move some courts to give lighter sentences—on the grounds that choosing otherwise would be especially difficult for a given individual—while the very same information could move courts in the opposite direction—to give stiffer sentences, on identical grounds that this person is especially dangerous precisely because, due to genetics, he can't stop himself.

Both Schaffner and Edgar would agree that more than the facts—or even interpretations—of science influence judges and the criminal justice system. Sociologist Troy Duster voiced the concerns of several social scientists, who see the potential for harm when preexisting social injustices and vulnerabilities based on racial and ethnic discrimination collide with developing molecular genetics technologies. Such concerns are, of course, based in historical precedent, including the recent public receptivity to, for example, Herrnstein and Murray's *The Bell Curve*. Duster's chapter discusses the ongoing collection of DNA samples from those in prison or arrested, or even questioned, in regard to crimes. He fears the uses to which such large genetic databases, which will disproportionately include the DNA of African Americans and other individuals of color, might be put. For example, researchers might wish to use such a database of the putative "criminal population" to search for molecular markers of a propensity for violence or impulsivity. It would be likely that some DNA markers might be found that correlated significantly both with being African American and being a violent criminal. One need only think about earlier claims that the greater than chance representation of males who had an extra Y chromosome in the prison population indicated that this XYY genotype made one violent. Ultimately, it turned out that this was a marker of a disorder that led to mild mental retardation and not at all to violent criminal behavior. Sadly, before this was sorted out much mischief had been done and there are likely many individuals in the general population who remember XYY and its link to criminality—not later corrections and retractions.

In essence, what Duster and others in our working group were concerned about was that the "new" behavioral genetics would be used just as the "old" behavioral genetics had been—to stigmatize individuals and groups by reinforcing hierarchies, arguing that they are rooted in nature. These concerns were not lost on the genetic scientists in the working group, many of whom agreed that this danger creates an obligation incumbent perhaps first of all on the researchers who do this work to try to set the record straight.

In fact, in the wake of Jensen's inflammatory work on race and IQ, behavioral geneticist and working group member Irving Gottesman was invited in February 1972 to testify before Walter Mondale's Senate Select Committee on Equal Educational Opportunity. Gottesman takes seriously the genetic influence on intelligence and thinks that IQ tests can be a useful measure of an individual's cognitive ability. He agrees with Jensen that IQ tests are like a thermometer: you don't throw it away because it tells you that you have a fever and you don't want one. We should not simply ignore the fact that, on average, black kids are scoring worse on IQ tests than white kids. But, in his testimony, Gottesman (1972) painted a more complex picture:

> There are at least two situations I can imagine where you would not take action as a result of the thermometer reading. If, unknown to the examiner, a child had been sucking on ice cubes or drinking hot tea before testing, you would be obtaining accurate but misleading information. I would suggest to you with respect to the IQ testing of many disadvantaged children, that the readings reflect an intellectual diet of ice cubes between the time of conception and entrance to elementary school.

In 2003, thirty-one years after Gottesman's testimony before the Mondale committee, he, Eric Turkheimer, and their colleagues published a study that addresses the influence of socioeconomic status (SES) on IQ scores (Turkheimer et al., 2003). The new study, based on data from an earlier study by Paul Nichols and Elving Anderson, found that whether genetics helps to explain differences in IQ scores depends on the SES of the persons taking the tests. Genes appear to help explain the differences in test scores among high SES children, but not among low SES children. This study is an example of how behavioral genetics can be wielded in support of progressive social interventions. It provides scientific support for programs like Head Start, which aim to put all children on a level playing field.

Yet the possibility of potential bad uses, or inaccurate perceptions, of behavioral genetics work was not the only concern expressed by the social scientists in the working group. Basic methodological concerns remained as well. Social scientist Nancy Press believes, for example, that behavioral genetics has not solved problems with the definition of the phenotypes for which genetic underpinnings are sought. Like the equal environments assumption mentioned earlier, this is a challenge to behavioral genetics that has been acknowledged and addressed by the field. Yet Press believes that the solutions have been overly reliant on psychology and psychiatry, which are themselves bedeviled, in her anthropologist's view, by an insufficient attention to the way culture affects how we parse and judge various behaviors in various times and places. She avers that this creates problems for molecular behavioral geneticists by leading to spurious correlations that are then not replicated. She also has concerns that the very act of undertaking a search for genes predisposing to some trait—say, shyness—reinforces the view that they are real, bounded entities "out there" in nature. And, as behavioral genetics is viewed as a branch of medicine, these traits thus become medicalized, bringing what might better be seen as normal variation interacting with the pressures and concerns of a quite specific cultural time and place under the rubric of disease; thus *shyness* becomes *social anxiety disorder.*

Indicative of the shape of our conversations, some of the humanists and social scientists who shared Press's concerns—that is, agreed that such medicalization would be a problem—were also eager to point out how behavioral genetics inquiry could at least in principle also be used to resist efforts at medicalization. Parens, for example, appealed to a distinction made by Robert Plomin between the "species typicality perspective" held by most scientists and the "individual differences perspective" held by behavioral geneticists (Parens, 2004). That is, researchers in many fields seek to discover what is typical or normal for a member of the human species with respect to some trait. In traditional neuroscience, for example, researchers seek to understand what typical, or normal, or average human cognition consists in. Behavioral geneticists, however, ask not about what is typical or normal for a species, but rather about why members of a population are *different* from each other with respect to some trait (and how a genetic difference helps to explain a phenotypic difference). For example, they seek to understand why individuals score differently on IQ tests. Insofar as the individual differences perspective proceeds from the premise that we should always expect variation with respect to most traits, insofar as it teaches us that variation is "natural," Parens sees that it could be an ally to those who would criticize views that privilege the normal or typical. Just as there is a continuum of heights within a population, one would expect a continuum of novelty-seeking behavior, food intake, memory retention, and so on. That sort of insight is already being used by people on the so-called autism spectrum, who are saying, Yes, we know we're not "normal," but we don't need your medical interventions; we're quite happy with our place on the sociality spectrum (Harmon, 2004).

So Press and Parens share an awareness of and concern about the history of behavioral genetic findings being used to shore up hateful views about between-group differences. And they share the worry that the individual differences perspective will be used to intensify the medicalization process. They disagree, however, about whether it makes sense to hope that the individual differences perspective will be used to resist that same process. The luxury of being in a working group and talking over time is that friends get to carefully identify where they agree and disagree. But it's not just academics in a working group who have to participate in this sort of conversation.

Public Conversation about Behavioral Genetics

Given that research aimed at understanding the genetic influence on complex human traits and behaviors is inherently interesting, given that such research promises to make a contribution to the reduction of human suffering, and given our country's widely shared commitment to the freedom of scientific inquiry, behavioral genetics is not going away. Nor, again, does it seem that the desire to give scientific accounts of why those with social power deserve it and why those without power deserve to be without will disappear any time soon. Given the promise of the research and the persistent danger that attends it, our only real option is to learn to talk together about it. We need to learn to talk together to distinguish between real and hyped-up findings, real and hyped-up benefits, and real and hyped-up dangers. Doing that will not be easy. As David Wasserman and colleagues at the University of Maryland discovered in 1995, when they convened scientists and critics of the science to discuss the genetic contribution to criminality, talking together about these matters can be exceedingly difficult. In spite of Wasserman's Herculean efforts to balance the voices of enthusiasts and critics, the conference was interrupted by protestors who were angry that anyone would dignify the question, What, if any, role do genes play in influencing criminal behavior? by holding a conference about it. It is not clear, however, what would be achieved by remaining silent about a line of research that is going forward and will go forward, whether it's publicly discussed or not.

When we called our project "crafting tools for public conversation," we first meant tools in the sense of basic concepts and distinctions: our project aimed to identify the sorts of basic concepts and distinctions that one needs to have in hand if one is going to talk productively about what findings by behavioral geneticists do and don't mean for important ethical and social ideas. Our public conversation will be only as good as our grasp of the basic concepts of behavioral genetics. We believe that the first part of this volume, which introduces basic methods in classical and molecular behavioral genetics, will give the lay reader a sense of those basics.

When we talk about *public conversation,* however, what precisely do we mean? The term *public* can be used to describe a place, as in: in fifth-century Athens, community members met in the public space of the Agora to debate matters of common concern; they did not meet in the private space of any one individual. The same term can be used to describe people, as in: participants in the conversation were nonexperts and experts alike. Nonexperts are members of the public vis-à-vis the special knowledge of a given group of experts. There is, of course, an infinite number of publics in the latter sense of nonexperts with respect to behavioral genetics. For example, there is the "public" of people who read newspapers or watch TV and are moved to think about what the latest behavioral genetics finding means for how they conceive of themselves and others; there is the public of lawyers and judges who need to understand whether the latest findings should affect how they think about criminal culpability; there's the public of people in health care who want to know whether the latest findings are of any clinical relevance; there's the public of people who write to their congresspeople to urge them to vote to fund or not fund research who want to understand the value of the research; and so forth.

How then, amid all this diversity of interests, knowledge, and preferences, can we approach crafting a public *conversation?* In the United States, there is one sophisticated and highly developed theory, devoted to understanding what it takes to engage in a specialized public conversation, which is often called "rational democratic deliberation." According to this body of theory, which builds on the work of political philosopher John Rawls, if people are willing to give reasons for their views and to work through a state of internal conflict and even confusion, then they can reach a consensus about some contested public policy matter. Indeed, one member of our working group, Leonard Fleck, has led two National Institute of Health (NIH)-funded projects aimed at creating public conversations of exactly this sort on topics in genetics.

In fact, our project writ large one of Fleck's key questions: how much knowledge of the science do participants need in order to conduct a meaningful conversation about policy and values? Ultimately, Fleck decided the answer was that people need enough factual, scientific information to really understand the complexities of the issue; people giving gut feelings based on scientifically improbable scenarios isn't going to move the conversation forward. This meant that Fleck had to get a commitment from those involved in his rational democratic deliberation projects to come to multiple meetings and learn some science. Given the experience of our working group, the editors of this volume would concur. However, we also know firsthand how difficult such an approach can be, even when the group involves individuals whose work life comprises just such endeavors.

But even if time and effort were available in endless supply, problems would remain. One problem is that many people have a preference for simple answers, and there are advantages for both scientists and the media to give those simple answers. Sometimes it is in the interest of researchers, who are in constant need of funds, to exaggerate the significance of their findings. As Rick Weiss, a science writer for the *Washington Post* and member of our working group, has noted, journalists too benefit from exaggeration. The more exciting the findings sound, the easier it is for journalists to sell a story idea to their editors and to have their article well placed. "Researchers Find Gene for Bipolar Disorder" is much more arresting than "Researchers Identify Gene That May Have Small Role in Bipolar Disorder; Results Await Replication." Nor do bioethicists escape the temptation to exaggeration. When journalists write their stories about gene discoveries, it spices up the story to have a bioethicist pronounce that the finding will transform our understanding of what it means to be human, will lead to an overhaul of the health care system, and so on.

One example of how good science can lead to bad media representations involves the work of Avshalom Caspi, Terrie Moffitt, and colleagues. This exciting work looks at genes that come in various forms, or alleles, and examines whether the interaction of environmental stressors with different alleles produces different reactions. They have published several findings from a prospective study of a cohort of New Zealanders, age 3 through their 20s. One paper, published in 2002 in the journal *Science*, reported on an interaction between childhood abuse and a gene for an enzyme (monoamine oxidasae A [MAOA]) involved in the regulation of several neurotransmitters, including serotonin (Caspi et al., 2002). The researchers discovered that boys who were abused as children and who had a form of the gene that predisposed them to produce low levels of the MAOA enzyme were twice as likely to become antisocial as were those boys who were abused but whose genotype predisposed them to produce high levels of that enzyme. Since MAOA is involved in neurotransmitter regulation, the work also proceeded from a plausible hypothesis about how, physiologically, a genotype might affect a phenotype. While not without its critics, and as always, in need of replication, this work demonstrated great subtlety in looking at the interaction between genotypes and environmental variables. This is the good news.

The bad news is that this study was the subject of a piece in *Popular Mechanics* titled "Criminal Genes" (Wilson, 2002) and in *Time* titled "The Search for a Murder Gene" (Lemonick, 2003). Though both reporters told subtler stories than the titles announced, the idea that "some kids [are] simply born bad" persists. Even though the Caspi and Moffitt MAOA study is about the interaction between genes and the environmental pathogen that is child abuse, the story titles in the popular press suggest that genes "cause" criminality. Especially given that when Americans talk about criminality they often have in mind strung-out poor teenagers, and, as Troy Duster would point out, teenagers of color, this "criminal genes" language is at best dangerous. It risks being co-opted by those who want to justify why some groups enjoy more power than others. That danger was around in Galton's time and it's around in ours, and given the fact that the vast majority of people get their information about science from the popular press, many of our project members saw this as a significant and disheartening problem.

However, some working group members had a more optimistic view of what the public already believes about genetics, finding them less swayed by all this hype and holding more sophisticated understandings of genetics than one might suppose. For example, Celeste Condit, Roxanne Parrott, and Tina Harris reported on their empirical research, which explores the intellectual resources members of the lay public already have to wrestle with such complicated scientific and ethical questions. They argue that the lay public has more resources than it is given credit for. That is, although the participants in Condit et al.'s focus groups were unfamiliar with the details of molecular genetics and the methodologies of twin studies, their accounts of human behavior incorporated a wide range of variables, including both genes and environmental factors. Moreover, their perception that genes play a significant role did not correlate with deterministic frameworks. Some working group members were frankly a bit skeptical about the encouraging nature of Condit's group's results. But it should be noted that Condit's group is the only we one we know of that is trying to "connect the dots" between an analysis of what is written in the popular media about genetics (Conrad, 2001; Peterson, 2001) and what the public actually knows and thinks. Like Caspi and Moffit, and all other good, suggestive, and disputed science, replication will be required.

If we, as editors of this volume, have learned one lesson, it is that public conversation is an exceedingly complex enterprise, as much so in its own way as the science of behavioral genetics itself. We hope, therefore, that this volume will be able to impart sufficient information about the science for those who want to undertake their own conversations about behavioral genetics, and sufficient stimulation to motivate readers to want to keep talking. In the end, we trust that the best of behavioral genetics will have much to teach us about the interaction of genes and environments as it helps us to grasp the permanent fact of human variation. Of course, the science of behavioral genetics, as a science, will not teach us to affirm the positive value of human genetic— or cultural—variation. That task falls to all of us. There is perhaps no larger or more important a task for public conversation.

What You'll Find in the Volume

This book is divided into three sections. The first (chapters 1–5) is intended to help readers understand what behavioral geneticists do and why they do it. The second (chapters 6–11) introduces the fundamental ethical, social, and conceptual issues raised by research into the genetic influences on complex human behaviors. The third (chapters 12–14) explores the prospects for a productive public conversation, informed by the science, about the ethical, social, and conceptual issues raised by behavioral genetics.

Part I opens with two chapters by philosopher Kenneth Schaffner, who offers an extended introduction to the basic concepts of behavioral genetics. He introduces the terms and methodologies that nonscientists need to follow the scientific debates and discussions in the rest of the volume. By using the trope of a conversation with a hypothetical judge, Schaffner presents some of the social and philosophical dilemmas behavioral genetics raises and that will be discussed by authors in Parts II and III. The next two chapters offer lengthier explorations of some critical questions raised by Schaffner. Beginning from a historical perspective, molecular geneticist Jonathan Beckwith focuses on a critique of the foundational equal environments assumption. Although Beckwith acknowledges that some recent behavioral genetic investigations of gene-environment interactions may be harbingers of an important shift in the field, he maintains that behavioral geneticists have largely neglected serious study of environmental influences on complex traits. In chapter 4 Eric Turkheimer again raises the issue of the environment and increasing contemporary attempts to examine the nature of gene-environment interactions. Turkheimer presents the "gloomy view" that even the most dedicated attention and conceptual sophistication will not be able to yield predictive or even explanatory clarity regarding those interactions. In the final chapter of Part I, Steven Hyman, speaking as the former director of the National Institute of Mental Health, presents an overview of what the science of behavioral genetics has achieved so far and what he hopes will be the positive and long-term consequences of bringing molecular genetics to bear on understanding and treating complex mental disorders such as schizophrenia, depression, and autism.

Part II begins the exploration of the broader social, legal, and philosophical issues raised by behavioral genetics. Chapters 6, 7, and 8 focus on societal implications. Nancy Press considers the challenges raised for the behavioral genetics enterprise by the social construction of phenotypes, while Troy Duster discusses the dangers that may occur when value-laden phenotypes converge with the investigations of genetic differences among socially disadvantaged population groups. Harold Edgar then picks up the threads of Schaffner's dialogues with Judge Jean in considering in depth the potential effect behavioral genetics might have on criminal justice decisions. In chapter 9, Dan Brock explores the various meanings of social and political equality and justice in the face of a more speculative aspect of behavioral genetics—the possibility of genetic enhancements. In chapters 10 and 11, Gregory Kaebnik and Robert Wachbroit shift the conversation to the broadly philosophical and moral issues raised by behavioral genetics: Kaebnick offers a summary of the major strains of philosophical thought on causation and moral responsibility and the challenges that behavioral genetics may—or may not—pose to our views of our own freedom. Finally, Wachbroit provides a framing consideration of the various meanings of the concepts of the normal and the natural and investigates how sorting out the variety of the meanings of these terms can help clarify the broad set of claims made about the implications of behavioral genetics.

Part III begins to explore what it would mean to have a constructive public conversation about behavioral genetics given the complexities explored in Parts I and II. It shows, in three very different empirical modes, how the public may be wrestling with behavioral genetics. In chapter 12, Leonard Fleck begins by providing a model of a public conversation on this topic, based on Rawlsian rational democratic deliberation, in which he has been engaged. He lays out, in an instructive, programmatic fashion, precisely what sorts of factors need to be in place to make deep and engaged public conversation possible and successful. In chapter 13, speech communication scholars Celeste Condit, Roxanne Parrott, and Tina Harris report on their empirical research, which provides an optimistic view of the intellectual resources members of the lay public may already possess in their consideration of these complicated scientific and ethical questions. In chapter 14, Rick Weiss, veteran science reporter for the *Washington Post,* tells the story of how his profession has gone from an original state of rather uncritical enthusiasm for the new science of behavioral genetics to a more mature state of critical appreciation of what the science has thus far achieved—and not achieved. It is a cautionary tale, but a hopeful one, and, we trust, ends the volume with the message that behavioral genetics is a fascinating, profound, and complex topic in which the lay public, as well as the specialist scientist, can and needs to be involved.

REFERENCES

Caspi, A., et al. (2002). "Role of Genotype in the Cycle of Violence in Maltreated Children." *Science* 297: 851–54.
Caspi, A., et al. (2003). "Influence of Life Stress on Depression: Moderation by a Polymorphism in the 5-HTT Gene." *Science* 301: 386–89.
Conrad, P. (2001), "Genetic Optimism: Framing Genes and Mental Illness in the News." *Culture Medicine and Psychiatry* 25(2): 225–47.
Gottesman, I. I. (1972). "Testimony Submitted to United States Senate Select Committee on Equal Educational Opportunity." U.S. Senate Select Committee on Equal Educational Opportunity.

Gould, S. J. (1996). *The Mismeasure of Man*. New York: W.W. Norton.

Hamer, D. (2002). "Rethinking Behavioral Genetics." *Science* 298: 71–72.

Harmon, A. (2004). "The Disability Movement Turns to Brains." *New York Times* (May 8).

Herrnstein, R. J., and C. A. Murray. (1994). *The Bell Curve: Intelligence and Class Structure in American Life*. New York: The Free Press.

Jensen, A. R. (1969). "How Much Can We Boost IQ and Scholastic Achievement?" *Harvard Educational Review* 39.

Kevles, D. J. (1985). *In the Name of Eugenics*. New York: Knopf.

Lemonick, M. (2003). "The Search for a Murder Gene." *Time* (January 20).

Parens, E. (2004). "Genetic Differences and Human Identities: On Why Talking about Behavioral Genetics Is Important and Difficult." *Hastings Center Report Special Supplement* 34(1): S1–S36.

Paul, D. B. (1995). *Controlling Human Heredity, 1865 to the Present*. Atlantic Highlands, N.J.: Humanities.

Peterson, A. (2001). "Biofantasies: Genetics and Medicine in the Print News Media." *Social Science and Medicine* 52(8): 1255–68.

Plomin, R., et al. (2001). *Behavioral Genetics*. New York: Worth and W. H. Freeman.

Rutter, M. (2002). "Nature, Nurture, and Development: From Evangelism through Science toward Policy and Practice." *Child Development* 73(1): 1–21, at 4.

Turkheimer, E. (1998). "Heritability and Biological Explanation." *Psychological Review* 105(4): 784.

Turkheimer, E., et al. (2003). "Socioeconomic Status Modifies Heritability of IQ in Young Children." *Psychological Science* 14(6): 623–25.

Wilson, J. (2002). "Criminal Genes." *Popular Mechanics* (November).

I / Basic Scientific Concepts and Debates

CHAPTER ONE

Behavior

Its Nature and Nurture, Part 1

Kenneth F. Schaffner, M.D., Ph.D.

This is the first of two chapters intended to serve as a selective overview of the field of behavioral genetics. Though my discussion focuses on a variety of genetic methods and results, I do not mean to suggest that we should think of genetics as the fundamental cause in the analysis and explanation of behavior. My approach to what has traditionally been called the nature-nurture debate sees genetics as part of a larger constellation of causes that crucially includes environments, which work jointly with genetics.

The nature-nurture issue is a perennial one, with its modern roots dating back to Galton's writings in the late nineteenth century. After the rediscovery of Mendel in 1900, the issue and ensuing debates have usually been couched in terms of genes versus environments and their respective influences on the organism. Themes revolving around nature and nurture have been especially contentious when behavioral and mental traits (and disorders) are at issue. ("Psychiatric genetics" is widely viewed as a part of the field of behavioral genetics.) This contentiousness arises not only in our society at large, where the specters of discrimination and eugenics are quickly raised, but also in the social sciences and psychiatry.

The past 30 years have seen a shift from an earlier period in which behavioral or psychiatric disorders were seen as primarily environmental, due to poor parenting, for example, to the contemporary view that amalgamates both genetic and environmental influences as major causal determinants. This shift, which has not been without controversy (Rowe and Jacobson, 1999, 2, 34), reflects broader shifts in psychosocial studies of nature and nurture (Reiss and Neiderhiser, 2000).

In these two chapters, I review some of the recent empirical methods and results of studying genes and environments in behavioral (and psychiatric) genetics, and I also touch on a few more general issues including genetic determinism and complexity. Because of the breadth of studies dealing with nature and nurture in behavioral studies and in psychiatric disorders, I focus on several *prototypical* examples. Prototypical examples are concrete exemplars that will help us to grasp the roles of genetics and environment by providing specific instances of how genes and environmental factors are believed to work. Frequently I employ schizophrenia as a prototypical disorder, but I also deal with normal mental functions, including "general cognitive ability"—a notion often related to the more contentious terms *intelligence* and *IQ*. In addition, I consider the trait of novelty seeking and, to some extent, the concept of impulsivity. I approach impulsivity primarily in connection with another prototypical disorder, attention deficit hyperactivity disorder (ADHD).

These two chapters contain three dialogues between a behavioral geneticist and an appeals court judge who wishes to find out more about behavioral genetics. The first dialogue introduces the basic notions of the more traditional quantitative (often called epidemiological or classical) approaches to understanding the influence of genes on behavior. The second dialogue (in the following chapter) introduces the newer, molecular approaches to understanding the genetics of behavior. In the third dialogue, I introduce two hypothetical legal cases involving testing for genes implicated in IQ and ADHD, to focus much of the discussion from dialogues 1 and 2. Finally, I conclude with a projection of where the current debates and new methodologies may lead regarding genetics and the understanding of human behavior in a combined nature-nurture perspective.

Basic Terms

Though concepts like *gene* and *environment* are widely used both in science and in public discourse, they sometimes have special meanings in behavioral genetics. To begin, we will understand behavior in a very broad sense, to include the reactions and interactions of an organism to its environment, including other organisms. Because we will focus on human behavior, this broad meaning will also include people's (reported) thoughts and feelings as well as their observable bodily movements (compare BSCS 2000, 19). Genetics is the science that deals with the inheritance of those characteristics that are physically passed on from parent(s) to offspring, and includes the simpler forms of classical Mendelian genetics of pea plants that some readers may remember from high school. The field of genetics includes, as well, later developments such as the study of chromosomes and the molecular basis of the unit of inheritance, the gene, constituted by DNA sequences (or RNA in some viruses such as the AIDS virus, HIV).

Millions of DNA sequences, linked together in a chain and partially covered with special proteins, constitute the chromosomes, of which there are 23 pairs in human females (males have 22 pairs and an X and a Y sex chromosome). Genes come in different forms at their typical position, or locus, along a chromosome, and those forms are called alleles. The genotype of an organism sometimes refers to all of the genes (or more accurately, alleles) in that organism and sometimes refers to all of the alleles that are found at that particular locus. For example, a gene that helps determine whether pea color is yellow or green has two alleles, Y and G. The genotype for a pea plant at the pea color locus thus could be YY, YG, or GG. The observable effects of the genes are called the phenotype, for example, the yellow or green color of the aforementioned peas.

The genes that affect a trait may have a dominant form, which means that only a single allele at a given locus is needed to produce a particular phenotype. For example, if the Y allele is dominant for yellow pea color, then a YG genotype produces a yellow pea. (A YY genotype would do the same.) The genes that affect a phenotype may also have a recessive form, which means that two alleles of the same type must be present at a given locus for a trait to be expressed. If green pea color is recessive, then only a GG genotype will produce a green pea. In a number of cases the alleles are co-dominant, which means they blend to produce an effect that is midway between the two pure allele forms.

Observable features are also called traits. Traits can be virtually any described or measured feature of an organism, including behavior. Whether those features are unambiguously determined by any single allele or even combinations of alleles, however, must always be discovered through empirical genetic research. A trait that varies continuously, like height, is called a quantitative trait, and a gene that helps determine such a trait is termed a quantitative trait locus (or QTL); the plural is quantitative trait loci (QTLs).

Behavioral geneticists understand the term *environment* very broadly. As Robert Plomin et al. (2000, 91) write,

> In the field of [behavioral] genetics, the word environment includes all influences other than inherited factors. This use of the word environment is much broader than is usual in psychology. In addition to environmental influences traditionally studied in psychology, such as parenting, environment includes prenatal and nongenetic biological events after birth, such as illness and nutrition.

As we will see later, the prenatal, *in utero* environment may exert an extremely important influence on highly prized phenotypic traits.

Behavioral geneticists recognize two forms of environment, called the *shared environment* and the *nonshared environment*. Intuitively, included in the shared environment are those things experienced in common in a family and that make family members similar; included in the nonshared environment are those things that are experienced differently and make individuals different, whether experienced within the family or through outside-the-family interactions. In fact, that is not exactly what behavioral geneticists mean when they use that distinction. Toward the end of this chapter, I discuss some of the subtle and perhaps odd technical aspects of this distinction that are so important for behavioral genetic studies.

Finally, though environment is broadly conceived in behavioral genetics, there is no "theory of the environment." This stands in stark contrast with genetics, which can appeal to the framework of genes, chromosomes, and general knowledge about gene actions and interactions discovered by classical and molecular biology (BSCS, 2000). The lack of such a theoretical orientation or environmental framework will prove important at several points later in this chapter. Toward the close of this chapter, I return to several research projects that address various aspects of the environment concept, and in the following chapter I introduce the concept of the *envirome* to describe such projects.

Quantitative (or Epidemiological) Approaches to Nature and Nurture

Behavioral geneticists use two broad approaches to study the influences of nature and nurture. The first approach is called quantitative (or often epidemiological or classical) and the second is called molecular (Plomin et al., 2000). As we will see in detail below, epidemiological or quantitative approaches use twin, adoption, and family studies to investigate the influence of genetic and environmental factors. Molecular approaches use the tools of molecular genetics to identify specific genes implicated in a given behavior. An overview of methods can be found in Neiderhiser (2001) and a systematic analysis in Plomin et al. (2000).

In this chapter I introduce some of the quantitative types of studies, and then move to an interlude—the first of three dialogues—in which we probe how and why some of the methods work—and do not work. Later on we return to consider the second class of methods for analyzing behavioral genetics, namely, various molecular approaches.

Quantitative methods are used to distinguish nonspecific genetic and environmental contributions to traits or features of individuals or, more accurately, to assess correlations and interactions between genetic and environmental factors that account for differences between individuals.[1] In any given study, all individuals have the trait of interest, but they have the trait to different extents. Quantitative approaches study collections of individuals or populations and typically do not examine individual identified genes or individually identified environments. Rather, these methods examine what proportion of the phenotypic differences between individuals is due to genetics or environment (or interactions between the two). Behavioral geneticists who employ the quantitative methods use fairly simple equations to infer the effects of genes and environments on the (mostly) quantitative traits. The methods of quantitative behavioral genetics include family, adoption, and twin types of study, and each of these can be coupled together with the other types.

Types of Studies

Family studies look to see if a trait or a disorder runs in families. Individuals in the family with the trait or disorder are identified, and then other family members are screened for the presence of the trait or disorder. Usually first-degree relatives (parents, siblings, and offspring) are examined, but second-degree relatives (aunts and uncles, cousins, and grandparents) may also be included in a study (Neiderhiser, 2001). Family studies can suggest that a trait or disorder is genetic, but since both genes and environments are shared by family members, contributions of nature and nurture cannot be disentangled in family studies. Different types of studies are thus needed.

Adoption studies examine genetically related individuals in different familial environments, and thus can prima facie disentangle contributions of nature and nurture. If a trait or disorder tends to be present in both adopted-away children and their biological parents, then researchers suspect the existence of an important genetic influence. (At least, at first blush it appears to be genetics—not environments—that the biological parent and adopted-away child share.) If, on the other hand, adopted children and their adopting parents tend to share a trait or disorder, then researchers suspect the existence of an important shared environmental influence. (After all, the adopted child and adopting parents are genetically quite different.) This reasoning depends on several assumptions that can be questioned. For example, it is usually assumed that there is no selective placement that would create a correlation between traits of the biological parents and the adopting parents, such as socioeconomic status or intellectual capacity. If this assumption is violated, the interpretation of the study results needs to be corrected. It is also assumed that the parents and offspring studied represent the population as a whole, which is questionable. Also, the possible effects of the prenatal environment need to be considered. If, say, prenatal (and thus preadoption) nutrition might affect an offspring's trait or disorder, this effect might be erroneously ascribed to genetic causes. We will discuss this issue specifically in dialogue 3, where we consider IQ and the maternal environment. (For a further discussion of these assumptions and ways of dealing with them, see textbox 5.2 in Plomin et al., 2000.)

The first adoption study of schizophrenia conducted by Heston in 1966 resulted in the then startling finding that shared rearing environment has little, if any, effect on the risk of developing schizophrenia. It was also found that being adopted had no effect on the risk of developing schizophrenia (Heston, 1966). This study was the first nail in the coffin of the idea of the "schizophrenogenic mother," an environmentalist concept articulated at the time by psychoanalyst Frieda Fromm-Reichmann. These results were confirmed by other later adoption studies. Adoption studies, however, are increasingly difficult to conduct in contemporary society. This is because there are fewer adopted children, and also because the confidentiality of adoption records makes it difficult to assess the traits and disorders of biological parents accurately.

Twin studies, the third and final study type, compare identical and fraternal twins, both within the same familial environment and (in adoption studies) in different familial circumstances. Twin studies have been used extensively in behavioral genetics and in psychiatry to understand the extent to which a trait or disorder is influenced by genes or environments. One of the simplest ways to report the results of twin studies uses concordance rates. A concordance rate can be thought of as a risk factor for the second twin of having a trait or a disorder given a diagnosis of the first twin.[2] As an example, concordance studies of twins reported by Gottesman and his associates over many years, including several new ones, indicate that the risk of developing schizophrenia is ~45 percent for monozygotic (MZ) twins, 17 percent for dizygotic twins (DZ), and 9 percent for siblings, if the other has been so diagnosed (Cardno and Gottesman, 2000; Gottesman and Erlenmeyer-Kimling, 2001). (The risk for developing schizophrenia over a lifetime assuming no affected relatives is about 1%.) This concordance pattern suggests that schizophrenia is caused by many genes, which interact in a complex, non-Mendelian fashion; it also suggests that the environment has a major (>50%) effect.

Twin studies are also used to obtain heritability estimates for behavioral traits. Heritability estimates, which we explore in some depth shortly, are meant to indicate how much of the phenotypic variation in a population is due to genetic variation. The bigger the heritability estimate, the more researchers think that genetic differences help to explain why people are different with respect to a trait. Heritability estimates tend to run about 30 to 50 percent for personality traits, and for most major psychiatric disorders heritabilities range from about 30 percent (e.g., depression) to about 70 percent for schizophrenia, though one recent review estimates schizophrenia's heritability at about 85 percent (Cardno and Gottesman, 2000). But it is important to know that approximately 63 percent of all persons suffering from schizophrenia will have neither first- nor second-degree relatives diagnosed with schizophrenia (Gottesman and Erlenmeyer-Kimling, 2001), reinforcing the idea that genetic and environmental contributions to the disorder are complexly related.[3] Readers may wonder how quantitative behavioral geneticists can consider schizophrenia to be a continuous or quantitative trait when it looks so discontinuous, like you either have it or you don't. The key to understanding this is to bear in mind the difference between a continuum of phenotypes and a continuum of liability to express a categorical (present or absent) trait like schizophrenia (SZ). When behavioral geneticists say that schizophrenia is a quantitative trait, they have not traditionally meant that there is a continuum of phenotypes between, say, no schizophrenia and flagrant schizophrenia as there is a continuum between those who are very short and those who are very tall (or those who are prone to have the occasional blues to those who are prone to major depression). They have meant, instead, that there is a continuum of liability or risk for SZ: individuals only exhibit SZ if they pass some threshold of risk (much like a bridge breaks only if it is subject to some threshold of stress). This liability approach is represented in what is called a threshold model, first introduced by Falconer (Falconer, 1965) and then developed and applied by Gottesman to schizophrenia in a long series of influential papers as well as in his book.

Because heritability is such a confusing concept, and because the models that estimate it serve as the foundation for quantitative (or epidemiological) genetics, I introduce that concept and those models through an imagined dialogue between an inquisitive judge and a behavioral geneticist. Judge Jean is an imaginary member of the Ohio State Supreme Court. She expects she may be asked to hear cases in the near future that will appeal to the results of behavioral genetics, both in its traditional quantitative forms and its newer molecular forms.[4] This is the first of three dialogues that are intended to be fairly simple introductions to the basic concepts and methods of behavioral genetics. More details can be found in the notes referenced within the dialogues, and also in the text preceding and after the dialogues.

Dialogue 1: A State Supreme Court Judge and a Behavioral Geneticist Talk about Heritability and Twin Studies

Judge Jean (JJ): I keep seeing in news stories about behavioral genetics that they have been able to calculate "heritabilities" for all sorts of human behaviors, from personality traits, IQ, and even criminal behavior, to severe psychiatric illnesses, like schizophrenia. What does this word mean? Why should I care about it?

Behavioral geneticist (BG): *Heritability* is a term behavioral geneticists have adopted from quantitative genetics. The idea had its original applications down on the farm, as it were, improving crop strains and breeding better farm animals, like cattle. The general idea is that a heritability estimate tells you how much of the total phenotypic variation in a trait (i.e., the variation due to both genetics and environment) can be explained by genetic variation alone. Another way to put it would be: a heritability estimate is supposed to tell you how good a prediction of the phenotype you can make if you know the genotype. I will be more precise about the definition as we talk more. *Quantitative* here means the traits of interest continuously vary, like height and weight do among people. (Geneticists do not estimate heritabilities for traits like the yellow or green color of Mendel's peas, because they would be trivially 1, meaning that the phenotypic differences among the plants would depend completely [100%] on the plants' genotypes.) Heritability is symbolized by H^2. It's a squared term for reasons relating to statistics that we need not be concerned with at this point.[5] Heritability is important because for quantitative traits we can estimate how much of the phenotypic variation in a population is maybe influenced by genetics and how much by the environment. And if a trait appears to be highly genetically influenced in terms of its variation, maybe we can identify the genes that causally influence that trait.

JJ: Wait a minute! You just said H^2 estimates how much the trait is maybe influenced by genetics, and then you said maybe we can identify the genes that influence that trait. Why the two maybes here?

BG: The first *maybe* is because usually we have no direct evidence of genetic influence on the trait's range. (There are rare cases where we know what the underlying genotype is that affects the trait, and we are able to genotype the individuals in the population and get direct evidence of influence.) But when we don't have direct evidence, that is, we don't know the real genotype and cannot measure it, we can still use a wonderful experiment of nature to make a good indirect guess at how much of a trait's variation is genetic. We'll talk about that natural experiment a little later.

I used the second *maybe* because it is still very controversial whether high heritabilities indicate that we will be able to find a specific molecular genetic basis for the trait (or a disorder) with that high heritability. For today's discussion we will concentrate on getting a clearer idea about how quantitative genetics defines heritability and obtains heritability estimates. Another day (in dialogue 2) we will look at how molecular methods work. At that point we will consider what the relationship might be between the heritabilities that are given to us by quantitative genetics and what molecular studies tell us, and whether the quantitative results can really assist the molecular research programs.

JJ: Okay, let's put aside the molecular approaches for now. But in response to my very first question you told me that heritability estimates give you a sense of the extent to which genetics explains the variation that is observed in a population with respect to a particular trait. Then you told me that "maybe" heritability estimates help you determine the extent of the genetic influence on a trait. Please clarify exactly what is explained by the quantitative approach.

BG: Remember that a quantitative trait, like height or weight, in any collection of individuals we look at usually varies. By the way, a collection of individuals that we examine is usually called a population. The scores of the trait of interest, like height, are plotted along an X axis and the number or percent of individuals with that score is plotted along the Y axis. Often the figure that results looks like a bell-shaped curve. You've seen curves like this for Scholastic Aptitude Test (SAT) scores and for IQ scores. The figure is also called a distribution, since it tells us how the scores are distributed. Every distribution has an average or mean, and also a spread around the mean. The spread tells us how much variation there is in the scores, and it can be made precise by the notion of a variance, but I won't ask you to learn about the mathematical definition of variance.[6] Heritability is a measure of how much of the differences among the individuals in a population is estimated to be genetic and how much is estimated to be environmental.

One has to be very careful with this heritability concept. As three geneticists recently put it in their lingo: "heritability does not describe the quantitative contribution of genes to . . . any . . . phenotype of interest; it describes the quantitative contribution of genes to *interindividual differences* in a phenotype studied in a particular population" (Benjamin et al., 2002, 334)[7] [my emphasis]. That is, a heritability estimate may tell us something about how much of the phenotypic differences between individuals is due to genetic differences among those individuals, but it cannot tell us anything about how much genes affect the phenotype of a given individual. One of the surprising features of the heritability concept is that if, for example, there are no interindividual differences in a trait, then the heritability of that trait is zero. Of course, that isn't to say that genes don't influence that trait in a given individual! I'll give you some examples of this subtle but critical distinction in a bit.

JJ: I think examples would help, because I'm confused. Can you go over that again? Maybe you can describe individual differences and what's genetic and what's environmental variation in another way?

BG: Sure. There are a few rare cases for which we know exactly what the underlying genotype is and what the phenotype and its distribution look like. Here is a good example based on the writings of the geneticist Richard Lewontin, who used data from a study by Harry Harris. Work with me on it for a bit. Lewontin's (1995) example uses some real data involving a human trait, red blood cell acid phosphatase activity, which is governed by three different gene forms or alleles. But because the function of acid phosphatase is not well understood, though it can be measured for any individual in the lab, I am going to modify the example, just as I do for my students, to try to give you a more intuitive grasp of the concepts. We will actually use the same data and the same figure and summarizing table as Lewontin, but now we will interpret the trait as the height of hypothetical ornamental rubber tree plants, or, better, a population of hypothetical rubber trees that a tree breeder is studying. These particular rubber trees, like Mendel's pea plants and like humans, are diploid (they have two copies of every chromosome),[8] and, as was found in red cell acid phosphatase, these rubber plants have three alleles (A, B, and C) that are known to affect this trait. Thus, any given rubber tree must have one of six possible genotypes (AA, AB, AC, BB, BC, or CC). Now Lewontin used data on the phosphatase activity phenotype and graphed the activity for each genotype (on the horizontal axis) and relative frequencies of the percentage of individuals with that activity (on the vertical axis) (Figure 1.1). For us the graph represents the heights of the rubber tree plants with the five or six different genotypes (genotype CC was actually too rare to graph) on the horizontal axis, and the vertical axis represents the number of the rubber trees that have that height.

Note that each genotype has a nearly bell-shaped curve distribution. The AA genotype has the least height, but it ranges from about 80 to 160 centimeters (about 32 to 64 inches), whereas AB runs from about 100 to more than 200 (40 to 80 inches), and other genotypes have their own distributions as shown (again, CC is not graphed because too little is known about this very rare genotype to have any data). Each genotype has a range or variance for its height, and, of course, each of those variances has a mean or average. Since the five or six genotypes are fixed in the plant studies, all of the phenotypic variance (i.e., variation in height) associated with each genotype is due to environmental variance. The rubber trees' heights are environmentally affected by the climate and the soil in subtle and uncontrollable ways at this stage of our tree breeder's research. The different genotypes have those different means, however, and a part of the phenotypic variance in the population as a whole is because of the

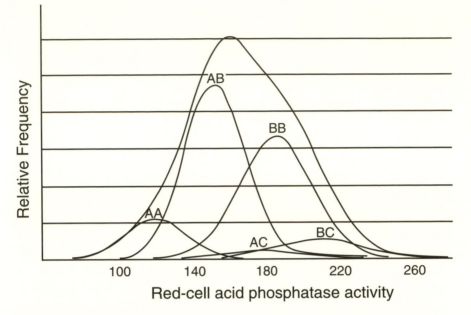

Fig. 1.1. The activity of red-cell phosphatase (and height in centimeters of hypothetical rubber tree plants). *Source:* Adapted from Harris, 1980, 196. Reprinted with permission of Elsevier.

variance of those five or six different genotypic means. But, again, this genetic variance does not account for all of the population's variance, because within each genotype there is variance that is due to those unknown environmental causes (Lewontin, 1995, 66). Thus, the population's phenotypic variance is a mix of genotypic variation and environmental variation.

It might be good to emphasize again that our hypothetical height genes here, the As, Bs, and Cs, do not by themselves provide the instructions for growing a plant of a specific height. Maybe one influences the concentrations of some plant hormone, and another affects water transport into a cell. But it takes thousands of genes working in concert with proteins and chemical environmental factors to grow a rubber tree plant. Each of the genotypes we show has a mean value associated with it, but the genotype does not produce that mean in anything but the most indirect sense.

JJ: Okay, I can see there are two different sources of variation, or, if you want, variance, in that figure. So what?

BG: Heritability is the ratio of the genetic variance to the total (phenotypic) variance. If you don't mind me writing the formula, the ratio is $Vg/Vp = H^2$.

Vp is also just equal to Vg + Ve. (These variances or measures of the range of individual differences in the heights—the spread-outness—can be read off from the figure, or more accurately calculated from the data that were used to graph the distribution. Specific values are presented in Table 1.1 based on Harris's measurements.) In Figure 1.1, the curves labeled with the letters show the environmental variation for each genotype, and the unlabeled (top) curve shows the total phenotypic variation. This ratio (Vg/Vp) is the average of the genotypic variance divided by the variance of the total (phenotypic) distribution. Remember: what we're trying to figure out is how much of the total phenotypic variation is due to genetic variation. In this case, we know that for each genotype all of the phenotypic variance is due to environmental variance. Because by definition the total phenotypic variance is equal to the sum of the environmental and genetic variances (Vp = Ve + Vg), we can calculate the genotypic variance by subtracting the average of the environmental variances for each genotype from the total phenotypic variance (Vp − Ve = Vg). If you want to trust me, I'll tell you that when you do the numbers, it turns out that about 49 percent (which we can round up to 50 percent for discussion purposes) of the total phenotypic variation is due to genetic variation. Thus, the heritability of rubber tree height in this plant population is said to be ~50 percent. If you don't trust me, take a look at Table 1.1 and do the calculations for yourself.[9] Again, this ratio, or heritability estimate, is thought to be a measure of how much of the variation in the height in this rubber tree population in this environment is influenced by genetic variation.

JJ: That's a strange graph. If I knew only about the unlabeled curve value for someone, I could not figure out exactly what genotype that individual had.

BG: You are exactly right. If the phenotypic value for an individual was low, say, about 120 centimeters, that individual probably would have genotype AA, but not necessarily. And for a plant height up around 160, the rubber plant could have *any* of the underlying genotypes.

JJ: Another thing. If the rubber trees (or people in the original phosphate example) in this population were to change, I mean, if for some reason there were none of the B or C genes around, it looks like the unlabeled curve would be the same as the AA curve. And if I followed you, there would be no genetic variance at all, because all variance would be environmental, even though the genotype AA is clearly of major influence here. And doesn't that mean a heritability of zero even though the AA genotype is exerting all the influence on the trait?

BG: You got it! But to impress on you just how tricky this heritability no-

Table 1.1. *Red Blood Cell Activity of Different Genotypes of Red-Cell Acid Phosphatase in the English Population*

Genotype	Mean Activity	Variance of Activity	Frequency of Population
A/A	122.4	282.4	0.13
A/B	153.9	229.3	0.43
B/B	188.3	380.3	0.36
A/C	183.8	392.0	0.03
B/C	212.3	533.6	0.05
C/C	~240	—	0.002
Grand average	166.0	310.7	
Total distribution	166.0	607.8	

Source: Harris, 1980, 194. Reprinted with permission from Elsevier.

Note: Averages are weighted by frequency in population. The "grand average" 310.7 is the average of the environmental variances *within each genotype*. The total phenotypic variance is 607.8 and is measured in the population as a whole. The genetic variance is 607.8 − 310.7 = 297.1, since there are only two sources of variation, and genetic variance plus environmental variance = total variance. Thus the heritability of the trait of red-cell acid phosphatase activity in this (English) population = Vg/Vp = 297.1/607.8 = 49%.

tion can be, let me ask you to think about another example. What would you say the heritability of a human having a brain is?

JJ: Well, if all humans have a brain, or, as you geneticists would say, if there's zero variation among humans with respect to having a brain, then I guess the heritability ratio would be given by zero divided by some environmental variation—maybe due to toxins, for example, that could produce anencephalic infants—so the heritability would be zero. Wouldn't that mean that, even though our genes are crucially involved in the fact that we have brains, the heritability of having a brain is zero?

BG: Again you got it! Variance is a very tricky notion to reason with, and when you are reasoning about genetic and environmental variance, you really have to keep your eye on the ball—or, rather, on the genes, and everything else at once. It is very easy to make the wrong inferences even if you are trying very hard. Part of the problem is due to the fact that the definition of heritability is computed from measurements on a specific population in a particular environment, and, strange as it may seem, *if the environment changes, the heritability will almost certainly change.*

Many scientists who work with the heritability concept think it would be clearer if we used a different way to represent the influences of genes and environments on the phenotype that would make this very labile nature of heritability explicit. One popular alternative is called a "norm of reaction." A norm of reaction graphs the value of the phenotype for different genotypes in different environments. A good illustration of norms of reaction is from a widely cited example of another type of plant called *Achillea*. Seven different strains or genotypes of the plant were raised at three different elevations on a mountain, with the results shown in Figure 1.2. One can even look at the differences in expression of phenotypes over time by introducing a third dimension. In this case, the reaction norm becomes a reaction surface. We can look at an example and a picture of a reaction surface later on.

JJ: That variation in the plants due to both genotypes and environments is astounding. I look forward to coming back to reaction norms and surfaces later. But talking just about heritability again, you said the rubber plant—or, more accurately, the blood phosphatase—case you showed me was rare. Why was it rare, again?

BG: Because in the cases that behavioral geneticists usually study, we do *not* know what alleles and genotypes underlie the trait, and of course then we do not have distributions of genotypes we can directly test for and plot out, like we did for those curves that underlie the total population's distribution.

JJ: So what do the behavioral geneticists do, then? How do they get information about how much genes might influence a trait—or, more accurately, how genetic variation might influence phenotypic variation?

BG: They use twins. They study both identical twins and fraternal twins, and they look at those types of twins both in the same family and in the different families into which they were adopted. Twins are a wonderful "experiment of nature"—identical twins have identical genotypes, and fraternal twins, though they are born about the same time, have only about 50 percent of their genes alike.

JJ: Just 50 percent? Where did you get that number? I once heard Dr. Francis Collins say that humans were about 99.9 percent identical as regards their DNA. How can any random pair of humans be 99.9 percent identical with respect to their DNA, but fraternal twins have only 50 percent of their genes alike?

BG: You have to remember this: Francis Collins was saying that at only one in a 1,000 points (base pairs) along our chromosomes, we're different. The thing is, small differences at those points make for different alleles (or versions) of the same gene. Behavioral geneticists are interested in the percentage of *alleles* the twins share. It is a little complicated to explain this, but see if you can follow the argument here. If not, or you want to think more about this later, fine, but maybe you can trust me in the meantime. We start from the fact that everyone has two parents, at least biologically. We are not cloning humans yet! And

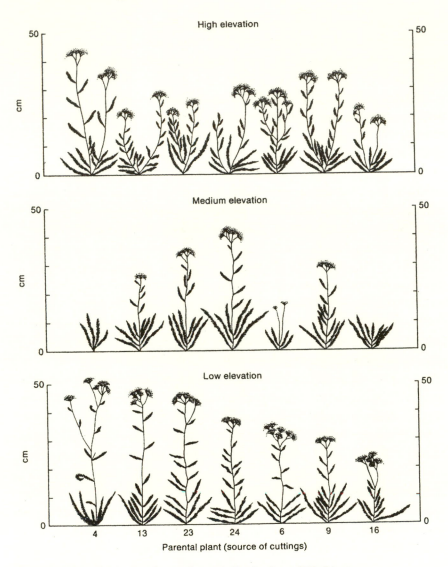

Fig. 1.2. Norms of reaction. *Source:* Carnegie Institution of Washington.

everyone has two copies of a gene (two alleles), and that goes for Mom and for Dad. Mom gives one of her alleles to each sibling and so does Dad.

Some elementary probability arguments show on average (nonidentical twin) siblings share the same allele at a given locus 50 percent of the time and identical twins share the same allele at the same location 100 percent of the time. Further, it is assumed that, if on average siblings share only one allele at a given location, then, with respect to the relevant trait, they will resemble each other about half as much as twins, who share two alleles at the same location.[10]

Note that we are assuming a very simple linearity here; that is, one dose of gene sharing gives one unit of resemblance and two doses give two units. Additive genetic variance is that portion of the total genetic variance that can be attributed to the straightforward addition of the effects of single alleles. This additivity assumption is important, because without it we can't use the numbers of ½ for fraternal twins versus 1 for identical twins, and those numbers function in absolutely central ways in obtaining heritabilities from twin studies.[11] Heritability estimates based on this simplifying, additivity assumption are called narrow sense heritability estimates, as distinguished from broad sense heritability estimates, which allow for more realistic gene-gene interactions. Heritability in the narrow sense is a component of heritability in the broad sense. Some behavioral geneticists say that the narrow heritability component will do just fine and we can confine our focus to narrow heritability, but others say the distinction is important and should not be ignored. We will come back to this distinction several times later.

JJ: This "narrow sense" still seems pretty complicated to me, but even granted it's not as complex and realistic as it all could be, and we can talk about that later maybe, what do behavioral geneticists do with these 100 percent and 50 percent figures?

BG: First, they measure quantitative traits in identical twins and in fraternal twins, comparing scores within a family, and then aggregating twin pairs from a number of families. It often turns out that the identical twins are more alike on a trait that's measured than are the fraternal twins. Like height, and maybe like IQ or disposition to a disease such as heart disease or schizophrenia. If so, that's at least a hint that the trait has an important genetic component. It's only a hint, because the identical twins could be more alike than the fraternal twins because they were treated more alike. But behavioral geneticists assume there is no difference in the way the two types of twins are treated that affects the traits they want to study. This is called the equal environments assumption, or EEA, and though it is controversial, behavioral geneticists claim they have reasonable empirical evidence for this assumption.[12]

JJ: What's next? How do you get from these measured differences between identical and fraternal twins to the heritability estimates I read about in the New York Times and Washington Post?

BG: We need to appeal to a correlation coefficient here. Correlation measures how similar the deviations in one variable are to deviations in another variable. I say deviations because remember that we are looking at variances that track together, or *covary*, often referred to as covariance. (For example, if one twin is 5 feet, 10 inches, then what's the likelihood that her twin will have the same height?) I think I can make the correlation coefficient idea simple. We symbolize this correlation coefficient by r, and it ranges from +1 (perfect correlation or perfect predictability) through zero (no correlation) to −1 (perfect reverse correlation). A high correlation coefficient (say, r = 0.75) can be depicted graphically as a fairly tight cloud of points along a line (like an airplane's contrail). And that cloud narrows into a straight line as the correlation becomes higher and goes to 1.0. If we are looking at the covariances between phenotype and genotype, such a high coefficient indicates a high heritability. And, as an aside, it's worth noting that the correlation coefficient between phenotype and genotype can give us the heritability—all we have to do is square the correlation coefficient! That's because the statisticians tell us that the square of the correlation coefficient gives us a percentage of how much the one variable (the genotype's variation) predicts (or accounts for) the phenotype's variation. (See Figure 1.3 for the four graphs representing zero, low, medium, and high correlations.)

Getting back to the twins, the correlation coefficient can be used to give a number, usually between zero and 1, which indicates how much the groups of twins are alike, in the sense of how closely they covary, on their measured scores.

JJ: Hmmmmm . . . Maybe that squaring of the correlation coefficient to get a heritability can help me understand that concept better, but let's not move so fast! I think I might be getting lost in all the math. Let's just talk about twins and what's correlating with what again, and what happened to the two different types of twins.

BG: Okay, let's start with the identical twins first—but remember this is a *population* of identical twins so they have a range of scores, and we look at how closely one twin in a pair resembles the other one in a large collection of twin pairs, maybe hundreds, say half of which are identical twins and half of which are fraternal twins that we will consider in a moment. Let's assume the identical twins correlate pretty well on a verbal reasoning test score, say, about 0.75, like that last figure in the correlation graphs. Reasonably enough, behavioral geneticists argue that these identical twins resemble each other because of genetics and environment. The genetic or heredity influence (variance) is represented by H², as always. The environment influence is represented by c^2 (for common environment). As we will discuss later, the common environment is defined by behavioral geneticists to be that which contributes to the similarity of the trait under consideration (as opposed to the unshared environment, which, by definition, does not contribute to that trait similarity). Then the correlation between identical twins is just the sum of those two influences, H^2 and c^2; in the case of the 0.75 correlation among the identical twins on the verbal reasoning score, we could write: $0.75 = H^2 + c^2$. If you will let me write this as a more general equation:

$$r_{MZ} = H^2 + c^2 \qquad \text{(first equation)}$$

JJ: Okay, so that's how we bring in the identical twins—I guess the MZ stands for monozygotic? But what about the other type of twins?

BG: The dizygotic, or DZ, twins share only one half their genes—remember, you agreed to (partly) trust me on this 50 percent number—so the joint effects of genetics (or heredity) and common environment that produce the correlation are $h^2/2$ and c^2. (Remember from grammar school fractions: 50% of H^2 is the same as $\frac{1}{2} \times H^2$, which can be represented as $H^2/2$.) We are assuming the common environments (c^2) work the same for both types of twins, and again this is known as the equal environments assumption (EEA). Let's assume the DZ twins' correlation on the verbal reasoning test score is 0.50, like in the third correlation graph. They are not as similar as the sets of MZ twins on verbal reasoning scores. Thus $0.50 = h^2/2 + c^2$. And the DZ twins general equation is:

$$r_{DZ} = h^2/2 + c^2 \qquad \text{(second equation)}$$

JJ: Where is this going? Are you ever going to get to how we can compute a heritability? And don't try to pull any fast ones on me—I saw that you wrote the heritability for the MZ twins as a broad heritability (H) and the heritability for the DZ twins as a narrow heritability (h), and earlier you had pointed out that these two concepts were different.

BG: You are one sharp-eyed judge. What most behavioral geneticists say is that for this kind of simple model, we are just interested in the narrow heritability, so we can assume that $H^2 = h^2$, for the time being. If we can accept this, we are actually where we can compute heritabilities. All we have to do is take those two equations and solve for h^2. I hate to remind you about high school algebra, but you can subtract the second equation from the first after we have rewritten H^2 as h^2 for the MZ twins, and you would get

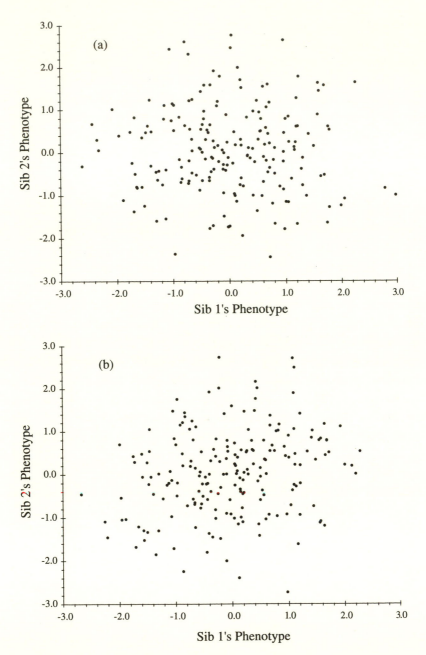

Fig. 1.3. Correlation coefficients of values 0, .25, .50, and .75 (for panels *a* through *d,* respectively). *Source:* Carey, 2003, 282–83. Reprinted with permission of Sage Publications.

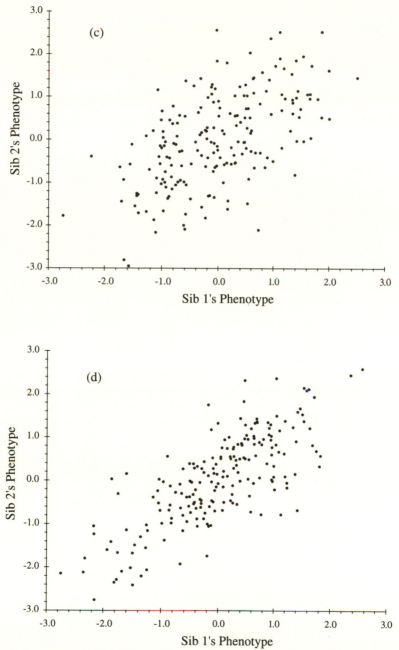

$r_{MZ} - r_{DZ} = h^2 - h^2/2 + c^2 - c^2$, so you can drop the c^2s since they subtract away, and then we have $r_{MZ} - r_{DZ} = h^2/2$ or multiplying both sides of the equation by 2:

$$h^2 = 2 (r_{MZ} - r_{DZ})$$

So, if we substituted in those sample correlations of 0.75 and 0.50 from the verbal reasoning case that we talked about earlier, the heritability for this trait is 50 percent:

$$2 (0.75 - 0.50) = 2 (0.25) = 0.5 \text{ (or 50\%)}$$

JJ: I get it. I think I get it! Generally heritability is twice the difference between the similarity of the identical twins compared to the fraternal twins.

BG: You got it, but wait—there's more!

JJ: Why do I need more? I now understand heritability and twin studies.

BG: We need to talk more about the environmental effects. We can get a measure of c^2 from our first equation, just by moving h^2 to the other side and making it a minus, so $c^2 = r_{MZ} - h^2$. But behavioral geneticists are interested not only in the common environment or shared environment. They're also interested in the nonshared environment—what makes people different.[13] We can get this into the picture very easily. The only factors we consider in this simple model are heritability, shared environment, and nonshared environment.[14] This last term we will abbreviate as e^2. We can state this idea as, if you will excuse me, another (third) equation:

$$1 = h^2 + c^2 + e^2 \qquad \text{(third equation)}$$

This holds because h^2, c^2, and e^2 are each proportions, and proportions must sum to one. (The genetic influence, plus the influence of the shared environment, plus the influence of the unshared environment is said to equal the total influence on the trait.)

And because we already know how to get h^2 and c^2, we can get e^2 as well from this equation. And all these values come *just from the observed similarities (expressed as correlation coefficients) of the monozygotic and the dizygotic twins!* I will not do the algebra with you, but it's simple enough, and it turns out that:

$$e^2 = 1 - r_{MZ}$$

JJ: All right! But let's go back to the beginning and see where this long argument has led us. Can you summarize?

BG: Twin studies give us a way to infer genetic and environmental contributions to quantitative traits, like heights, weights, and verbal reasoning scores. Typically we do not have any identified genes or genotypes that we can directly assess in the latter cases. We used the amount of shared genetic variance found in identical versus fraternal twins and their scores on some quantitative trait of interest to portion out how much was genetic, and how much was common environment and nonshared environment.

But in the argument we made lots of assumptions. Two big ones were equal environments ($c_{MZ}^2 = c_{DZ}^2$) and additivity of gene effects (both in obtaining the ½ figure and asserting that $H_{MZ}^2 = h_{MZ}^2$). There are other assumptions, too, that we did not fully make explicit, such as denying that there are any correlations between genes and environments, and interactions between genes and environments, but those are complex issues we can largely skip for the moment. But also remember that heritability estimates can change, depending on the populations and environments that are tested. Please don't forget that graph we discussed in connection with norms of reaction studies in plants! And norm of reaction studies for humans have not been done and cannot, for ethical reasons, be done in any well-controlled way. (We can't breed human beings to be genetically identical and then place them in different environments to study the relative importance of genetics and environment for a given trait.) But for the population studied in the specific environments examined, if we have a high heritability, many behavioral geneticists think we may have a good pointer to an underlying genetic architecture. But that is actually still to be proven. I will discuss this later (in dialogue 2).

The twin model is a start, and the version we have discussed is a very oversimplified one at that. Behavioral geneticists can make more complex models that deal with some of these complexities and measure the effects, such as broad and narrow heritabilities. But that's for another day.

JJ: Another day is fine, but before we break, maybe you can quickly tell me if this strange heritability concept is ever used outside the human area, where it seems so hard to study. Is it ever used in animal studies?

BG: The answer is yes, and interestingly, in animal and plant studies, heritability is extensively used in the narrow sense that we found we had to move to in the twin study analysis. (Remember that narrow sense heritability assumes linear or additive relationships among genes.) But in the animal and agricultural world, investigators are mainly interested in breeding programs, so as to improve the weight of offspring of cattle, for example. These researchers use narrow heritability as a breeding value coefficient to predict how much change they will see in the next generation, because narrow heritability represents the genetic source of the resemblance between parents and offspring. If the narrow heritability is 100 percent (i.e., if all variation is genetic), then the value of the trait of interest, such as height, in the offspring will be exactly midway between the trait values in the two parents. Thus, it is the narrow heritability that is relevant to any evolutionary effects that genes have, and this is an important point to remember in any eugenics discussion.

JJ: Uh oh! The concept of a "breeding program" related to behavioral genetics scares me, as does the eugenics concept. But do the animal breeding programs really work on behaviors? Can you give me an example?

BG: The classic study was done in mice, in which populations were measured for fearfulness, which was tested for by putting the mice in a brightly lit box called an "open field." Fearful mice froze and lost excretory control—they were scared s——less, as one prominent neuroscientist has indelicately put it.[15] Brave mice, on the other hand, actively explored their surroundings. Mice from the brave and the fearful lines were interbred over 30 generations, and as controls the two lines were also crossbred. The results of the breeding program on open-field activity is shown in Figure 1.4.

JJ: Interesting! Though the lines zigzag around a bit, I can imagine roughly straight lines though the three sets of points, so I guess that allows for predictability of what you'll see in each successive generation. But exactly how does heritability come in?

BG: Maybe it would help to use a simpler example, say, one involving our rubber plants again, but now breeding them to increase their height. We will now assume, like in virtually all cases involving quantitative genetics, and especially behavioral genetics, that we do *not* know about those A, B, and C alleles, but only about the heritability of height. (Quantitative geneticists have means of estimating heritabilities from phenotypic resemblance between parents and offspring, and also using resemblances among other relatives.) Look at Figure 1.1 again. Note that the plant height varies all the way from a minimum of some around 2½ feet (80 centimeters) up to the really tall almost 9-foot rubber plants at the other extreme. The average height in this entire collection of plants is about 160 centimeters (~5 feet). Suppose our plant breeder anticipates orders for a large number of big rubber trees for some new malls. If he can interbreed just very tall parents (that he selects from those that have heights about 260 centimeters) and if the heritability of height in this population is 50 percent, then the average height of their offspring will be about 210 centimeters (about 6 feet, 10 inches), well above the average of the origi-

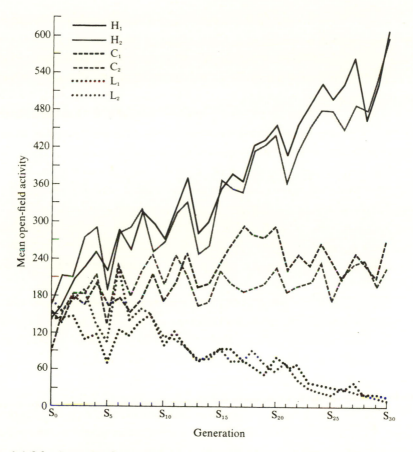

Fig. 1.4. Selecting traits. *Source:* DeFries, Gervais, and Thomas, 1978, 67. Reprinted with permission of Springer Science and Business Media.

nal population. (This comes from taking 50% of the average deviation of 100 [the difference between the average height of the tall plants (260) and the average height of the original population (160)] and adding this figure of 50 centimeters to the average height of 160 for the original population.) In case you're interested, the equation that predicts this response is given in standard textbooks of quantitative genetics as

$$R = h^2 S,$$

where the response (R, the increase above the average in the offspring) is equal to the heritability estimate (h^2) times the selection difference value (S, the amount above the average) in the breeding parents.[16]

This easy prediction using the narrow heritability concept, however, assumes that there is no nongenetic cause of resemblance between parent and offspring that would affect height, like nutritional or climate differences. (This is assumed as part of the derivation of the equation above as found in genetics texts.) The prediction also assumes that the underlying genes, which are in truth veiled from us now, act to sum together in terms of their effects on height (as before, this is called additive genetic variation), so that one dose of the allele results in the addition of one unit of a trait, two doses of the allele yields two units, and so forth, just like in our shared resemblance units for human twins. Additive genes are stipulated to not have more complex nonlinear interrelations that would confuse the selection and breeding process, such as the gene dominance effects or gene-gene interaction effects. Though the genes are veiled from us, selection experiments can provide some evidence of additivity of gene contributions through multigeneration breeding experiments, as we saw with the mice.

Finally, you might be interested in knowing that one of the critics of quantitative behavioral genetics, Douglas Wahlsten, wrote in a classic article in 1990 that "the only practical application of a heritability coefficient [h^2] is to predict the results of a program of selective breeding" (1990, 119).

JJ Final Comment: Well, that's very interesting. I can actually grasp intuitively how the heritability estimate works here a bit better—as a partial predictor of a characteristic in the next generation—than I could either looking at the picture of those rubber trees (acid phosphatase activity) or at those twin study equations. And though I appreciate Wahlsten's viewpoint, after all of our discussion today and all the qualifications about heritability, I imagine many behavioral geneticists see it quite differently. But now we really have to stop.

The Twin Study Model and the ACE Path Diagram in Behavioral Genetics

Now that we have the rudiments of the heritability concept and understand how shared and nonshared environments can be appealed to, we should note that the twin-study model can be represented graphically in the ACE model. The graphical picture may help some readers imagine how twin studies work, and also might assist them in reading other papers in the field. (Readers familiar with ACE diagrams or just in a hurry might skip to the next section.)

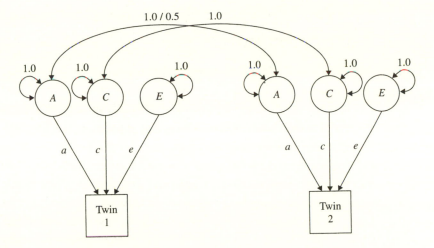

Fig. 1.5. ACE path. *Source:* Plomin et al., 2001, 360.

This model can be depicted graphically in a path diagram, as in Figure 1.5, for MZ and DZ twins. The straight arrows represent causal influence, and the curved arrows correlations.

There are easy and straightforward ways to obtain the three equations given above in the dialogue on twin studies with Judge Jean directly from these diagrams, but the reader must be referred to other sources for these techniques (Plomin et al., 2000). This model uses h^2 to represent heritability, and since most often behavioral geneticists assume they are working only with additive genotypic variance, they underscore this additivity by using a^2 in place of h^2, and call this kind of diagram an ACE model, capitalizing the a, c, and e factors that influence a trait. It should be stressed that the circles around A, C, and E indicate that these are theoretical or unobserved variables, in contrast to the observed, empirical, or measured variables represented by the squares for twin 1 and twin 2. The long, curved double-headed arrow labeled with a value of 1.0 (MZ) or 0.5 (DZ) between the As represents the values for shared additive genetic correlation that the behavioral geneticist derived for Judge Jean above. The other long, curved double-headed arrow labeled with a value of 1.0 between the Cs represents that value that is based on the equal environments assumption (EEA) discussed earlier.

Environmental Complexities and Startling Results from Quantitative Genetics

The c^2 (shared) and e^2 (nonshared) components of the environment that were discussed earlier in this chapter, and that appeared in the dialogue and just now reappeared in the ACE model, represent critically important distinctions that are at root somewhat nebulous. I have noted earlier that many people would probably assume that those things twins experienced in common in a family would be considered part of the *shared* environment, and that those things they did not experience in common would be considered part of the *nonshared* environment. But recall that in the derivation of the equations for the twin model, c^2 was defined as all those things that make the twins alike (correlated). Similarly, e^2 is defined as all those things that make the twins different. The notions can escape from empirical circularity by being further specified and qualified, but this is where the somewhat nebulous character of the concepts becomes apparent. Ultimately, I will suggest, the distinction between shared and nonshared becomes almost a term of art, to be determined in each specific study. That can lead to some problems, such as a reintroduction of circularity, which I note below.

The most explicit discussion of what else needs to be known for an environmental effect to be termed *shared* is by Rowe and Jacobson (1999, 16–17), who note that "four conditions must be satisfied for an environmental effect to count as shared" (all quotes come from these two pages).

These conditions are that (1) near universals found in a culture from which the subjects are drawn do not count because they would be common to all families. For example, the use of the English language among second-generation Americans is such a near universal. Also, (2) the environmental exposures must be common to all siblings. Rowe and Jacobson say that parental divorce would typically count as shared for the involved children, but this is an example we will need to return to again. Another condition (3) requires that "the environmental exposure must have a directional effect on a given trait to be considered an environmental influence on that trait." Directional here seems to mean "plausibly causal and relevant," a meaning that raises a question of circularity (since we are trying to establish causal properties).[17] Finally (4), in what seems to be a variant of the third condition, "environmental effects can be shared environmental influences only to the extent that they reliably change a trait in a *constant* direction." Here the divorce example is returned to, but it is qualified so that if divorce affects siblings differently (say different sibs have distinct emotional/behavioral reactions), then divorce would count as a nonshared environmental influence. To add to the potential complexity, Rowe and Jacobson add that as regards this latter type of factor, "the number and variety of potential nonshared environmental influences are nearly limitless." How to specify such nonshared factors and assess their significance reliably turns out to be a very difficult problem for behavioral geneticists, as I note in the next subsection.

The bottom line, for this observer, is that the distinction between what counts as shared and what counts as nonshared becomes a term of art, to be specified only in the individual study. (By *term of art,* I mean that context and judgment are involved in drawing the distinction, and they may well depend on special data available in particular studies, and not admit of any easily generalizeable rules.) But because the individual study is establishing the environmental factors as causal and as either shared or nonshared, circularity may be introduced, which may weaken the empirical force of the study. For such key concepts to have such prima facie vagueness and potential circularity may point to the reasons behind what I'll soon call the "gloomy hypothesis" regarding the nonshared environment.

Shared and Nonshared Environments: A "Gloomy Prospect"?

Twin studies, incorporated within more sophisticated "biometric"[18] path models like the ACE model I mentioned above, use the shared and nonshared environments distinction with the qualifications I just mentioned. Perhaps surprisingly, quantitative studies of normal personality traits (as well as mental disorders) indicate that of all the environmental factors, the nonshared ones have the major effect.[19] As noted earlier, it is estimated that about 15 percent of the variance of the schizophrenia trait is due to the nonshared environment and little, if any, to the shared environment (Cardno and Gottesman, 2000). However, a meta-analysis of 43 studies by Turkheimer and Waldron (2000) indicated that though nonshared environmental factors were responsible for 50 percent of the total variation of behavioral outcomes, identified nonshared environmental factors accounted for only 2 percent of the total variance. In this meta-analysis, Turkheimer distinguished two senses of nonshared: objective and effective. An environmental event is objectively nonshared if it is (verifiably, measurably) experienced by only one sibling in a family, irrespective of the consequences it produces. An event is effectively nonshared if it makes siblings different, rather than similar (this is how the term is typically defined), irrespectively of whether it was experienced by one or both.

The significant claim about the role of the nonshared environment, originally made by Plomin and Daniels in 1987, was that children in the same family are as different as they are because measurable differences in their environments made them that way. But, contrary to that claim, the meta-analysis I just mentioned found that, although 50 percent of the variance in behavioral outcomes was accounted for in the effective nonshared sense (the children *were* different), "the median percentage accounted for by objectively definable nonshared event is less than 2%" (Turkheimer, 2000, 163). That is, the nonshared environment may help to explain about 50 percent of the phenotypic variance, but the specific factors that constitute the nonshared environment typically are not measured and so thus far only seem to account for 2 percent of explained variance.

A related article (Turkheimer, 2000) infers that these nonshared differences are nonsystematic and largely accidental or random, and thus have been and will continue to be very difficult to study. This possibility had been considered earlier by Plomin and Daniels (1987), but dismissed as a "gloomy prospect." That "gloomy prospect" now looks more plausible, though Plomin and colleagues have offered a more optimistic gloss, as well as recommendations for further research in this area (Plomin et al., 2001). The gloomy results regarding specific environmental factors may in part result from the fact that we have no general theory of the environment, as noted earlier in this chapter. Without some fairly detailed general backdrop view that can suggest how to decompose the environment and measure it reliably, gloomy results may continue. There are only glimmers of hope that this problem will be remedied in the short run.[20] At least one team of investigators in the IQ area declined to explicitly factor in the effects of the nonshared environment, and instead treated the nonshared environment as part of the error term, rather than treating them as distinct terms (Devlin et al., 1997).

On the more positive side, quantitative investigations have identified two important ways that genetic variables and variables in the shared and nonshared environments interact to influence phenotypes. The first, genotype-environment correlation (usually written as G·E but occasionally as G→E), represents possible effects of an individual's genetics on the environment (e.g., via that individual's evoking different responses from or selecting environments). Such effects were found for both normal and pathological traits investigated in the large Nonshared Environmental Adolescent Development (NEAD) study, described in detail in *The Relationship Code* (Reiss et al., 2000). Second, different genotypes have different sensitivities to environments, collectively called genotype×environmental interaction (G×E). A classical example is phenylketonuria (PKU), which can produce devastating mental retardation unless the diet is controlled for phenylalanine. There are two recent discoveries using molecular methods that involve early environment interacting with genetic dispositions to criminality (Caspi et al., 2002) and to depression (Caspi, 2003) that have stimulated additional interest in gene-environment interactions. (For a discussion of the Caspi et al. articles, see pp. 44–45, below, and Parens's special supplement to the *Hastings Center Report* [Parens, 2004].) Differential sensitivity is important in many models of genetic disorder, including the neurodevelopmental models of schizophrenia genetics mentioned later.

Testing the Models and Goodness of Fit

The ACE model I have presented is very simple. Contemporary behavioral genetics uses such simple models, but it also employs more complex, multivariate models that can represent common factor genes—genes that can account for correlations between different traits such as verbal and quantitative cognitive abilities. For additional discussion of a genetic contribution underlying several traits, see the following chapter, where the g factor will be briefly discussed. The more complex multivariate models can also represent additional family relationships that I haven't discussed (e.g., half sibs and unrelated sibs), and more sophisticated means of assessing family influences over time (i.e., longitudinal models). Given the plethora of conceivable models, assessing the best (or at least better) ones is of major importance. Behavioral geneticists can use multiple models and combine them, and test them jointly using empirical data to determine which models fit the data best. Goodness of fit tests use highly developed mathematical and computer techniques that are also widely found in other social sciences. An accessible account of how a goodness of fit determination is done for some simple ACE models involving MZ twins, related sibs, and unrelated sibs can be found in Rowe (1994). Though such goodness of fit tests are what Rowe called the "state of the art" in behavioral genetics, some behavioral geneticists such as Turkheimer (personal communication) have doubts as to whether these empirical tests can adequately control for the mix of additive and nonadditive genetic influences (as well as shared and nonshared environmental influences) involved in human studies. I give an example of a goodness of fit approach involving four models in the IQ section of dialogue 3 in the following chapter.

Largely traditional, quantitative, or epidemiological behavioral genetics produces evidence to suggest that a given trait *may be* importantly influenced by genetics. But to understand whether such a trait *is* specifically influenced by identified genes, researchers have to use newer, molecular approaches. In the following chapter, in a second dialogue between Judge Jean and the behavioral geneticist, we will turn to those molecular approaches. In a third and concluding dialogue with Judge Jean, we will examine the strengths and weaknesses of both the quantitative and the molecular methods by focusing on two specific, though hypothetical, cases of genetic testing for high IQ and for ADHD. The chapter will conclude with some speculations about the future direction of behavioral genetics research in elucidating the relations of nature and nurture.

ACKNOWLEDGMENTS

I want to thank Elving Anderson, Catherine Baker, Greg Carey, Lindley Darden, Megan Davis, Bernie Devlin, Harold Edgar, Ilya Farber, Irv Gottesman, Ken Kendler, Matt McGue, Erik Parens, Eric Turkheimer, and Bill Winslade for comments on portions of the draft manuscript of this chapter. However, the opinions expressed (and errors) are my own. Supported by the National Institutes of Health Ethical, Legal, and Social Implications of the Humane Genome Project (NIH ELSI) program (through HC-AAAS) and the National Science Foundation Science and Technology Studies (NSF STS) program.

NOTES

1. This emphasis on individual differences in quantitative genetics is an important point. It has analogies with philosophers' emphasis on the roles of Mendelian genes as makers of phenotypic difference, rather than phenotype makers. See Waters, C. K. (1994). "Genes Made Molecular." *Philosophy of Science* 61: 163–85. To explain how to make a phenotype, a developmental explanation is needed—a huge undertaking. See

Kitcher, P. (1984). "1953 and All That: A Tale of Two Sciences." *Philosophical Review* 93: 335–73. Some critics of behavioral genetics demand a developmental explanation in all cases, whereas behavioral geneticists argue they can provide important results that bypass such demands, and explore differences in a trait in a population at the more abstract level, similar to what Mendelian geneticists do although quantitative genetics does not seek single-locus prototypical Mendelian traits. A developmental explanation separates the effects of genes and environments only with great difficulty.

See Schaffner, K. F. (1998a). "Genes, Behavior, and Developmental Emergentism: One Process, Indivisible?" *Philosophy of Science* 65(June): 209–52. Behavioral genetics can make a good case that such gene-environmental effect separation can be done analytically for differences. See Plomin, R., J. C. DeFries, G. E. McClearn, et al. (2000). *Behavioral Genetics*. New York: Worth: 87–88.

2. Technically this is true only of the "probandwise concordance rate," a detail that need not concern us. Also, concordance rates can be extended to other family members' risk as well, such as parents, children, and sibs.

3. Relatedly, less than one-third of the patients recently seen in early detection (prodromal and first-episode psychosis) programs have first-or second-degree relatives diagnosed with a psychotic disorder. Schaffner, K. F., and P. D. McGorry. (2001). "Preventing Severe Mental Illnesses—New Prospects and Ethical Challenges." *Schizophrenia Research* 51(1): 3–15 [L. J. Phillips, T. H. McGlashan, personal communications].

4. It was Mark Frankel's suggestion that I imagine the audience for this chapter as including a judge. (Relatedly, Franklin Zweig has, for a number of years, been educating judges in genetics as part of his Einstein Institute programs, largely supported by Department of Education [DOE] grants.) I decided to put much of the material in these two papers into dialogue form after multiple attempts to write more traditional simple text explanations. Traditional exposition did not work in a natural way since the concepts had to be revisited a number of times to make them clear. A dialogue format seems to do that more easily and more readably.

5. The dialogue starts with what is termed broad heritability (symbolized by H^2), and later distinguishes it from narrow heritability (h^2). The use of the squared term seems to come from the fact that statistics defines a correlation measure symbolized by r (dealt with in the dialogue below), and also introduces a statistic r^2 that can be interpreted as the proportion of variance in the dependent variable that is contained in the independent variable. r^2 is misleadingly, perhaps, called the "coefficient of determination"—misleadingly, since it's only hypothetically a causal, rather than a correlational notion, and at values less than 1 it is probabilistic, and not deterministic. Later in the dialogue, after the concept of the correlation coefficient is introduced, another way to understand heritability in terms of r^2 will be discussed.

6. For those who wish to be reminded of their elementary statistics course, the variance of a population is the average of the squared differences between the mean of the population and the individual values of the measured variable.

7. This comment, though helpful, cannot be strictly true, since if the genes were entirely irrelevant to the trait of interest, they would not affect the variance of the trait either. Perhaps it's more accurate to say such genes can have vanishingly small, or empirically undetectable, effects on the mean.

8. Except males have one X and one Y chromosome.

9. The variance of the total distribution is 607.8 from all of the phenotypic data. But

the average of the environmental variances within each genotype is only 310.7 Thus v_g is equal to $607.8 - 310.7 = 297.1$, and $h^2 = 297.1/607.8 = 49\%$.

10. The arguments are shown explicitly in Plomin et al. (2000), Appendix, page 348, and how additive effects work in a linear way is detailed on pages 343–44 of the same.

11. There are more intricate models that can check for dominance but more complex forms of gene interactions such as epistasis are harder to model.

12. Critics of genetic influence often question this EEA assumption, but it has been defended using empirical data. On the critical side, see Lewontin, R. C., S.P.R. Rose, and L. J. Kamin. (1984). *Not in Our Genes: Biology, Ideology, and Human Nature*. New York: Pantheon; and Joseph, J. (2001). "Separated Twins and the Genetics of Personality Differences: A Critique." *American Journal of Psychology* 114(1): 1–30, who argue we need a better set of controls. See also Jonathan Beckwith's chapter in this book. Compare this view with the defense of EEA by Kendler, K. S., M. C. Neale, R. C. Kessler, et al. (1993). "A Test of the Equal-Environment Assumption in Twin Studies of Psychiatric Illness." *Behavioral Genetics* 23(1): 21–27; Kendler, K. S., M. C. Neale, R. C. Kessler, et al. (1994). "Parental Treatment and the Equal Environment Assumption in Twin Studies of Psychiatric Illness." *Psychological Medicine* 24(3): 579–90; Hettema, J. M., M. C. Neale, and K. S. Kendler. (1995). "Physical Similarity and the Equal-Environment Assumption in Twin Studies of Psychiatric Disorders." *Behavioral Genetics* 25(4): 327–35. Perhaps the most persuasive data supporting the EEA come from twin studies in families that have misidentified the zygosity of their twins and treated monozygotic twins as dizygotic, and vice versa , see Kendler et al. (1993), above. Though a systematic and in-depth unbiased general review of the EEA would be extremely useful, this author is unaware of any such review authored by a disinterested party—that is, one who has neither ideological nor genetically based research-program interests involved. (A point-by-point debate of the EEA would be a good alternative to an unbiased review, but I do not know of any parties that have done this either.) Prima facie, the EEA issue seems to be of critical importance, since if overlooked environmental correlations are truly responsible for observed similarities in identical twins, then this will result in higher reported concordances and an overestimation of the true genetic effects. But the difference if EEA does not hold is estimated not to be a huge change in heritabilities, probably a reduction from 50 to 35 percent (for an h^2 of 0.5) (Kendler, personal communication). This estimate needs to be quantitatively verified, however, using some empirical data.

13. More needs to be said about the prima facie tautological character of the characterizations of shared and nonshared environments, and about some ways that tautology can be clarified to have empirical content. This is covered toward the end of this chapter.

14. The nonshared environmental term also includes an implicit error term—an important point that will be noted again toward the end of this chapter and also in the discussion of Devlin et al.'s (1997) article on IQ in dialogue 3.

15. See LeDoux's discussion of the similar fearful rat phenotype in relation to neuroscience in [emotional brain], 135.

16. This comes from Falconer and MacKay, chapter 11, 186.

17. This condition seems not to distinguish shared from nonshared effects but rather to stipulate a general plausibility condition for any environmental trait.

18. A reference to why the model is called biometric—it is within the "biometric" tradition—follows further below.

19. There are some exceptions to this remarkable conclusion, including such variant ones as interest in music and delinquent behavior where c^2 is high, see Rowe and Jacobson (1999, 44) and also Moffitt—see Caspi, A., A. Taylor, T. E. Moffitt, et al. (2000). "Neighborhood Deprivation Affects Children's Mental Health: Environmental Risks Identified in a Genetic Design." *Psychological Science* 11(4): 338–42.

20. In preparation for a AAAS-sponsored presentation to two U.S. congressional members (Reps. Slaughter and Morella) and their staffs on genes and environments, related to Rep. Slaughter's bill on genetic discrimination, I conducted a Medline search of citations with the breast cancer gene (*BRCA1*) in its title or abstract, and another search with *BRCA1* and environment in the title or abstract. The hits were about 2500 for the first search and 44 for the second search (repeated June 24, 2002). This suggests the major focus is on the genetics, not on the gene-environment interaction in breast cancer studies, even though there is strong evidence for environmental effects in breast cancer. A further look for programs that were prioritizing environmental studies in cancer showed that the NCI has identified this as an "extraordinary opportunity" area for special attention in 2003: see www.plan.cancer.gov/scipri/genes.htm (accessed June 24, 2002).

REFERENCES

Benjamin, J., R. P. Ebstein, and R. H. Belmaker. (2002). *Molecular Genetics and the Human Personality.* Washington, D.C.: American Psychiatric Publications.

BSCS, ed. (2000). *Genes, Environment and Human Behavior.* Colorado Springs: Biological Sciences Curriculum Study (BSCS).

Cardno, A. G., and I. I. Gottesman. (2000). "Twin Studies of Schizophrenia: From Bow-and-Arrow Concordances to Star Wars Mx and Functional Genomics." *American Journal of Medical Genetics* 97(1): 12–17.

Carey, G. (2003). *Human Genetics for the Social Sciences.* Thousand Oaks, Calif.: Sage.

Caspi, A., J. McClay, T. E. Moffitt, J. Mill, J. Martin, I. W. Craig, A. Taylor, and R. Poulton. (2002). "Role of Genotype in the Cycle of Violence in Maltreated Children." *Science* 297(5582): 851–54.

Caspi, A., A. Taylor, T. E. Moffitt, et al. (2000). "Neighborhood Deprivation Affects Children's Mental Health: Environmental Risks Identified in a Genetic Design." *Psychological Science* 11(4): 338–42.

DeFries, J. C., M. C. Gervais, and E. A. Thomas. (1978). "Responses to Thirty Generations of Selection for Open-Field Activity in Laboratory Mice." *Behavior Genetics* 8: 3–13.

Devlin, B., M. Daniels, and K. Roeder. (1997). "The Heritability of IQ." *Nature* 388(6641): 468–71.

Falconer, D. S. (1965). "The Inheritance of Liability to Certain Diseases, Estimated from the Incidence among Relatives." *Annals of Human Genetics* 29: 51–76.

Falconer, D. S., and T. MacKay. (1996). *Introduction to Quantitative Genetics.* Englewood Cliffs, N.J.: Prentice Hall.

Gottesman, I. I., and L. Erlenmeyer-Kimling. (2001). "Family and Twin Strategies as a Head Start in Defining Prodromes and Endophenotypes for Hypothetical Early-Interventions in Schizophrenia." *Schizophrenia Research* 51(1): 93–102.

Harris, H. (1980). *The Principles of Human Biochemical Genetics*. 3rd ed. Amsterdam: North Holland.

Heston, L. L. (1966). "Psychiatric Disorders in Foster Home Reared Children of Schizophrenic Mothers." *British Journal of Psychiatry* 112(489): 819–25.

Hettema, J. M., M. C. Neale, and K. S. Kendler. (1995). "Physical Similarity and the Equal-Environment Assumption in Twin Studies of Psychiatric Disorders." *Behavioral Genetics* 25(4): 327–35.

Joseph, J. (2001). "Separated Twins and the Genetics of Personality Differences: A Critique." *American Journal of Psychology* 114(1): 1–30.

Kendler, K. S., M. C. Neale, R. C. Kessler, et al. (1993). "A Test of the Equal-Environment Assumption in Twin Studies of Psychiatric Illness." *Behavioral Genetics* 23(1): 21–27.

Kendler, K. S., M. C. Neale, R. C. Kessler, et al. (1994). "Parental Treatment and the Equal Environment Assumption in Twin Studies of Psychiatric Illness." *Psychological Medicine* 24(3): 579–90.

Kitcher, P. (1984). "1953 and All That: A Tale of Two Sciences." *Philosophical Review* 93: 335–73.

LeDoux, J. E. (1996). *The Emotional Brain: The Mysterious Underpinnings of Emotional Life*. New York: Simon & Schuster.

Lewontin, R. C. (1995). *Human Diversity*. New York: Scientific American Library [distributed by W. H. Freeman].

Lewontin, R. C., S.P.R. Rose, and L. J. Kamin. (1984). *Not in Our Genes: Biology, Ideology, and Human Nature*. New York: Pantheon.

Neiderhiser, J. M. (2001). "Understanding the Roles of Genome and Envirome: Methods in Genetic Epidemiology." *British Journal of Psychiatry* (suppl. 40): S12–S17.

Parens, E. (2004). "Genetic Differences and Human Identities: On Why Talking about Behavioral Genetics is Important and Difficult." *Hastings Center Report* 34(1): S4–S35.

Plomin, R., K. Asbury, and A. Dunn. (2001). "Why Are Children in the Same Family So Different? Nonshared Environment a Decade Later." *Canadian Journal of Psychiatry* 46: 225–33.

Plomin, R., and D. Daniels. (1987). "Why Are Children in the Same Family So Different from One Another?" *Behavioral and Brain Sciences* 10: 1–60.

Plomin, R., J. C. DeFries, G. E. McClearn, and P. McGuffin. (2000). *Behavioral Genetics*. New York: Worth.

Reiss, D., and J. M. Neiderhiser. (2000). "The Interplay of Genetic Influences and Social Processes in Developmental Theory: Specific Mechanisms Are Coming into View." *Developmental Psychopathology* 12(3): 357–74.

Reiss, D., J. M. Neiderhiser, E. Mavis Hetherington, et al. (2000). *The Relationship Code: Deciphering Genetic and Social Influences on Adolescent Development*. Cambridge, Mass.: Harvard University Press.

Rowe, D. C. (1994). *The Limits of Family Influence: Genes, Experience, and Behavior*. New York: Guilford.

Rowe, D. C., and K. C. Jacobson. (1999). "In the Mainstream: Research in Behavioral Genetics." In R. A. Carson and M. A. Rothstein, eds. *Behavioral Genetics: The Clash of Culture and Biology*. Baltimore: Johns Hopkins University Press,: 12–34.

Schaffner, K. F. (1998). "Genes, Behavior, and Developmental Emergentism: One Process, Indivisible?" *Philosophy of Science* 65(June): 209–52.

Schaffner, K. F., and P. D. McGorry. (2001). "Preventing Severe Mental Illnesses—New Prospects and Ethical Challenges." *Schizophrenia Research* 51(1): 3–15.

Turkheimer, E. (2000). "Three Laws of Behavior Genetics and What They Mean." *Current Directions in Psychological Science* 9: 160–61.

Turkheimer, E., and M. Waldron. (2000). "Nonshared Environment: A Theoretical, Methodological, and Quantitative Review." *Psychological Bulletin* 126(1): 78–108.

Waters, C. K. (1994). "Genes Made Molecular." *Philosophy of Science* 61: 163–85.

CHAPTER TWO

Behavior

Its Nature and Nurture, Part 2

Kenneth F. Schaffner, M.D., Ph.D.

The previous chapter introduced basic terms, ideas, and methods of behavioral genetics, both discursively in the early sections and in the form of a hypothetical dialogue between a behavioral geneticist and Judge Jean. Specifically, I introduced basic concepts at work in the classical, quantitative, or epidemiological approaches to understanding human behavior. This chapter focuses on the more recent molecular approaches of behavioral genetics. First, I introduce the background to the "molecular turn" in behavioral (and psychiatric) genetics, and then I resume the dialogue format between Judge Jean and the behavioral geneticist. In what I call dialogue 2 (dialogue 1 is in the previous chapter), I discuss linkage and association methods, summarize results of novelty-seeking behavior and Alzheimer disease studies, and raise some questions about how quantitative and molecular research programs are related. In dialogue 3, I describe two hypothetical cases involving genetic testing for IQ and for attention deficit hyperactivity disorder (ADHD). Judge Jean learns how much is known about both the quantitative and the molecular aspects of IQ and ADHD, and she is introduced to a promising but skeptical vision of the future of behavioral genetics in the context of neuroscientific complexity.

Molecular Methods

Classical (or quantitative) studies discussed in the previous chapter can indicate that genes may contribute to complex human behaviors, but they do not identify specific genes or how genes contribute to behaviors. McGuffin, Riley, and Plomin wrote that such approaches can no longer be seen as an end in themselves, and that the field must move to specific genes assisted by the recently completed draft versions of the human genome sequence (McGuffin et al., 2001). In fact, my review of the recent literature on the nature-nurture issue (Schaffner, 2001) indicates that most research in psychiatric genetics has taken a "molecular turn."

It is now widely acknowledged that most genes playing etiological and pathophysiological roles in behavioral traits and in psychiatric disorders are not single-locus genes of large effect following Mendelian patterns (McGuffin et al., 2001). Hyman recently noted that mental disorders will typically be heterogeneous and be affected by multiple, partially overlapping sets of genes (Hyman 2000 and in this volume). Mental disorders will thus be "complex traits," technically defined as conforming to non-Mendelian inheritance patterns. A classic, though difficult, article on genetics and complex traits appeared in 1994 by Lander and Schork. The article is still essential reading for those wanting to familiarize themselves with this notion of a complex trait, which does not deny Mendel's accomplishments, but enriches traditional genetics by moving beyond the study of monogenic traits, which result from mutations of a single gene.

Two general molecular methods are widely used to search for genes related to behavioral traits and mental disorders: linkage analysis and allelic association. Linkage analysis is the traditional approach to gene identification, but it works well only when genes have reasonably large effects, which does not appear to be the case in behavioral (or psychiatric) genetics.[1] Allelic association studies are more sensitive, but at present they typically require candidate genes to examine familial data.[2] To introduce these molecular methods, we return to the dialogue format used earlier and reintroduce the inquisitive Judge Jean.

Dialogue 2: Molecular Hopes and Problems

Judge Jean (JJ): Our conversation the other day helped me understand how heritability works and how twin studies can give us some estimates of the roles that genes and environments play. But what I really want to know about are the molecular advances. I know that the sequence of the entire human genome has been completed, and over the last several years I've heard about various genes for novelty seeking and anxiety, as well as about genes that cause Alzheimer disease and maybe even predispose people to criminality. This molecular area has to be where results about genes could affect my decisions. What can you tell me?

BG: Unfortunately, there has been an awful lot of hype in the molecular area, though there have been some stunning advances as well. We have two versions of the entire human genome, one created by a publicly funded consortium and the other by a privately owned company, which were completed in 2001.[3] But these identify only the sequence of the base pairs of the genomes that the two research groups studied. Information about those DNA sequences is very valuable, but there's still much that we do not understand, such as how much of the DNA codes for genes and how much is nonfunctional, or exactly how many genes there are, and especially how most of the coding sequences work to produce phenotypic effects. Also, it is very hard to tie even general types of behaviors to genes, though some progress has been made, as you mentioned, in the area of Alzheimer disease. Maybe we should start with that novelty-seeking gene you mentioned and I could explain how it was identified and also some problems with it.

JJ: Great! Novelty seeking isn't exactly the sort of "impulsive" behavior that the people who come before me engage in, but maybe that case can give me a sense of how behavioral geneticists try to understand complex behaviors at the level of the gene.

BG: Some researchers do think they have discovered a correlation between a particular allele (or form of a gene) and novelty-seeking behavior. That correlation was found by comparing two groups of people. In the first few studies, one group had a short form of an allele (called *DRD4*)[4] that codes for a receptor for the neurotransmitter molecule dopamine, which I will explain in a moment. The second group had a long form of the same allele. Using a standard psychological questionnaire, the researchers compared how the first group's level of novelty seeking compared with the second group's. The researchers found that in comparison with the first group, the second group exhibited greater novelty-seeking behavior.

That kind of genetic study is called an association study, because it looks to associate a variation in the gene's alleles with a variation in the behavioral phenotype (in this case, the level of novelty seeking). The *DRD4* gene was examined because a prominent psychiatrist, Dr. Robert Cloninger, argued that dopamine is one of the important chemicals used by nerves to communicate either among themselves or with muscle cells, especially about novelty-seeking behavior. This kind of chemical is called a neurotransmitter. Cloninger's argument was based on his studies using rats and other animals. In association studies, typically you first need to have a plausible candidate gene from some other study, maybe from an animal study, or from a theory about how a certain gene might be related to a behavior. Then you look for the correlations between the alleles and the behavior.

JJ: That seems straightforward enough. So this gene was a good candidate and it makes more of a chemical that makes the person with this allele seek out novel experiences?

BG: I don't think they thought that precisely about making more of a chemical, but they did expect an effect related to the biochemistry, which might involve gene regulation, which can be complex. And initially there were two different genetic studies that supported an effect for the long form of the allele of *DRD4* on novelty-seeking behavior. But then there were some disconfirming studies, and the results have gone back and forth between positive effects and no effects. It has turned out that it is very hard to confirm, or replicate, molecular studies in the behavioral area. There have been several review articles that pooled the various studies together in what is called a meta-analysis. One by behavioral geneticist Matt McGue concluded that there is a "significant" but quite small effect. ("Significant" here only means not due to chance alone.) The genetic difference at that one locus (the genetic variation) appears to help explain about 4 percent of the difference in novelty-seeking activity between the two groups (the phenotypic variation). While interesting, such a finding was thought to be of doubtful clinical value (McGue, 2001). McGue also has some doubts about the underlying biological explanation of the effect, though remember that Cloninger thinks he has a theory of how this might work. But then there were two more meta-analyses that suggested the net effect of *DRD4* might be even less than McGue estimated, possibly approaching zero.[5]

JJ: Does anyone know why different scientists get such different, even inconsistent, results in this area?

BG: The reasons are partly technical, having to do with statistics. It turns out that to get a solid confirmation you need to look at many more subjects than you looked at in the initial discovery study (Lander and Kruglyak, 1995).

Doing such large studies is hard to arrange since you need to recruit many subjects (or find the information in a database), and it can be very expensive. But part of the problem is that there is a lot of human variation and we don't really understand whether the same allele has different effects in different groups. It's possible, for example, that a *DRD4* allele has one effect in the U.S. and Israeli groups that were studied, and a different effect in, say, the Finnish group that was studied. Also, remember the *DRD4* long allele effect was pretty small even in populations where it had detectable effects. Cloninger has suggested that standard meta-analysis approaches may incorrectly pool different populations together and mask the *DRD4* effect (personal communication, May 2004). But more important, ignoring different environments in such studies can also mask potentially large genetic effects. In a very recent, but so far unreplicated study in Finland, a group of behavioral geneticists found that several of the alleles of *DRD4* had a pretty large effect on increasing novelty-seeking behavior, but only if the subjects had experienced a "hostile" childhood-rearing environment (Keltikangas-Jarvinen et al., 2004) The researchers defined a "hostile" environment as being emotionally distant, with low tolerance of the child's normal activity and with strict discipline. This result is an example of what is called a gene-environment interaction effect, and it's been expected, based on classical quantitative results in some areas, but it now seems to be showing up in some recent molecular studies.

JJ: That's very interesting! What are those other studies that show this gene-environment interaction?

BG: There are two I know of, and possibly another that may be announced soon (Caspi et al., 2002, 2003). And one of them will be of particular interest to you since it relates to aggression and the increased likelihood of having a criminal record. That study, as well as the second one, was done by an English group headed by Avshalom Caspi and Terrie Moffitt, who had access to the records of a New Zealand population going back over 20 years. Caspi and Moffitt looked at two alleles of the monoamine oxidase A, or MAOA, gene. Monoamine oxidase A is an enzyme that metabolizes neurotransmitters, and the short allele form does not metabolize as well as the long allele. Individuals who had the short allele were much more likely to develop antisocial behaviors, including a record of criminal convictions, but only if they had been abused in childhood. Those with the long allele did not display these increased antisocial behaviors, even though they also likely suffered childhood abuse.

JJ: Wow! That seems to accord with what you just told me about gene-environment interactions in the DRD4 case. What about the other result you mentioned?

BG: It, too, is similar, and involves an increased likelihood of becoming depressed, but only if those becoming depressed experienced an increased number of stressful life events (Caspi et al., 2003). This result was also based on the same New Zealand population studied in the MAOA case, but I should stress that it is very hard to get such a resource of data that goes back all the way to childhood and to study the environment so as to reveal these genetic effects.

JJ: That's fascinating. So we really need to try to study the environment as well as we study the genetics. But, as you say, that is very hard to do. Are there other examples of genes that have a substantial and consistent effect on behaviors that seem to do so independently of these hard-to-study environmental influences?

BG: You need to understand that these days behavioral geneticists are expecting that almost all genes that relate to behaviors, including some of the major psychiatric disorders, are likely to be ones that have small effects, and that there are likely to be many of them. Also, it's likely that different mutations in different families or population groups might produce the same phenotype, a notion known as genetic heterogeneity. So, each allele working at many different locations or loci has a small effect on a quantitative trait such as novelty seeking, and these, as I've mentioned before, are called quantitative trait loci, or QTLs.

But that said, there is a QTL that affects Alzheimer disease (AD), which has had strong and consistent replications in most though not all ethnic groups. This is the famous apolipoprotein E4, or epsilon4, allele that we usually abbreviate by APOE4. It is probably the only example of a broad-based and replicated allelic finding that is related to a "behavioral" phenotype in humans that is not dependent on difficult-to-study related environmental studies, and some other well-confirmed gene effects in AD have been found in addition.[6] Maybe I should also mention that there is a well-confirmed protective effect against alcoholism of some genes related to alcohol metabolism, but that seems restricted to some Asian populations.

JJ: So is this really the only example that seems to hold that broadly? That must be discouraging for behavioral geneticists. But what does this APOE4 gene do? Does it make a different fourth type of neurotransmitter receptor?

BG: No, it's not related to a neurotransmitter. The *APOE4* gene makes the APOE4 protein. This and other forms of this kind of protein seem to have at least two different roles to play in humans, one in cholesterol metabolism that can affect a disposition to heart attacks, and the other in Alzheimer disease. In AD the protein may bind to some brain cell receptors, but exactly how the protein works is not yet understood. What is known is that humans have three different alleles for this protein, confusingly called *E2*, *E3*, and *E4*. Since we have a double dose of chromosomes—remember our discussion of the red cell acid phosphatase the other day?—there are six possibilities (3×2) for any given individual's genotype. People with one or more of the *E4* alleles generally have six times the risk of developing AD than people with no *E4* alleles, who might have two *E3* alleles or an *E2* and *E3* or even two *E2*s.

JJ: So the E4 alleles act like a risk factor, just like my brother's high cholesterol increases his risk of a heart attack, but do not determine AD?

BG: Right! It's a "risk-factor allele," if you will, though geneticists usually call this a "susceptibility gene," and it is also a QTL because it quantitatively affects AD risk, and it is just one among others that does so.[7]

JJ: Was this very interesting result found by an association study?

BG: Yes, eventually the *APOE4* result was produced by an association study. But initially researchers tried to do a linkage study in their search for what turned out to be *APOE4*.[8] Even though the linkage approach didn't work in that case, I should take a minute to explain it. After all, you're looking for an introduction to some of the major molecular approaches to understanding human behavior, and linkage analysis has been the traditional one.

Remember, when researchers do an association study, they begin with a candidate gene that they have reason to believe is implicated in the behavior under consideration, and then they see if people who carry that allele exhibit the trait to a greater (or lesser) extent than those who carry a different allele at the same location. If you want, I guess you can think of linkage studies as moving in the opposite direction: in linkage approaches, researchers begin with people who exhibit the behavior and then see if they can identify a shared allele. More specifically, in the linkage approaches, researchers look at the history of a family with a particular disease and construct what is called a pedigree—actually a number of families' pedigrees—a family tree, as it were. Geneticists then look for evidence that some allele called a "marker" that they can test for shows up most of the time in those individuals affected by the disease. They look for co-transmission of the disease and a marker allele. That allele may well not be causative of the disease, but if it tracks well with the disease, that tracking is evidence the allele is genetically linked to the causative gene, in the sense of being fairly near it and certainly on the same chromosome. Thanks to advances in human molecular genetics we can now identify lots of these genetic markers along the chromosomes, which makes it easier to make better maps of the chromosomes. The better those maps become, the easier it will be to zero in on the gene that is causally related to the disease under investigation. Researchers hope that once they finally locate the causally related gene and make copies of it, they'll be able to see what it does, maybe what kind of protein it makes that differs in normal and diseased persons.

JJ: Sounds great! Have linkage studies produced any clinically useful results?

BG: Linkage studies have produced some clear results in single-gene types of diseases, like cystic fibrosis and Huntington disease, and some kinds of cancer, and even special forms of Alzheimer disease called early-onset AD that I briefly alluded to earlier. But if the linkage approach is going to work, the genes to be identified need to have a large effect (probably at least 10% of the total phenotypic variance)—and the genes implicated in most complex traits just won't have such big effects. Another problem with the linkage approach is that it requires researchers to make big assumptions, like about whether the genes of interest act in a dominant or recessive manner. In fact, a linkage study for schizophrenia, which made some of those assumptions, produced false results—results that even got published in the 1980s.

There is a kind of linkage study, however, called allele sharing, that can work well with quantitative traits. A special form of allele sharing known as Affected Pedigree Member—and that we need not go into—was in fact employed by Allan Roses's group at Duke University. They used this method to relate late-onset AD to a region of chromosome 19, later determined to be the *APOE4* allele (more accurately, the apoliprotein e epsilon-4 allele).

JJ: OK, if linkage studies aren't so great for identifying alleles involved in common, complex diseases, then what kind of method did give us this fascinating Alzheimer disease result—that APOE4 allele? And also please clarify about these early- and late-onset forms of AD, if you can.

BG: Let me start with your second question. One form of Alzheimer disease appears unfortunately early—often in a person's 50s—so it is called early-onset. It now seems this kind is caused by any one of three different types of gene mutations. Whereas late-onset AD appears to be affected by many alleles of small effect, early-onset AD (like, for example, Huntington disease) is quite rare and is caused by highly penetrant, dominant mutations. The more common kind of AD—the late-onset type that struck President Reagan—is the form related to *APOE4*. To distinguish this late-onset AD form, we sometimes use the abbreviation LOAD.

And again, the *APOE4* discovery was first made using an association study design, just like the novelty-seeking *DRD4* discovery. Roses's group at Duke University suspected that the apolipoprotein gene might play an important role in AD, and therefore would make a good candidate gene in an association study.[9] And they got a positive result. It was pretty controversial at first, but is now well confirmed, as I suggested earlier.

JJ: This association design now looks very attractive. Can't it be used for other behavioral traits with results as good as were found for AD?

BG: Remember that it was an association study design that was used for novelty seeking and it had those mixed results. But association designs are increasingly attractive to behavioral geneticists, and two geneticists, Neil Risch and Kathleen Merikangas, have championed association studies as the best research method in behavioral genetics. But there are some problems with the method. One of the most famous is the chopsticks problem. Two other molecular geneticists, Eric Lander and Nicholas Schork (1994), introduced this in that wonderful though very complex paper I mentioned earlier. They write:

> Suppose that a would-be geneticist set out to study the "trait" of ability to eat with chopsticks in the San Francisco population by performing an association study with the HLA complex [a set of immune response genes that frequently vary between ethnic groups]. This would-be geneticist suspects that immune response genes, that he believes are involved in the autoimmune disease multiple sclerosis, may also affect manual dexterity in normals. The allele *HLA-A1* would turn out to be positively associated with ability to use chopsticks—not because immunological determinants play any role in manual dexterity, but simply because the allele *HLA-A1* is more common among Asians than Caucasians. (1994, 2041)

Lander and Schork urge caution regarding the use of association analyses because of this problem, and offer some guidelines about ways that additional controls and tests might help. Good studies use those additional controls.[10]

JJ: Got it! The association between a gene—or better, an allele—and a behavioral trait can be just coincidentally true and really due to another common factor like ethnicity. So caution is advised. If, based on an association study, someone claimed a gene "influenced" some trait, I'd certainly want to obtain the services of a good critical methodologist to make sure appropriate controls and tests were in fact used, even

if that someone said it made additional sense because it involved one of those neu-
rotransmitters.

BG: That's very wise, especially given the hype that so often surrounds behavioral genetic results.

JJ: So how do these molecular methods differ from the quantitative or epidemio-
logical results we discussed the other day? Do the classical results help identify where
the molecular-oriented scientists should look?

BG: Well, the studies we have been talking about today involve specific,
identified genes that we could actually test individuals for. In the twin studies
we were talking about yesterday, we almost never had had any idea what specific genes might be involved. Remember, in those heritability studies, we were
making inferences about the percentage of genetic influence on a trait. Now
you would think that traits with high heritability would be the ones that we
would find specific underlying genes or alleles for, but it has not yet worked
out that way. In fact, one prominent geneticist whose work I just mentioned,
Neil Risch (2001, 739), wrote that, and I quote him:

> Heritability estimates should . . . not necessarily be viewed as a good predictor of
> the ease with which molecular genetic analysis can identify the actual suscepti-
> bility genes involved. In fact, looking historically, one would draw the conclusion
> that molecular genetic success is either independent of or negatively correlated
> with estimated heritability from twin studies.

On the other hand, another prominent psychiatric geneticist has suggested
that if a research program is searching for specific genes (alleles) that affect a
trait (or disorder), it makes more sense to look at those traits or disorders that
have high heritability, since those with low heritability are likely to be mostly
environmentally influenced. But a high heritability as I have mentioned
before might be the result of thousands of genes of tiny effects on many different chromosomes acting in complex ways, and such gene effects would be
virtually invisible to any current genetic methods (Kendler, personal communication, April 2003).

So the jury is still out. Maybe classical heritability studies with high h^2 values
will point the way for molecular behavioral genetics, but there's no good evidence as yet. Twin study methodologies, however, might find new ways of application in molecular studies, since twins can be used to control for some com-
plicating circumstances, like different years of birth and familial environments.

But those strengths can also mask the differences in effects due to interacting genes and environments, so careful designs and controls are needed here too.

JJ: Before we end, is there some kind of overall perspective you could share with me that ties all of this together?

BG: A prominent psychologist-geneticist, Irving Gottesman, has used the diagram in Figure 2.1 (Gottesman, 1997) to bring together some of the recent results in cognitive behavioral genetics with that variability of response of a genotype that depends on the environment such as we saw in the diagram that depicted blood acid phosphatase activity. Gottesman's diagram looks complicated at first. But it's worth studying for a minute. The lower portion of the graph depicts QTLs (apoEe4, FMR1, etc.), which are thought to influence intermediate phenotypes or endophenotypes. These endophenotypes are structures or traits (like lipoprotein receptors or synaptic plasticity) that are thought to in turn influence the larger phenotypic trait under consideration (which, in the diagram, is general cognitive ability).

To wrap your mind around this new terminology, maybe it would help to think of it this way. You mentioned that your brother's doctor told him that his good (HDL) and bad (LDL) cholesterol counts put him at risk for a heart attack. If his heart attack risk is the phenotype, then you can think of his cholesterol counts as endophenotypes, or intermediate traits that influence his chances of getting a heart attack. Presumably there are also genes of small effect that influence his cholesterols, and these would likely be QTLs. Gottesman's diagram suggests that it might help to think of QTLs as early causes in the chain leading to endophenotypes and endophenotypes as intermediate causes of the complex phenotypes that are the disorders of interest.[11]

Of course, the premise of behavioral genetics is that how a given trait appears in an individual will be importantly affected by that person's particular complement of genes (or QTLs). But as Figure 2.1 suggests, how that trait appears also will be crucially affected by other variables, such as the age of the individual (a child and an adult with the same genome appear differently!) and that individual's environment (orchids don't grow well in the desert).

Take another look at Gottesman's diagram. Do you see in the top portion the two intersecting planes, with the one plane parallel to the page you're reading and the second at a 90 degree angle to the first? Gottesman uses that second plane to represent the age and environmental ranges that affect the phenotype, cognitive ability. Notice that the age range is depicted with the line parallel to the first plane and the range of environments (from stifling to fa-

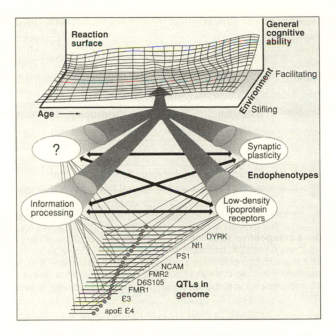

Fig. 2.1. Reaction surface. *Source:* Gottesman, 1997, 1522. Reprinted with permission of AAAS.

cilitating) is depicted by the line perpendicular to that plane. Cognitive ability is thus conceived of as a function of one's age, environment, and genetics. The reaction surface represents in a three-dimensional way the simple but important idea that different genotypes will have different phenotypes, depending on age and environment.[12] That might not sound very exciting, but it's actually an important step in beginning to appreciate how complex the interactions are, not only among QTLs, but among genes, environment, and time. I should add that though the Gottesman diagram depicts many complexities, it does not depict any downward arrows from the environment affecting which alleles (QTLs) might get turned on and off in response to different environmental conditions. This two-way possibility is, however, acknowledged by Gottesman, and is increasingly stressed by writers who favor what is called a developmentalist perspective (see Moore, 2002; Ridley, 2003).

This concludes the second dialogue between Judge Jean and the behavioral geneticist.

At this point the reader should have a pretty good sense of the general strengths and weaknesses of both quantitative and molecular genetics. But it would be useful to develop the issues a bit more, and do so in a way that the hypothetical judge might find relevant to her legal concerns. To do that, I introduce two more examples, one involving attention deficit hyperactivity disorder (ADHD) and the second involving IQ. Both areas have been extensively researched using quantitative techniques, but ADHD has had far more molecular studies directed against it than has IQ. This difference in the number of studies is probably due to the difficulty of doing molecular studies of a high-level and complex phenotype like IQ or general cognitive capacity (g). Another possible factor is that genetic research on IQ is more socially controversial than ADHD research, which might yield pharmacological interventions. Possible pharmacological interventions affecting general cognitive capacities might raise an issue of enhancement in addition to issues of ethnic and racial discrimination—a problem that has periodically plagued genetics and IQ studies, as is noted in the following dialogue.

Dialogue 3: IQ and ADHD Genetic Testing

JJ: I called for your advice one more time because I have heard that there are two emerging cases involving genetic testing that I suspect I might see on appeal. While our recent discussions are still fresh in my mind, I'd like to discuss these two case areas with you before actual cases really emerge.

It seems that two families who each have a child in a very progressive science-oriented elementary school have sued the school board. One family's child, whose name I have heard through the grapevine is Adam, is described as a bit on the wild side. The school nurse wants him genetically tested for ADHD. If this test and other interviews with Adam's parents and teachers are positive, he will be placed in a special education class—something his parents do not want. The school board supports the nurse as "doing the right thing for the child and other children at the school."

The other family's child, in the same school, is named Iquena. Reportedly she is extremely bright, but before she can qualify for a special gifted students' program, she (and any of her peers who want to be admitted to that program) has to be tested for the presence of high IQ genes. The presence of these genes, the school board says, will ensure students are routed into the most appropriate tracks. By the way, Iquena's family happens to be African American; Adam's family is of eastern European descent.

Both families have retained the services of a prominent Columbus, Ohio, lawyer who has filed suits in both state and federal courts on equal protection grounds. The lawyer claims in preliminary papers that both of these students are being discriminated against on the basis of an unverified genetic reductionism and determinism.

What can you tell me about the genetics of ADHD and IQ, and these notions of genetic reductionism and determinism?

BG: Well, I think both of these cases are wildly premature. Some might even go so far as to say that, in this context, the science is "junk." But I can give you an overview of these areas if you like.

JJ: Please do. And even if some think this type of testing is "junk science," others clearly seem to disagree. And, since I am in a court that follows the Frye rule regarding evidence, and I also worry about the Daubert decision,[13] I will need to know about how to decide if this kind of science was legally admissible. (See, we lawyers have pretty elaborate terminologies, too!) Also, there is legal precedent for courts to consider the heritability of IQ (Johnson v. Calvert No X 63 31 90 at 7(Cal. Super. Ct 1990) so I think I need to be familiar with this kind of thing.[14]

BG: Let's start with the genetics of IQ. The concept is a bit more familiar because everyone has taken an IQ test at sometime in her or his life, or taken tests like the SAT, which produce scores that track IQ test results fairly closely. And, as you just mentioned, at least one court has already considered IQ and its heritability. ADHD is a bit more complex, since it's a disorder and the definition of it is a bit complicated, so we can come back to that later.

I am sure you know that just the concept of the *genetics of IQ* is controversial. Partially this is because IQ seems to be important for how one does in life. The idea that such an important aspect of a person is constrained by her or his genes doesn't sit well with our democratic instincts. Further, some controversial scholars have argued the putative 15-point IQ gap between blacks and whites is largely genetic, and that social attempts to close that gap are doomed to fail (Herrnstein and Murray, 1994; Jensen, 2000). I would not be surprised if Iquena's family was especially sensitive to genetic testing requirements given this backdrop.

JJ: I remember the controversy about Herrnstein and Murray's Bell Curve book in the mid-1990s, and think I recall that this was the second time in the last couple of decades or so that such an IQ and genetics controversy roiled the Academy. But sometimes bad news for an individual or a group has a basis in fact. Is IQ genetic?

BG: Remember our discussion about heritability from a few weeks ago? Just as the genetics of schizophrenia that we talked about then has been investigated using twin and adoption studies, so IQ and related cognitive abilities have been extensively examined in humans. Remember our simplified example of the heritability of verbal reasoning? The behavioral geneticists, and many psychologists, prefer to talk not about IQ but rather about general cognitive ability, or g. Someday you might want to get into the details of psychological tests and what g means and what its validity is. But for now, since IQ measurements are a good index of g (Chorney et al., 1998), we'll just stick with talking about IQ.

You probably remember that when we used the rubber tree plants' heights (acid phosphotase levels) to explain the heritability concept, we saw that the activity associated with each genotype (and with the sum of those activities) could be depicted by a bell-shaped curve. Well, the distribution of IQ levels among humans can also be depicted by such a curve. Figure 2.2 shows IQ distribution and describes what kinds of occupations individuals with different ranges of IQ typically hold. Now this is a phenotypic distribution, and to get to a measure of how much of these individual differences is genetic requires that we go back to our earlier discussions about quantitative or epidemiological genetics.

JJ: Okay, but are there no molecular genetic results in the IQ area?

BG: In the molecular area, the IQ results have been checkered, and those vagaries may well be important for your case of Iquena, so we will discuss it in a minute. But essentially all the behavioral genetics work on IQ (or g) has actually been of the quantitative, nonmolecular sort. And these quantitative studies have been somewhat controversial themselves. The typical value given for the heritability of IQ is about 50 percent. But some writers have suggested it may be as high as 80 percent (Jensen, 2000), and others have pinned it at about 30 to 35 percent (Cavalli-Sforza and Feldman, 1973) (Devlin et al., 1997).

JJ: Remind me what heritability means again, and did we not distinguish two types of heritability—the broad and the narrow kinds—when we talked a few weeks ago? Is that not important here?

BG: As you'll recall, heritability is the percentage of the phenotypic variation in a trait that is estimated to be attributable to genetic variation. This is broad heritability. And you remember the distinction correctly. The difference between the two types of heritability—broad and narrow—may well be important for some policy decisions of a general sort, though not for testing individuals like Iquena. I'll explain why a bit later. But first let me stress again that we are dealing with populations in epidemiological genetics, not specific individuals. Heritability is a characteristic of a group—and only of *that* group in *that* tested range of environments and at *that* time. Thus, inferences to other groups at different times in different circumstances cannot be made using the heritability estimates found for another group at a different time.[15]

JJ: I remember your cautions, but on what kinds of studies does this 50 percent fig-

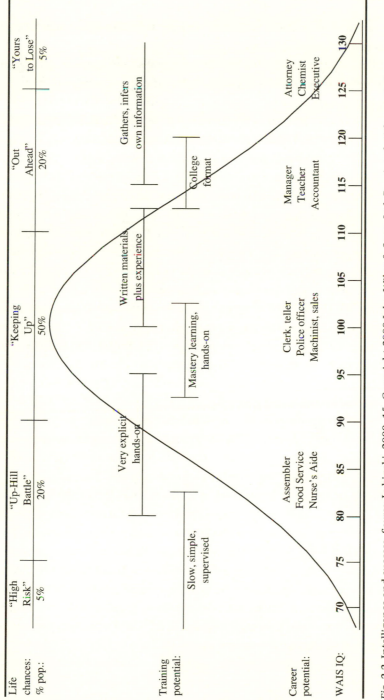

Fig. 2.2. Intelligence and success. *Source:* Lubinski, 2000, 15. Copyright 2000 John Wiley & Sons, Ltd. Reprinted with permission.

ure for heritability you cited earlier rest? And do the studies tell us anything really pragmatically useful?

BG: The results are useful but only in a general sort of way—maybe for stimulating further scientific advances—and I'll come back to the notion of usefulness in a moment. The idea of studies of the heritability of IQ really goes back to the founder of modern debates about nature and nurture, Sir Francis Galton, who wrote about the familiality of genius way back in 1869. Studies of IQ and its genetic and environmental bases were conducted throughout the twentieth century, though it has been claimed that the data in some of those so-called studies were made out of whole cloth (see Jonathan Beckwith's essay in this volume). But again, if you look at all of the twin, adoption, and family studies aimed at calculating the heritability of IQ, you'll find that the average comes out to about 50 percent. It's not clear, however, what to make of that 50 percent figure. Is some ways, it's a nice figure because it's small enough to satisfy many environmentalists and big enough to satisfy many geneticists. The problem is that it's a compromise, which can mask some very deep disagreements.

As I mentioned a little earlier, some researchers think a good heritability-of-IQ estimate for "the" general, contemporary U.S. population is closer to 0.8 and others think it's closer to 0.3 or 0.4. Matt McGue and colleagues, for example, examine much of the data collected during the twentieth century and conclude that by the time we are adults, about 80 percent of the variation with respect to IQ is due to genetic variation.[16] We don't have time to talk about the details, but let me say this. McGue and colleagues think that as we get older, what they call "shared environment" becomes less important in explaining IQ differences. That is, they think environmental variables that tend to make siblings in the same family similar earlier in life exert a smaller influence later in life. Plomin thinks that because individuals seek out environments that reflect their genetic endowments, over the course of a lifetime genetic variables are increasingly important in explaining why people act and appear differently. Put bluntly, according to this theory, individuals who are genetically well endowed seek out environments that stimulate cognitive activity and individuals who are badly endowed seek out environments that do not stimulate cognitive activity; stimulated abilities tend to flourish and understimulated abilities tend to whither (Plomin et al., 2001).

JJ: Wow, 80 percent! If you accepted that figure, you might think testing makes a whole lot of sense.

BG: Right, but like I said, some first-rate researchers think that figure is much too high (Devlin et al., 1997; Plomin et al., 2001, 175). They argue that you only get to 80 percent (or even 50%) by neglecting important environmental factors. In several articles, Feldman has maintained that many twin studies of IQ are flawed because they do not take cultural transmission influences into account and also ignore the special character of the twin relation. (Remember our discussion of the equal environments assumption, which Feldman argues does not hold [Feldman et al., 2000]. And, again, see the Beckwith essay in this volume.) Taking those corrections into account, Feldman estimates that the heritability of IQ is about 33 percent (74–75). His analysis suggests that cultural transmission also accounts for another 33 percent of the variation with respect to IQ, with the remaining 33 percent due to the noncultural environment. Cloninger and colleagues do a similar analysis, which also arrives at a heritability-of-IQ estimate of 33 percent. Plainly, these studies suggest that the familial and larger cultural environments have a significant effect on IQ.

More recently, Devlin and colleagues did a meta-analysis of more than 200 studies that estimated the heritability of IQ. Those studies included twin, family, and adoption studies, and involved more than 50,000 pairs of relatives. Devlin and colleagues reached a heritability-of-IQ estimate of 34 percent, almost identical to the figure arrived at by Feldman and Cloninger. But in the Devlin analysis it was not special twin effects or cultural transmission that were viewed as confounding for the mainstream studies' estimates. Rather, Devlin argued that mainstream studies ignored the maternal, or more accurately the womb, environment as a factor.

JJ: Womb environment? How was that studied? Are we still talking about that "simple" twin study model we explored when we first started our conversations—the one with those three equations?

BG: Yes, we are talking about Devlin and colleagues' analysis of 200 studies that involved twins. They wanted to see whether the fetus's environment had an important effect on the intelligence of the person that fetus would become.

To see whether the *in utero* environment was an important variable in explaining the phenotypic variation in a population, Devlin and colleagues created four models, each of which postulated that different factors affected variation in IQ.[17] These sets of factors were just extensions of the ones allowed for by the simple models we discussed earlier. Devlin's models allowed for nonadditive genetic effects (i.e., effects that are dependent on other alleles), as well as for variations in the kinds of environments. The most complex or richest of these models, which they happened to call model IV, allowed for "additive and non-additive genetic effects, twin and singleton maternal effects, and familial environmental effects for twins, siblings and parent-offspring." But this model IV, which was richest with respect to number of variables it allowed, did not fit (or help account for) the data as well as their model III. That best-fitting model estimated that the maternal environment accounted for 20 percent of the IQ variance between twins and 5 percent between (nontwin) siblings. Since twins share the same womb at the same time, and siblings share it at different times, it was not surprising to find the difference between the 20 percent and 5 percent figures. This maternal effect is a quite startling finding, since maternal effects are typically ignored in the traditional IQ analyses.[18]

JJ: That's very interesting. And Devlin's models do seem more nuanced than the models we discussed a couple of meetings ago, though I don't want to ask for the details of how they work. I'll have to trust you on that for the moment at least. Did using these richer models produce anything else of interest?

BG: As a matter of fact, yes. Devlin and colleagues suggest that the maternal environment better helps explain IQ variation than does the age-related hypothesis I mentioned earlier, which assumed that the effects of a common environment waned and/or that there was an interactive snowballing effect. I should emphasize that Devlin estimates that the broad-sense heritability for IQ is about 48 percent,[19] and that the narrow-sense heritability is only 34 percent. It is the narrow sense of heritability that is important for any evolutionary or next-generation effects—for reasons that you might remember from our discussion of breeding values. So the Devlin article both identified important maternal effects and estimated the most relevant type of heritability as much less than most behavioral geneticists. It's worth quoting the conclusion of this article to you because of the importance of both points. Devlin et al. (1997) wrote:

> These results have two implications: a new model may be required regarding the influence of genes and environment on cognitive function; and interventions aimed at improving the prenatal environment could lead to a significant increase in the population's IQ. Moreover, some of Herrnstein and Murray's conclusions regarding human evolution such as the development of cognitive castes and IQ dysgenics, arise from their belief that IQ heritability is at least 60%, and is probably closer to the 80% values obtained from adoption studies. Our results suggest far smaller heritabilities: broad-sense heritability, which measures the total effect of genes on IQ, is perhaps 48%; narrow-sense heritability, the relevant quantity for evolutionary arguments because it measures the additive effects of genes, is

about 34%. Herrnstein and Murray's evolutionary conclusions are tenuous in light
of these heritabilities. (470)

I should add, speaking of Herrnstein and Murray, that those authors make a
lot of the 15-point gap in IQ results between U.S. African Americans and
whites, though they do not explicitly attribute the difference to genetics—they
only imply that. Jensen, on the other hand, seems to explicitly attribute a substantial portion of the group difference to heredity (Jensen, 2000) using his de-
fault hypothesis. But there is a serious question whether the gap even exists,
since one large study ignored by both Herrnstein and Murray and by Jensen
found the difference only to be 4 IQ points, and actually within the margin of
error of that study when SES corrections were made (Nichols and Anderson,
1973). There is a lot of misinformation, and misinterpretation, about IQ, especially involving racial differences. Iquena's parents are probably reacting in
part to this, though they have other excellent grounds to distrust any genetic
test for IQ genes.

*JJ: Okay, even though now I'll be suspicious of anybody who claims to understand
"the genetics of IQ," and am sensitive to the social dimensions of this issue, tell me
how this all affects genetic testing and about any molecular studies of IQ. Why should
Iquena's parents distrust molecular studies?*

BG: Robert Plomin, whose work I have mentioned before, has a large ongoing project that has been looking at specific genes of small effect that addi-
tively may contribute to high IQ. The rationale for the project is not to provide means of testing for such genes, but rather to identify QTLs and then
specific genes that may indicate the neurophysiological basis of human cognitive behaviors—genes that make us human, if you will. Two years ago Plomin's project believed it had a sound replication of one gene that related to
high IQ, but then that result did not stand up to a further study. But that project continues and another replicated result was just recently published.

*JJ: I'm confused. Could you be a little more specific? What exactly is the situation
now?*

BG: Initially a gene, or more accurately the allele, was found on chromosome
6 and is an insulin-like growth factor-2 receptor. The gene is called *IGF2R*, and
two forms or alleles were examined known as Allele 4 and Allele 5. This gene
was thought to be involved in brain neurophysiology, but exactly what it does
is not known yet. The study was an association study. The difference between
the two alleles in the population was small, accounting for approximately 2 per-

cent of the variance of IQ, or 4 IQ points, but Plomin's expectation is that such genes will typically have these kinds of small effects. The allele was found in one small (N≈50) high IQ population—interestingly enough, from your state, Ohio—and was replicated in a larger study (N≈100) by Plomin's group. So far, there have not been any further replications, and unfortunately for this allele, Plomin's group failed to replicate the *IGF2R* result in another more recent study (Hill et al., 2002). There have been a couple of additional QTLs or specific genes found in two other IQ projects of about the same effect size, around 1 to 3 percent of the variance, but neither of these has yet been replicated (see Plomin, 2003 for discussion and references). And in May 2004 Plomin announced his research group had found another allele that contributes to IQ. This gene codes for an enzyme with the complicated name of succinate-semialdehyde dehydrogenase (SSADH). Plomin has also indicated that additional results from this project are expected in the near future (personal communication, March 2004), but nothing is really firm yet (Plomin et al., 2004).

JJ: Well, now I understand why you said when we started today that testing for IQ genes was wildly premature, but the science does not seem to be "junk science"—just science in an early stage.

BG: That's what I meant—it's only "junk science" in the context of a genetic testing program directed at Iquena and other students in that progressive school you mentioned. And the results thus far are quite weak, but more solid results may come.

JJ: Enough about IQ. Let's talk about Adam's case and the ADHD area. First tell me about this disorder to refresh my memory.

BG: ADHD is a cluster of behavioral symptoms typified by a persistent pattern of inattention and/or hyperactivity-impulsivity. Persistent means the behavior is seen in more than one setting and also over time. Since everyone is inattentive sometimes and gets a little hyper as well, the psychiatrists emphasize that this pattern is more severe and frequent at comparable age levels in those diagnosed with ADHD. Symptoms also need to have begun before the age of 7 and have lasted at least six months. By the way, ADHD used to be, and still sometimes is, called attention deficit disorder, or ADD.

ADHD has been reported to occur in about 7 percent of young children in the United States, which means that just in the United States alone 1.6 million children between the ages of 6 and 11 are affected sometime between those ages. The disorder is, unfortunately, overdiagnosed in some populations, typically well-to-do suburban children, and underdiagnosed in poorly health-served areas, including the inner city. Though some behavioral therapies have been effective, especially family-based therapy, the usual treatment is with a stimulant such as Ritalin. And sometimes, in clear cases, Ritalin should be the first-line treatment. The disorder can be debilitating, and have negative effects on development. It not infrequently persists into the teen years, and can continue into adulthood. About 10 percent of children diagnosed with ADHD are in special education classes, but if there are learning disabilities associated with the disorder, that number goes up fivefold (see the May 2002 CDC report of Pastor and Reuben).

JJ: Is genetic testing for ADHD any closer to being useful than testing for IQ?

BG: Studies have tended to suggest high estimates for the heritability (h^2) of ADHD, about 80 percent, but there is a lot of variation across the studies that have looked at heritability in various subtypes (see Waldman and Rhee, 2002; Kirley et al., 2002). The molecular situation in ADHD is somewhat like the state of novelty-seeking gene research that we talked about at our last meeting. In fact, the novelty-seeking allele we considered, the 7-repeat allele of the dopamine receptor *DRD4* gene, is one of the alleles implicated in ADHD etiology. But the studies on *DRD4* in ADHD have been inconsistent. Though there is a general view that *DRD4* has an effect on ADHD, it is quite small, probably increasing the risk about 8 percent, and almost certainly will not be found in all populations.[20]

There is also another gene, a dopamine transporter gene called *DAT1,* which has a form—an allele—that also seems to affect ADHD. Again, this is a weak effect, about the same magnitude as *DRD4,* and the results have not been consistent (see Waldman and Rhee, 2002). While the studies are promising, larger ones are needed and are planned, including linkage studies that seem to work well in this disorder. There are some mouse models of both *DRD4* and *DAT1* for ADHD as well, that might better help us to understand how the genes work (see Waldman and Rhee, 2002 for current studies information as well as mouse model citations).

JJ: Well, in spite of the future promise, it does not sound like genetics will help much at this point in ADHD. But getting back to the 7 percent figure and that huge number of children that are diagnosed with the disorder, you said something about over- and underdiagnosis? Wouldn't genetics help here?

BG: The genetics, at some point, might actually help make diagnoses more accurate, but a lot more research at a number of levels needs to be done first, and is going on. Some of that research is attempting to define the disorder more specifically and accurately in the clinic, including various subtypes of the disorder. And the genetics *may* help with this at some point. Better definitions of subtypes of ADHD, such as a predominately hyperactive-impulsive or a predominately inattentive type are being evaluated, as are more refined classifications.

JJ: Okay, I take your point about how genetics might someday help clinicians make better diagnoses. But for now, it looks like the bottom line is that just as in IQ, genetic tests for ADHD are certainly not ready for use in making potentially momentous decisions about what track children like Adam and Iquena should be put on. I do recognize that Adam might be better placed in a special education situation, but not on any genetic grounds. Given these genetic facts, it's likely that there will be a resolution of this suit even before trial. Nonetheless, I now feel a bit better prepared for this type of case if one materializes. But we have not yet talked about the aspect of the Adam and Iquena cases where the plaintiffs' lawyer is alleging discrimination based on an "unverified genetic reductionism and determinism." Exactly what do behavioral geneticists mean by these terms?

BG: These are not really behavioral genetics terms but are more philosophical ideas, though the terms possibly have legal consequences. Behavioral geneticists do sometimes discuss these kinds of implications of their results. Reductionism means many different things—there is a discussion of about a dozen different senses in Schaffner (1993, chapter 9). But the core idea of reduction is simplifying something complex by explaining it in terms of the actions of its smaller parts. Often such a simplifying explanation suggests it is the parts that are the real things, and the real causes of what happens. In line with this, genetic reductionism would be attributing all behaviors to the actions of genes. If the genes acted so as to ensure 100 percent predictability of behavior based on knowledge of the genes, you would have genetic determinism—the genes would fully determine the behavior. Even in rare cases like Huntington disease, where we say that an allele is 100 percent penetrant, we are not 100 percent sure that the disease will be expressed, and we certainly do not know exactly when or how the disease will be expressed (Rubinsztein et al., 1996). Behavioral genetics research into common, complex behaviors does not support deterministic explanations. Most human behavior is the result of highly complex interactions among genes and environmental factors. Genes will likely have very small influences and result in small probabilistic changes in risk. Basing a decision such as class tracking for Adam and Iquena mainly on genetic test results is unsound and at best wildly premature.

Actually, I have heard of only one legal case where a defendant's lawyer claimed that the defendant, who had been judged guilty of murder, was less than fully responsible for his actions. This case involved an "aggression gene" found in an extended Dutch family. But that lawyer's request that his client be tested for the so-called aggression gene (in the hope of reducing his client's sentence) ultimately went nowhere. For some details of this case, see www.biojuris.com/crimlaw01.htm. The case does raise the perennial philosophical topic of free will, but you will have to read elsewhere on that topic, since I am not qualified to discuss it with you [see Kaebnick and Edgar chapters in this volume].[21]

JJ: Okay, maybe I'll look up those papers on free will sometime. But now that we have discussed many of the claims about genetics and behavior in our last three meetings, I have to say that I feel I have been overinfluenced by "genetics hype." Is anybody trying to battle the hype?

BG: Actually, a lot of different people, from a lot of different angles, are trying to offer subtler, more complex accounts of the role of genetics in human behavior. Some bioethicists and policy wonks and journalists have been concerned about the hype, though to be fair, many of them have engaged in it as well. Some researchers from within behavioral genetics have been concerned about the hype because they can see that the greater the expectations of the science grow, so grows the potential for disappointment. Some other researchers, outside of behavioral genetics—for example, from population genetics—have also been concerned about the hype in general, and the oversimplified reductionism and unwarranted determinism in particular. These other researchers, sometimes joined by sympathetic philosophers, are often referred to as developmentalists. A number of developmentalists are adversaries of behavioral genetics. (See Schaffner, 1998 for a discussion of developmentalism.)

JJ: I am used to adversarial relationships in the law but did not realize they were prevalent among scientists who study human behavior. That could make it difficult to figure out which expert testimony to trust. It's disappointing that there seem to be so few sound results in an area that has been written about so much and in which so much research has already been done. But maybe we are on the cusp of some real breakthroughs in behavioral genetics?

BG: A lot has been done and my field has come a long way, but it's a journey of a thousand miles, and we have just taken the first steps, to echo an old saying. We all need to remember just how complex an organism a human being is. Genes affect behavior largely by collectively building nerve cells, called neurons, and interacting with the organism's internal and external environments to knit the neurons together into networks, via connections called synapses. This can result in one huge network! And it is not accurate to characterize the genes as simply directing cell and pattern formations, since the causal and informational flow is two-way as genes are turned on and off by proteins and environmental conditions as the network gets built and self-regulates.[22] Much of this building and sculpting happens in the organism's development, but for humans, the nervous system grows until the person is an adult, with extensive remodeling during the teenage years. And there is also evidence of brain changes all the way through human life. Behavioral and psychiatric geneticists and molecular geneticists are both beginning to acknowledge the importance of mapping the environment—it's even been called the *envirome*—so in addition to mapping the genome, some are now calling for substantial enviromics studies (see Anthony, 2001). It is startling, and sobering, to compare Dean Hamer's articles (and books) written in the 1990s that were extremely optimistic regarding human behavioral genetics with his more recent comments on the subject.[23] Robert Plomin, whose work we discussed earlier, has also become much more cautious about what can be found easily in human behavioral genetics—(see Plomin, 2003, especially the introduction and conclusion).

It is difficult to overstate the complexity of the human brain and nervous system. Just the facts give a sense of the overwhelming numbers of cells involved. It has been estimated that the human brain has more than 100 *billion* neurons, which are so connected with each other that there are more than 100 *trillion* synapses. Groups of the connected neurons constitute circuits, probably each containing hundreds and thousands of neurons. These circuits probably have another thousandfold number of synapses each, which all work together in largely unknown fashion to produce mental and behavioral processes (WHO World Health Report on Mental Health, 2001, Advances in Neuroscience, at www.who.int/whr/2001/main/en/chapter1/001b1.htm, accessed June 21, 2002). The complexity of circuits and the difficulties with learning what is going on in them is just beginning to be appreciated by the geneticists and neuroscientists (see Cowan et al., 2002, esp. 28–29; Hamer, 2002).[24]

JJ: Goodness gracious! What will behavioral geneticists do in the face of that kind of complexity?

BG: Well, we behavioral geneticists seek to find useful, and hopefully robust simplifications in this vast network, so as to connect the inherited elements, the genes, with specific behavior types. With the help of neuroscientific tools, we need to at least partially decompose the huge network and localize functional parts.[25] Since this is very difficult to do, even with a very simple organism like the common soil worm known as *C. elegans* (Schaffner, 1998, 2000), we don't have any illusions about the difficulties we face. And this worm has only about 1000 cells, total, with exactly 302 neurons and approximately 5000 synapses (Schaffner, 1998, 2000).

There are new gene chips, known technically as microarrays, that monitor thousands of genes simultaneously that may help. The chips offer a lot of promise in cancer genetics, where they can discriminate the gene expression patterns of different types of cancer (Armstrong et al., 2002). And there are some tantalizing early results in schizophrenia using these chips (Mirnics et al., 2001a, 2001b) that actually have recently been replicated (Mirnics and Pevsner, 2004). But in basic physiology, development, and behavior, the chips have not yet been able to produce helpful simplifications—so far they have yielded vast amounts of data that are very hard to interpret. Preliminary results applied to behaviors in simple organisms, like this worm, offer promise, but even there the chips suggest that a lot more genes seem to be involved, and we do not yet know what most of the genes do, nor exactly how they affect the neurons and the circuits, though progress is being made.[26]

Maybe behavioral geneticists, working with neuroscientists, who can help identify those possibly promising endophenotypes I mentioned earlier, may be able to find genes or alleles of major effect that hold for diverse families and across diverse ethnic groups. In one sense, endophenotypes are at higher levels of aggregation, so they may give us some simplifications that we can understand and use, just like we can fairly easily understand the behaviors of a gas's temperature, pressure, and volume, even though the gas is composed of millions of interacting molecules. Maybe evolution designed us with behavioral modules, with only a few genes affecting them in major ways, which we can dissect out of behavioral patterns with stronger genetic methods and better neuroscientific tools. Maybe new studies involving what are called SNPs and haplotypes will help, though I can't go into exactly what these terms mean and how they might work better just now. There are a lot of promising possibilities. But it has been very difficult to get good results in behavioral genetics. And in spite of occasional optimism and frequent hype, and given the complexity of humans just noted, this will be really tough to bring off successfully. Maybe we will just have to get lucky.

This concludes the third dialogue, and also concludes, except for an overview summary and conclusion, this second essay.

Summary and Conclusions

The purpose of this chapter and the preceding one was to introduce the subject of behavioral genetics in a gradual manner, building on clear, albeit somewhat simplified, definitions, and then introducing the methods and some results. My intent was to demystify some of the basic ideas for people who are not behavioral geneticists, but who would like to know what the results of behavioral genetics do and do not mean. Some results, such as in Alzheimer disease research, have stood up under scrutiny. Even though some think that late-onset Alzheimer disease isn't squarely within the purview of behavioral genetics, it is a disorder that psychiatrists claim as one of their dementias and for which they have an entry in their *Diagnostic and Statistical Manual*. Also, it is a common, complex disorder, which may suggest some of the possibilities and problems that will be associated with research into other common, complex behaviors. Research on novelty seeking and on aggression (which are squarely within the purview of behavioral genetics) has also yielded some promising though limited results. But too often it looks like behavioral genetics results are pulled like a rabbit from a magician's hat. One way of looking at these two chapters is that they allow a peek inside the hat. That peek indicates that there are many assumptions that behavioral geneticists make, and also that the magnitude of their findings are often small ones, as well as hard to replicate. Characterizing the limitations in these disciplines and limits in what we can expect to infer from the disciplines' findings is the first step in a wise application of them.

Behavioral genetics will continue to pursue studies and new and exciting findings can be expected, if not daily, probably at least weekly. These will be hyped in the daily papers, on the evening news, and on the covers of weekly news magazines. I hope these two chapters will provide part of the information that readers can use to examine critically those frequently all-too-breathless stories. We can look forward to breakthroughs in new understandings of human complexity from these advances. I hope, also, both behavioral and pharmacological interventions will emerge that will assist those with behavioral and psychiatric disabilities, and provide some relief from them, with a chance to build a better life. Given the human complexity our behavioral geneticist outlined to Judge Jean in her closing comments, however, we should not expect any magic bullets, but we can anticipate some well-targeted rationally based interventions, including drugs, in the long run. And we can guard against simplistic genetic determinism and reductionism with an awareness and appreciation of the above-discussed limitations of behavioral genetics.

ACKNOWLEDGMENTS

I want to thank Elving Anderson, Catherine Baker, Greg Carey, Lindley Darden, Megan Davis, Bernie Devlin, Harold Edgar, Ilya Farber, Irv Gottesman, Ken Kendler, Matt McGue, Erik Parens, Eric Turkheimer, and Bill Winslade for comments on portions of this draft manuscript. However, the opinions expressed (and errors) are my own. Supported by the NIH ELSI program (through Hastings Center–American Association for the Advancement of Science [HC–AAAS]) and the NSF STS program.

NOTES

1. The field is constantly changing, so new methods and refinements of old methods are continually appearing. Both Lander's group and Roses have argued that recent explorations using single nucleotide polymorphisms (SNPs) and haplotypes—chunks of chromosomes with small amounts of genetic variation—may afford what is known as linkage disequilibrium studies more power. See Daly, M. J., J. D. Rioux, et al. (2001). "High-resolution Haplotype Structure in the Human Genome." *Nature Genetics* 29(2): 229–32. Roses, A. D. (2000). "Pharmacogenetics and the Practice of Medicine." *Nature* 405(6788): 857–65; a discussion of the differences between linkage and linkage disequilibrium is beyond this chapter.

2. An influential paper by Risch and Merikangas urged this strategy Risch, N., and K. Merikangas. (1996). "The Future of Genetic Studies of Complex Human Diseases." *Science* 273(5281): 1516–17, and more recently Risch presented additional refinements for this approach, which he views as being more congruent with the old Galtonian-Pearsonian biometrical approach than with a Mendelian tradition. Risch, N. J. (2000). "Searching for Genetic Determinants in the New Millennium." *Nature* 405(6788): 847–56.

3. Essential completion of the human genome project was announced on April 14, 2003, apparently timed to coincide with the 50th anniversary of Watson and Crick's discovery of the double helix—see www.ornl.gov/TechResources/Human_Genome/project/50yr/press4_2003.htm.

4. The same allele for this dopamine receptor of the fourth type is also sometimes referred to in the literature as D4DR; the long form is also referred to as the 7-repeat allele of the *DRD4* gene; later studies refer to 6, 7, or 8 repeats as "long."

5. There have been several more meta-analyses of DRD4 covering some 30 studies that have appeared in the literature including those by Kluger, A. N., Z. Siegfried, et al. (2002). "A Meta-analysis of the Association between DRD4 Polymorphism and Novelty Seeking." *Molecular Psychiatry* 7(7): 712–17, and also Schinka, J. A., E. A. Letsch, et al. (2002). "DRD4 and Novelty Seeking: Results of Meta-analyses." *American Journal of Medical Genetics* 114(6): 643–48. The first finds essentially no effect though the second analysis states that "although the associations between DRD4 and NS are small, our results suggest that they are real, at least for the long repeat and-521 C/T genotype" (at 647). (The latter genotype is a promoter variation but has only been examined in four studies.)

6. These other AD genes are discussed further below. Good recent reviews of gene effects in late-onset AD can be found in Bertram, L., and R. E. Tanzi. (2001). "Dancing in the Dark? The Status of late-onset Alzheimer's Disease Genetics." *Journal of Molecular Neuroscience* 17(2): 127–36, and in Nussbaum, R. L., and C. E. Ellis. (2003). "Alzheimer's Disease and Parkinson's Disease." *New England Journal of Medicine* 348(14): 1356–64. It should also be noted that there are well-confirmed genes (alleles) that have a protective effect in alcoholism (alcohol and aldehyde dehydrogenase polymorphisms, ADH2(2) and ALDH2(2), respectively), though this is largely confined to some subgroups with Asian ancestry.

7. Again, for a review of the various genetic contributions to AD, see Bertram and Tanzi, "Dancing in the Dark."

8. There is a brief history of these attempts in Thomas, A. M., G. Cohen, et al. (1998). "Alzheimer Testing at Silver Years." *Cambridge Quarterly of Healthcare Ethics* 7(3): 294–307.

9. Roses and his colleagues wrote: "several independent lines of evidence led us to examine apolipoprotein E in later onset familial Alzheimer's Disease [FAD]. We observed several proteins in CSF that bound to immobilized amyloid beta-peptide [found in AD-affected brains] with high affinity. Microsequencing and Western blotting techniques identified ApoE as one of these proteins. *APOE* was known to be localized to the region of chromosome 19, which in previous studies had shown possible linkage to late-onset FAD. Furthermore, antisera to ApoE stained senile plaques, neurofibrillary tangles, and cerebral vessel amyloid deposits in AD brains." Saunders, A. M., W. J. Strittmatter, et al. (1993). "Association of Apolipoprotein E Allele Epsilon 4 with Late-onset Familial and Sporadic Alzheimer's Disease." *Neurology* 43(8): 1467–72, at 1468.

10. The most frequently used control uses parental controls and is known as the TDT test (for transmission disequilibrium test). It is too technical a subject to develop in this chapter, but see Risch, N., and K. Merikangas. (1996). "The Future of Genetic Studies of Complex Human Diseases." *Science* 273(5281): 1516–17, and also McGue's meta-analysis of *DRD4* that indicates TDT was not used in all novelty-seeking studies. McGue, M. (2001). "The Genetics of Personality." In D. L. Connor, J. M. Rimoin, R. Pyeritz, and B. Korf, eds. *Principles and Practices of Medical Genetics.* London: Churchill Livingstone.

11. Endophenotypes are looked for in the schizophrenia area and are just beginning to be suggested in the Alzheimer disease area literature, for example, by the neuroscientist Michael Posner (see www.biomedcentral.com/1471-2202/2/14 for a Web published article proposing an attentional measure as an endophenotypes in AD studies).

12. See chapter 1 and the two-dimensional diagram of the reaction range, which showed that the same seeds would grow to different heights in different environments.

13. The U.S. Supreme Court *Daubert* decision—*Daubert v. Merrell Dow Pharmaceuticals, Inc.*, 113 S.Ct. 2786 ('93)—requires the trial judge to admit only reliable and accepted scientific evidence. The Frye rule, which is more limited, requires generally accepted evidence. The terms are not well defined and the legal discussion remains contentious.

14. The heritability argument was made by the trial court Judge (Parslow), who referred to the twin studies that attributed about 70 percent of the observed variation in IQ to genetic factors. Two subsequent appeal court decisions, however, utilized different nonhereditarian grounds in their reasoning. See Krim, T. M. (1996). "Beyond Baby M: International Perspectives on Gestational Surrogacy and the Demise of the Unitary Biological Mother." *Annals of Health Law* (5): 193–226, and also Annas's comments on this case in Annas, G. J. (1991). "Crazy Making: Embryos and Gestational Mothers." *Hastings Center Report* 21(1): 35–38.

15. Only the more complex reaction norm or reaction surface we considered in an earlier meeting can represent the broader range of differing environmental and genetic influences on a trait, such as IQ. And in virtually all cases we just do not have the data on humans to be able to produce the graphs for the reaction norms or surfaces.

16. A good introduction to the different studies can be found in a book chapter by McGue and colleagues. M. McGue et al. (1993). "Behavioral Genetics of Cognitive Abilities and Disabilities." In R. Plomin and G. McClearn, eds. *Nature, Nurture and Psychology*. Washington, D.C.: American Psychological Association: 59–76.

17. The Devlin et al. analysis also provides corrections for assortative or nonrandom mating and uses an advanced form of model fitting employing Bayesian inference. Details are not appropriate for discussion in the dialogue. An overview of the methodology can be found in the appendix to Daniels, M., B. Devlin, and K. Roeder. (1997). "Of Genes and IQ." In B. Devlin, S. E. Fienburg, D. P. Resnick, and K. Roeder, eds. *Intelligence, Genes, and Success: Scientists Respond to The Bell Curve*. New York: Copernicus Books: 45–70.

18. Devlin et al.'s analysis is not without its critics. One Web-published critique of the analysis by Bouchard is available at www.taxa.epi.umn.edu/bgnews/1997/msg00167.html (accessed May 24, 2004).

19. This can be tested using identical twin data; for specifics, see Devlin, B., M. Daniels, et al. (1997). "The Heritability of IQ." *Nature* 388(6641): 468–71.

20. The relative risk is about 50 percent in various meta-analyses, but the general population probability is only about 14 percent; see Faraone, S. V., A. E. Doyle, et al. (2001). "Meta-analysis of the Association between the 7-repeat Allele of the Dopamine D(4) Receptor Gene and Attention Deficit Hyperactivity Disorder." *American Journal of Psychiatry* 158(7): 1052–57, and Waldman, I. D., and R. Soo Hyun. (2002). "Behavioral and Molecular Genetic Studies of ADHD." In S. Sandberg, ed. *Hyperactivity and Attention Disorders in Childhood*. 2nd ed. New York: Cambridge University Press.

21. Other articles in this volume cover the free will topic. Readers should not be swayed to believe that the free will issue has been settled because the environment is involved, and not just genetics, or because "thoughts can turn genes on and off"—see Begley, S. (2002). *Wall Street Journal* (June 21): B1. Thoughts could be determined, too, but this gets into more difficult philosophical areas. For my views on this topic, see my "Neuroethics" essay in Marcus, S., ed. (2002). *Neuroethics: Mapping the Field: Conference Proceedings*. New York: Dana Foundation.

22. It is startling to discover that in yeast, with its 6000 genes, about 66 percent of them are turned on and off by the environment—factors involving temperature, salinity, and food supply. See Causton, H. C., B. Ren, et al. (2001). "Remodeling of Yeast Genome Expression in Response to Environmental Changes." *Molecular Biology of the Cell* 12(2): 323–37.

23. In 2002 Hamer wrote: "The results [in human behavioral and psychiatric genetics] have been disappointing and inconsistent. Large and well-funded linkage studies of the major psychiatric disorders including schizophrenia, alcoholism, Tourette syndrome, and bipolar disorder have come up empty-handed; not a single new gene has been conclusively identified. Most candidate gene findings have failed consistent replication, and even those that have been verified account for only a small fraction of total variation. Meanwhile, the statisticians who are supposed to be guiding and evaluating the research are unable to agree on how to design experiments or to interpret the results; their advice has proven as faddish (and useful) as the Hula-Hoop." Hamer, D. (2002). "Genetics: Rethinking Behavior Genetics." *Science* 298(5591): 71–72.

24. Hamer's 2002 diagnosis and treatment of the problems cited in note 23, above, are instructive. He wrote: "What's the problem? It's not the basic premise of linkage and candidate gene analysis; these approaches have identified dozens of genes involved in inherited diseases. Nor is it the lack of DNA sequence information; virtually the entire code of the human genome is now known. The real culprit is the assumption that the rich complexity of human thought and emotion can be reduced to a simple, linear relation between individual genes and behaviors (see the figure [in ibid.]). This oversimplified model, which underlies most current research in behavior genetics, ignores the critical importance of the brain, the environment, and gene expression networks" (71).

25. See Bechtel, W., and R. C. Richardson. (1993). *Discovering Complexity: Decomposition and Localization as Strategies in Scientific Research.* Princeton, N.J.: Princeton University Press, for some philosophical discussion of how this is done, and how difficult it might be to do in neural networks.

26. Zhang, Y., C. Ma, and T. Delohery, et al. (2002). "Identification of Genes Expressed in C. Elegans Touch Receptor Neurons." Nature 418(6895): 331–35. For the author's detailed views on the lessons we can draw from simple systems and the genetics-neuroscience interaction, see Schaffner, K. F. (1998). "Genes, Behavior, and Developmental Emergentism: One Process, Indivisible?" *Philosophy of Science* 65(June): 209–52.

REFERENCES

Annas, G. J. (1991). "Crazy Making: Embryos and Gestational Mothers." *Hastings Center Report* 21(1): 35–38.
Anthony, J. C. (2001). "The Promise of Psychiatric Enviromics." *British Journal of Psychiatry* (suppl. 40): S8–S11.
Armstrong, S. A., J. E. Staunton, L. B. Silverman, et al. (2002). "MLL Translocations Specify a Distinct Gene Expression Profile That Distinguishes a Unique Leukemia." *Nature Genetics* 30(1): 41–47.

Bechtel, W., and R. C. Richardson. (1993). *Discovering Complexity: Decomposition and Localization as Strategies in Scientific Research*. Princeton, N.J.: Princeton University Press.

Bertram, L., and R. E. Tanzi. (2001). "Dancing in the Dark? The Status of Late-onset Alzheimer's Disease Genetics." *Journal of Molecular Neuroscience* 17(2): 127–36.

Caspi, A., J. McClay, et al. (2002). "Role of Genotype in the Cycle of Violence in Maltreated Children." *Science* 297(5582): 851–54.

Caspi, A., K. Sugden, et al. (2003). "Influence of Life Stress on Depression: Moderation by a Polymorphism in the 5-HTT Gene." *Science* 301(5631): 386–89.

Causton, H. C., B. Ren, S. S. Koh, et al. (2001). "Remodeling of Yeast Genome Expression in Response to Environmental Changes." *Molecular Biology of the Cell* 12(2): 323–37.

Cavalli-Sforza, L. L., and M. W. Feldman. (1973). "Cultural Versus Biological Inheritance: Phenotypic Transmission from Parents to Children (a Theory of the Effect of Parental Phenotypes on Children's Phenotypes)." *American Journal of Human Genetics* 25(6): 618–37.

Chorney, M. J., K. Chorney, N. Seese, et al. (1998). "A Quantitative Trait Locus Associated with Cognitive Ability in Children." *Psychological Science* 9: 159–66.

Cowan, W. M., K. L. Kopnisky, and S. E. Hyman. (2002). "The Human Genome Project and Its Impact on Psychiatry." *Annual Review of Neuroscience* 25: 1–50.

Daly, M. J., J. D. Rioux, S. F. Schaffner, et al. (2001). "High-resolution Haplotype Structure in the Human Genome." *Nature Genetics* 29(2): 229–32.

Daniels, M., B. Devlin, and K. Roeder. (1997). "Of Genes and IQ." In B. Devlin, S. E. Fienburg, D. P. Resnick, and K. Roeder, eds. *Intelligence, Genes, and Success: Scientists Respond to the Bell Curve*. New York: Copernicus Books: 45–70.

Devlin, B., M. Daniels, and K. Roeder. (1997). "The Heritability of IQ." *Nature* 388(6641): 468–71.

Faraone, S. V., A. E. Doyle, E. Mick, et al. (2001). "Meta-analysis of the Association between the 7-repeat Allele of the Dopamine D(4) Receptor Gene and Attention Deficit Hyperactivity Disorder." *American Journal of Psychiatry* 158(7): 1052–57.

Feldman, M. W., S. B. Otto, and F. B. Christiansen. (2000). "Genes, Culture, and Inequality." In K. Arrow, S. Bowles, and S. Durlauf, eds. *Meritocracy and Economic Inequality*. New Delhi: Oxford University Press.

Gottesman, I. I. (1997). "Twins: En Route to QTLs for Cognition." *Science* 276(5318): 1522–23.

Hamer, D. (2002). "Genetics: Rethinking Behavior Genetics." *Science* 298(5591): 71–72.

Herrnstein, R. J., and C. A. Murray. (1994). *The Bell Curve: Intelligence and Class Structure in American Life*. New York: The Free Press.

Hill, L., M. J. Chorney, D. Lubinski, et al. (2002). "A Quantitative Trait Locus Not Associated with Cognitive Ability in Children: A Failure to Replicate." *Psychological Science* 13(6): 561–62.

Hyman, S. E. (2000). "The Genetics of Mental Illness: Implications for Practice." *Bulletin of the World Health Organization* 78(4): 455–63.

Jensen, A. R. (2000). "The G Factor: Psychometrics and Biology." *Novartis Foundation Symposium Series* 233: 37–47; discussion 47–57, 116–21.

Keltikangas-Jarvinen, L., K. Raikkonen, et al. (2004). "Nature and Nurture in Novelty Seeking." *Molecular Psychiatry* 9(3): 308–11.

Kirley, A., Z. Hawi, G. Daly, et al. (2002). "Dopaminergic System Genes in ADHD: Toward a Biological Hypothesis." *Neuropsychopharmacology* 27(4): 607–19.

Kluger, A. N., Z. Siegfried, and R. P. Ebstein. (2002). "A Meta-analysis of the Association between DRD4 Polymorphism and Novelty Seeking." *Molecular Psychiatry* 7(7): 712–17.

Krim, T. M. (1996). "Beyond Baby M: International Perspectives on Gestational Surrogacy and the Demise of the Unitary Biological Mother." *Annals of Health Law* 5: 193–226.

Lander, E., and L. Kruglyak. (1995). "Genetic Dissection of Complex Traits: Guidelines for Interpreting and Reporting Linkage Results." *Nature Genetics* 11(3): 241–47.

Lander, E. S., and N. J. Schork. (1994). "Genetic Dissection of Complex Traits." *Science* 265(5181): 2037–48.

Lubinski, D. (2000). "Intelligence: Success and Fitness." In G. Bock et al., eds. *The Nature of Intelligence*. Novartis Foundation Symposium 233. Chichester: Wiley: 6–35.

Marcus, S., ed. (2002). *Neuroethics: Mapping the Field: Conference Proceedings*. New York: Dana Foundation.

McGue, M. (2001). "The Genetics of Personality." In D. L. Connor, J. M. Rimoin, R. Pyeritz, and B. Korf, eds. *Principles and Practices of Medical Genetics*. London: Churchill Livingstone.

McGuffin, P., B. Riley, and R. Plomin. (2001). "Genomics and Behavior: Toward Behavioral Genomics." *Science* 291(5507): 1232–49.

Mirnics, K., F. A. Middleton, D. A. Lewis, et al. (2001a). "The Human Genome: Gene Expression Profiling and Schizophrenia." *American Journal of Psychiatry* 158(9): 1384.

Mirnics, K., F. A. Middleton, G. D. Stanwood, et al. (2001b). "Disease-specific Changes in Regulator of G-Protein Signaling 4 (Rgs4) Expression in Schizophrenia." *Molecular Psychiatry* 6(3): 293–301.

Mirnics, K., and J. Pevsner. (2004). "Progress in the Use of Microarray Technology to Study the Neurobiology of Disease." *Nature Neuroscience* 7(5): 434–39.

Moore, D. S. (2002). *The Dependent Gene: The Fallacy of Nature/Nurture*. New York: Times Books.

Nichols, P. L., and V. E. Anderson. (1973). "Intellectual Performance, Race, and Socioeconomic Status." *Social Biology* 20(4): 367–74.

Nussbaum, R. L., and C. E. Ellis. (2003). "Alzheimer's Disease and Parkinson's Disease." *New England Journal of Medicine* 348(14): 1356–64.

Pastor P. N., and C. A. Reuben. (2002). "Attention Deficit Disorder and Learning Disability: United States, 1997–98." *Vital Health Statistics* 10: 206.

Plomin, R. (2003). "Genetics, Genes, Genomics and G." *Molecular Psychiatry* 8(1): 1–5.

Plomin, R., J. C. DeFries, G. E. McClearn, et al. (2001). *Behavioral Genetics*. New York: Worth.

Plomin, R., et al. (2003). *Behavioral Genetics in the Postgenomic Era*. Washington, D.C.: American Psychological Association.

Plomin, R.D., D. M. Turic, et al. (2004). "A Functional Polymorphism in the Succinate-Semialdehyde Dehydrogenase (Aldehyde Dehydrogenase 5 Family, Member A1) Gene is Associated with Cognitive Ability." *Molecular Psychiatry* 9(6): 582–86.

Ridley, M. (2003). *Nature Via Nurture : Genes, Experience, and What Makes Us Human*. New York: HarperCollins.

Risch, N. (2001). "The Genetic Epidemiology of Cancer: Interpreting Family and Twin Studies and Their Implications for Molecular Genetic Approaches." *Cancer Epidemiology, Biomarkers and Prevention* 10(7): 733–41.

Risch, N., and K. Merikangas. (1996). "The Future of Genetic Studies of Complex Human Diseases." *Science* 273(5281): 1516–17.

Risch, N. J. (2000). "Searching for Genetic Determinants in the New Millennium." *Nature* 405(6788): 847–56.

Roses, A. D. (2000). "Pharmacogenetics and the Practice of Medicine." *Nature* 405(6788): 857–65.

Rubinsztein, D. C., J. Leggo, R. Coles, et al. (1996). "Phenotypic Characterization of Individuals with 30–40 Cag Repeats in the Huntington Disease (Hd) Gene Reveals Hd Cases with 36 Repeats and Apparently Normal Elderly Individuals with 36–39 Repeats." *American Journal of Human Genetics* 5(1): 16–22.

Saunders, A. M., W. J. Strittmatter, D. Schmechel, et al. (1993). "Association of Apolipoprotein E Allele Epsilon 4 with Late-Onset Familial and Sporadic Alzheimer's Disease." *Neurology* 43(8): 1467–72.

Schaffner, K. F. (1993). *Discovery and Explanation in Biology and Medicine.* Chicago: University of Chicago Press.

Schaffner, K. F. (1998). "Genes, Behavior, and Developmental Emergentism: One Process, Indivisible?" *Philosophy of Science* 65(June): 209–52.

Schaffner, K. F. (2001). "Nature and Nurture." *Current Opinion in Psychiatry* 14(September): 486–90.

Schinka, J. A., E. A. Letsch, et al. (2002). "DRD4 and Novelty Seeking: Results of Meta-Analyses." *American Journal of Medical Genetics* 114(6): 643–48.

Thomas, A. M., G. Cohen, et al. (1998). "Alzheimer Testing at Silver Years." *Cambridge Quarterly of Healthcare Ethics* 7(3): 294–307.

Waldman, I. D., and S. H. Rhee. (2002). "Behavioral and Molecular Genetic Studies of ADHD." In S. Sandberg, ed. *Hyperactivity and Attention Disorders in Childhood.* 2nd ed. New York: Cambridge University Press: 290–335.

CHAPTER THREE

Whither Human Behavioral Genetics?

Jonathan Beckwith, Ph.D.

Throughout its history, the field of human behavioral genetics has exhibited a tension between the search for genetic components of behavior and the awareness that environmental factors must be considered in that search. The difficulties in adequately dealing with the role of environment have repeatedly led to problems that have raised questions concerning the validity of behavioral genetic studies. While essentially everyone agrees that there are genetic contributors to variations in human behavior, the search for behavioral genes may be largely unsuccessful until familial, cultural, psychological, and other social and environmental factors are more fully integrated into such studies.

The past 15 years have brought revolutionary changes to the field of human behavioral genetics. With the development of a host of new molecular genetic techniques, the availability of a finely detailed human genome map, and the completion of the human genome sequence, it has seemed that the "holy grails" of the field—the identification of specific genes correlated with human behavioral variations and ultimately the specification of mechanisms—were at hand. These changes follow nearly a century of behavioral genetic studies of families, twins, and adopted children. Researchers carrying out these nonmolecular (classical or quantitative) studies reported that mental illnesses such as schizophrenia and bipolar manic depression, aptitudes (mainly intelligence as measured on IQ tests), and behavioral variations, including criminality, alcoholism, and homosexuality, showed strong genetic contributors. While the scientific community has largely accepted the conclusion that genetic variation is an important contributor to phenotypic variation for human traits, there is still debate as to how significant a role genes play in many of these behavioral traits. Nevertheless, the conviction that the conclusions of the earlier nonmolecular studies were valid has led many to assume that genes implicated for these socially important behavioral variations would be readily located by the new molecular genetic approaches.

But the hoped-for success has yet to materialize. Initial optimistic and widely publicized molecular genetic studies reporting genes predisposing to schizophrenia, bipolar manic depressive illness, alcoholism, homosexuality, risk taking, and others have either been retracted, rebutted, or have yet to be replicated successfully. The standards in the field for the valid identification of such genes have changed as a result (Lander and Kruglyak, 1995). Confirmatory replications of initial reports are considered essential before the community accepts such findings. Perhaps one of the most solid findings in this area comes from an unusual case of a single family in which a specific mutation is correlated with antisocial behavior (Brunner et al., 1993a, see below). In addition, genetic polymorphisms that cause defects in genes encoding enzymes of alcohol metabolism appear to be associated with increased risk of alcoholism, suggesting that the presence of the alcohol-metabolizing enzymes in people provides some protection against alcoholism (Osier et al., 2002).

In this analysis, I will leave out of consideration diseases such as Alzheimer disease that progressively affect brain function, outliers in cognitive function such as reading disabilities, and rare or relatively rare genetic conditions that include behavioral abnormalities such as Lesch-Nyhan's disease. In many of these cases, researchers have identified genes contributing to the behavioral variants. I will limit my analysis to behavioral traits such as mental illness and those considered significant for the evolution of social policy and social values.

As a consequence of the inability to locate genes for these latter traits, there has been considerable reexamination of the approaches used in the field of human behavioral genetics. A large number of review articles have discussed the problems, evaluated the reasons for them, and proposed new approaches or stricter standards for drawing definitive conclusions. The failure to find genes associated with many of these behaviors has been largely attributed by the practitioners of the field to the unanticipated genetic complexity of behavioral variation. It is proposed that multiple genes, each with small effects, interact in an individual in complex ways to cause the observed phenotypes. Perhaps by increasing the number of families or subjects involved in such studies, it is suggested, researchers will be able to tease out the individual genes. Or, choosing specialized subsets of populations (sib pairs, populations limited in ethnic diversity, etc.) may facilitate the gene hunts. Thus, the changes encouraged by these proposals focus mainly on technical improvements in genetic approaches, the subjects to be analyzed, and the statistical programs to be used to assure validity.

Given the emerging consensus on genetic complexity, we can ask whether technical improvements of the sort proposed are sufficient to allow definition of the sets of genes involved in these traits that are of such significant social interest. Could it be that, in addition to recognizing genetic complexity, there are other assumptions underlying this research that must be explored? I would argue that one such assumption can be found in the limited attention paid, since the inception of this research field, to the complexity of the interactions between genes and familial, social, psychological, cultural, and economic factors. A greater appreciation of the extent to which environmental factors have been neglected could actually lead to greater success in gene hunts than we have seen so far. Indeed, in the past few years, researchers have increased efforts to analyze and incorporate environmental factors into behavioral genetic studies (Kendler and Gardner, 2001).

At the same time, this new view of genetic complexity raises questions about the predictive value and utility of identifying genes correlated with human behavioral traits. According to current thinking, behavioral variations such as schizophrenia and aptitudes such as intelligence are influenced by numerous genes interacting with each other, each gene making only a small contribution to the trait. We already know that there is substantial variation in the degree of expression of disease symptoms in those many cases where mutations in only a single gene have been identified as causative. For example, a set of males carrying the same mutation in the cystic fibrosis gene exhibit a wide range of disease symptoms; some of them do not show any of the typical consequences of the gene mutation except for male sterility (Meschede et al., 1993; Donat et al., 1997). Imagine this degree of variation multiplied many fold in the cases of traits influenced by numerous genes, each subject to its own complexities of expression and interactions. Even if one were able to identify all of the genes that contribute to these traits, predicting the consequences of a particular genetic makeup and altering the expression of the traits under study may remain very difficult.

"Nature's Gift" to Behavioral Genetics?

Studies of genetically identical (monozygotic) twins have been one of the most important components of human behavioral genetic research over the past century. This "gift of nature" overcame a problem that differentiated human genetic studies from the study of genetics of other organisms (e.g., mice, fruit flies, plants, or bacteria). In nonhuman systems, it is possible to breed and mate members of species in a controlled fashion. For example, geneticists can generate inbred strains of these organisms that share all their genes or differ by only one gene. The existence of monozygotic (MZ) human twins appeared to provide a means of overcoming the limitations to human genetic research. But it was recognized early on that simply identifying shared traits among MZ twins was not, in itself, sufficient to allow researchers to conclude that a trait had a large genetic component. MZ twins might share traits because they grew up together in the same family environment, at the same time in the history of that family and of the outside world. The sharing of traits could be due to either shared environment, shared genes, or a combination of the two. Some sort of control for these studies was needed.

Behavioral geneticists pursued two possibilities for solving this dilemma. First, the existence of twins who were not genetically identical, fraternal (or dizygotic) twins, appeared to provide a direct control. MZ twins share, in principle, 100 percent of their genetic inheritance. Dizygotic (DZ) twins (like any two siblings of the same sex) share on average only 50 percent of their genetic inheritance. Yet, like MZ twins, DZ twins grew up in the same family at the same time, experiencing the same environment. The environmental influences for both types of twins were considered to be shared to the same extent. If the MZ twins were found to share a trait much more frequently than DZ twins did, then the researchers could conclude that that trait had a significant genetic component. The genetic contribution could be calculated from analyzing the degree of difference in the sharing of the trait between the two types of twins.

The second approach to controlling for environmental influences in the development of behavioral traits was to examine those cases in which MZ twins were separated from their parents at an early age and placed in different homes by the family itself or by adoption agencies. No longer was the study confounded by the fact that the twins were growing up in the same family and at the same time in that family. If twins, thus separated, still showed a high sharing of a trait, it was considered evidence for a significant genetic component.

The Equal Environments Assumption

For many years, identical twin studies of these types were carried out, conclusions drawn, and papers published, often achieving widespread attention both in the public and in academia, with little in the way of questioning. However, in the latter half of the twentieth century, challenges were raised about the assumptions behind these studies from both within and outside the field. In particular, some scientists questioned the fundamental assumption underlying studies comparing trait-concordance frequencies among MZ and DZ twins: that the degree of environmental similarity is about the same for the two types of twins. According to this equal environments assumption (EEA), DZ twins, between them, share environmental influences to the same degree as do MZ twins.

Challengers of the EEA raised the possibility (or likelihood) that MZ twins experienced much more environmental similarity than DZ twins *because* they were identical. In 1960, Jackson argued that a unique psychological bond between MZ twins, which did not exist for DZ twins, could potentially explain all the concordance results (Jackson, 1960). Furthermore, some suggested that parents and the outside world treated and interacted with MZ twins, because of their identical appearance, much more similarly than they would with DZ twins or ordinary siblings. Consider the potential influence of physical features on such social interactions. Children who are obese, for example, might suffer indignities that others do not. Children thought of as "attractive" might experience a very different world than those deemed "ugly." Both the suggested closer bond between MZ twins and the potentially similar responses of family and the surrounding culture to the identically featured MZ twins could well influence the behavioral development of the children in the direction of greater similarity.

Behavioral geneticists took these challenges seriously. From 1960 on, and continuing to the present time, a series of published studies sought to control for these factors. Questionnaires or interviews with parents and with the twins themselves attempted to quantify issues such as the degree of identical treatment of twins or degree of their closeness. A second approach was to study the impact of physical appearance on the behavior of DZ twins. Because DZ twins, on average, share only 50 percent of their genes, very few of them look physically similar enough to be mistaken for each other. But, of course, since (1) 50 percent is only an average and (2) the 50 percent figure does not specify which sets of genes are shared, some of the DZ twins could share more of their genes, or might happen to share those genes important for physical appearance. These DZ twins might appear as physically similar as MZ twins. If the EEA were not correct, these twins could elicit similar treatment by parents and others that was important for their development. They might then show concordances for behavioral traits higher than those seen with other DZ twins, giving results closer to those of MZ pairs. Researchers have studied this question by finding those DZ twins who tend to be mistaken for MZ twins.

While some researchers have argued that the results of these control studies have proven the validity of the equal environment assumption, others have been less persuaded by the conclusions (Rutter, 2002). Even those studies that appear to be unequivocally supportive of the EEA are questioned for methodological reasons (Joseph, 1998). In attempting to control for environmental influences on behavior, researchers make choices as to which influences are important for the development of the behavioral trait under study. For example, if they are studying the origins of schizophrenia or intelligence, they must decide which aspects of the closeness of the MZ and DZ twins should be measured and what features of parent-child interactions would be influential. But how do they decide exactly what these aspects and features might be? The assessment techniques vary from study to study, reflecting the lack of agreement over or knowledge of what factors are important. This is not surprising. Since the very purpose of studying the genetics of schizophrenia or intelligence is to understand what influences the development of a behavior or an aptitude, the researchers cannot be sure a priori which factors to examine for possible correlations with behavior. Our limited knowledge of those factors could significantly restrict the conclusions that can be drawn from those studies that appear to support the EEA.

Many of the researchers in twin studies have indirectly admitted the problems with the EEA. But they turn those problems into an asset for defining the genetic components of behavior in the following way. They agree that the environment of identical twins is more similar than that of DZ twins, but argue that this itself is a genetic phenomenon (Bouchard et al., 1990). They propose that, because of their identical genes, MZ twins seek out identical environments, creating a world for themselves that is more similar than that of DZ twins. According to this hypothesis, the traits influenced by the identical genes of the MZ twins may predispose the twins to choose environments or may elicit environments that then reinforce the genetic tendencies. For example, as I have suggested earlier, the physical features of twins may provoke certain common responses within the family and the society. This hypothesis, if true, would mean that the genetic influence becomes multiplied through the process. This proposal, while certainly a possibility, is problematic. First, it presents an ad hoc argument to get out of the contradictory findings of studies on the EEA. Second, it is an explanation that seems very hard to test. Third, it raises, at a different level, the question of whether this is an environmental or a genetic effect. But these interactions may merely be a reflection of the particular family or culture in which the twins develop and live. Changes in societal attitudes and responses could alter these interactions and, therefore, alter the behavioral manifestations. To group these effects with the genetic component of behaviors, as many researchers in the field do, can be seriously misleading. Arguing that this aspect of twin concordance be defined as a genetic component can give the impression that it is refractory to social and environmental change.

These comments are not meant to invalidate the field. Researchers have been creative in developing new theories, measuring tools, statistical programs, and so on. But, the constant retooling of approaches points to the extraordinary complexity of trying to dissect out the environmental, genetic, interactive, and stochastic parameters in the development of behaviors in human beings.

The Different Environments Assumption

The other major type of twin study compares the behaviors or aptitudes of twins separated at an early age. These studies can be divided into two types: those carried out in countries where national registries allow the identification of all twin pairs (e.g., Denmark) and those where twins are recruited via advertisements and other means (e.g., the Minnesota Twin Study).

One rationale for this type of twin study is to avoid the problems generated by the assumption that the environments of MZ and DZ twins are the same. If MZ twins are separated from each other at an early age, they are no longer subject to any joint equal treatment by parents. Furthermore, their family environments are now different, in general. Therefore, it is argued, if MZ twins raised in different families still showed high concordance for one or another behavioral trait, the trait must have a strong genetic component. A serious criticism of the rationale of these studies came to the fore when psychologist Leon Kamin, in the early 1970s, examined in detail records from the four major studies that used such an approach to assess the genetic contribution to intelligence (Kamin, 1974). Kamin argued that the supposedly different environments of the separated twins were not as different as the authors of these studies had assumed. First, he found that twins who were placed in new homes by adoption agencies tended to end up in similar environments; for example, the adopting families tended to be from the same social class. Second, in many cases the separated twins were placed by family members in the homes of relatives, so that they often went to the same school, and interacted with each other frequently. The only one of the four studies where members of twin pairs appeared to have been placed in homes of very different social class was that of the English psychologist Sir Cyril Burt. However, first Kamin, and then other researchers who attempted to evaluate Burt's data, suggested that the data had been made up and that the twins may never have existed. While debate has continued over Burt's data, his conclusions are generally no longer considered as valid support for those arguing for the strong genetic basis of intelligence. (Nevertheless, these questionable results became the mainstay of psychology and high school biology texts' discussion of twin studies for several decades.) In a 1995 book based on a symposium attempting to unravel the puzzle of Burt's data, psychologist Neil MacKintosh, the editor, stated "the cumulative data makes it difficult to maintain Burt's innocence" (MacKintosh, 1995, 142).

Kamin did not just point out these problems with the separated twin studies, he also reanalyzed the data to examine the correlation between the closeness of environments of separated twins and the degree of correlation of the measurement of intelligence. He argued that his reevaluation of the data supported a conclusion for strong environmental factors in the development of intelligence. While such analyses themselves could be criticized on the basis of which factors are taken into account, they again highlight how difficult it will be for behavioral geneticists to disentangle environmental and genetic factors.

Kamin's critique played a large role in forcing a more sophisticated look at the environments in which twins were placed and their degree of subsequent interaction. Because of Kamin, "behavior geneticists had to sharpen their arguments, design new, more careful studies, [and] obtain fresh evidence" (MacKintosh, 1995, 142) In more recent studies, researchers have made a significant effort to quantify and compare aspects of the home environments into which members of adopted twin pairs are placed. For example, they have assessed the adoptive parents' vocabulary and evaluated the nutritional environment. To gain a sense of the influences, intellectual and otherwise, they have counted the number of books in these homes, determined the availability of household facilities such as power tools, sailboat, telescope, unabridged dictionary, and original artwork (Bouchard et al., 1990; Rowe, 1994).

The problem is, how do we know what combination of factors both in the home and in the outside environment may provide the appropriate mix for development of the complex capabilities or behavioral problems that are being measured? (For more on this problem, see chapter 4.) How can researchers assess the less tangible features of such environments, such as the daily interactions between parent and child, that cannot be so easily quantified? While they have taken into account retrospective impressions of family environment by separated twins, such retrospective impressions are often thought to be subject to distortion.

In addition to dealing with the placement of identical twins, a feature of MZ twins already mentioned makes interpretation even more difficult. Aside from the environment in which they are raised, the identical appearance of such twins, even though they are separated, can mean that their interactions with the outside world are much more similar than for any two randomly selected people (see discussion above).

There are many other features of these studies and of twins themselves that add to the increasing complexity being recognized in the study of twins. For adoptive studies, there is little information reported on any differences in treatment of adopted children and biological children by adoptive parents. Also, new and unexpected developmental complexities peculiar to twins are being discovered (Spitz and Carlier, 1996). Indications of this complexity are to be found in recent reports of rare monozygotic twins of opposite sex (Somkuti et al., 2000; Wachtel et al., 2000); the variation in development of twins in the uterus depending on whether they coexist in the same chorionic sac or in separate sacs (Spitz and Carlier, 1996); and reanalysis of twin studies that reveal strong effects of prenatal and early postnatal environments (Devlin et al., 1997).

One last and perhaps most important point about the complexity of making arguments about genetics: a trait or behavior can be highly correlated with genetics, but, in fact, turn out to be largely due to environmental factors. As an example, consider a study that examines an essential aspect of IQ research—the tests of cognitive ability. Some U.S. researchers have reported that scores on tests of cognitive ability are, on average, correlated with skin color. But one study (Steele and Aronson, 1995) highlights the complex interaction between social, psychological, historical, and other factors that mix into the achievement of scores on such a test. These researchers administered tests of cognitive ability to mixed groups of black and white college students. In some cases they told the students that the tests would measure their abilities and in others that these tests were simply problem-solving tasks that were "nondiagnostic" of ability. To quote their conclusions: "Blacks underperformed in relation to whites in the ability-diagnostic condition but not in the nondiagnostic condition." They attributed this striking finding to what they called "stereotype vulnerability"—the fears that result from years of being exposed to an environment in which blacks are considered intellectually inferior to whites.

The main reason for referring to the study by Steele and Aaronson is to highlight the limitations of our knowledge of the mix of factors that influence how human behavior and human aptitudes are manifested. There are little-studied factors influencing the development of human behavior and of human capabilities, some of which we probably cannot even imagine at this point. At this stage of exploration, it is hard to see how the likely intricate interplay of so many societal, familial, and genetic factors with the ultimate score that is achieved on a test by an individual will be meaningfully linked to genetic factors. Attempts to quantify the environmental factors will incorporate the social and scientific assumptions or the limited knowledge that we bring to such an analysis. These complexities are relevant to both the attempts to reveal a genetic basis for a trait, as discussed above, and the attempts to find gene variants that are associated with behaviors, discussed below.

Molecular Genetic Approaches to Human Behavioral Genetics

Advanced molecular genetic techniques and vast amounts of information on the human genome sequence and map have accumulated over the past 15 years. One consequence of this revolution in human genome analysis is that a large number of biologists, clinical geneticists, and psychologists have begun to search for genes associated with human behavioral traits and aptitudes ranging from manic-depressive illness to intelligence. What factors have given these researchers the confidence to believe that their search has a significant likelihood of success? First, the rapid progress in finding genes associated with a host of human physical diseases encouraged efforts to extend these successes to behavioral traits. Second, an important stimulus may have been the belief in the conclusions from earlier family and twin studies that these traits were largely subject to genetic influences. For example, based on adoption studies investigating heritability of schizophrenia, Ingraham and Kety (2000, 21) state: "Despite our current ignorance of the mechanisms affected by genes related to schizophrenia, we can proceed with confidence that there are such genes to be found." (For an introduction to the *heritability* concept, see chapter 1.) If behavioral geneticists had not so deeply believed that the past century of research had demonstrated the predominant influence of genetic over environmental contributors to behavioral traits, they might have been less enthusiastic about their hopes for such gene hunts.

From the late 1980s through the early 1990s, a number of studies appeared, which claimed to have discovered genes or chromosomal loci for such traits as manic depressive illness, schizophrenia, attention deficit hyperactivity disorder, alcoholism, risk taking, and homosexuality. In nearly all of these cases, the claims were either subsequently retracted, were cogently criticized, or could not be replicated. While the earlier of these reports received widespread publicity—most of them were featured on the front page of papers such as the *New York Times*—their subsequent retractions led to more cautious reporting of later findings.

These setbacks have led to a series of review articles that question the assumptions, the approaches (genetic and statistical), and other aspects of the studies. These critical articles are nearly all written by researchers in the field who propose new methodologies to solve the problems. A list of some titles of these articles gives a sense of the concerns within the field: "Will Schizophrenia Be a Graveyard for Molecular Geneticists?" (Owen, 1992); "A Manic Depressive History" (Risch and Botstein, 1996); "Case-control Association Studies in Complex Traits—The End of an Era?" (Paterson, 1997); "Mapping Genes for Personality: Is the Saga Sagging?" (Baron, 1998); "The Frustrating Search for Schizophrenia Genes" (Tsuang and Faraone, 2000); and "Psychiatric Genetics:

Back to the Future" (Owen et al., 2000). In, for example, "A Manic Depressive History," geneticists David Botstein and Neil Risch state that "the distress engendered by the numerous reversals and non-replications has led many to rethink the paradigm being employed" (Risch and Botstein, 1996, 351). (While the authors argue for a new paradigm, they limit their conception of paradigms to the realm of genetics.)

Yet, despite the greater stringency in statistical approaches and other aspects of these studies, at the time of writing of this chapter, there are still no reports of genes for these socially relevant traits (see above for boundaries of this discussion) that are widely accepted as convincing within the field. What is the problem? The slow progress does not mean that researchers were wrong in assuming genetic influences on behavioral traits. Even though I have pointed out what I consider to be flaws in earlier nonmolecular studies, it still seems likely to me that, in many instances, genetic variation contributes importantly to some of the phenotypic variation in these traits. The review articles themselves have led to a consensus in the field that the inability to detect bona fide major loci is explained by the likelihood that these complex human traits are polygenic, that is, the result of interactions between many genes, each of which by itself has only a small effect. To detect these genes, according to this analysis, what is necessary is to look at larger population samples, use better statistical criteria, and perhaps novel sampling approaches. These proposals may well be necessary to ensure success.

But there is a growing recognition that other contributory factors should be considered in analyzing these problems (Anthony, 2001; Kendler and Gardner, 2001; Hamer, 2002; Rutter, 2002). That is, the degree to which attention has been paid to environmental influences on behavior—human social, psychological, and cultural complexity—may have been as much of a problem for contemporary molecular studies as it has been for the earlier nonmolecular studies (Alper, 2002). Turkheimer and Waldron suggest: "New methodological paradigms will no doubt evolve, but some aspects of the development of complex human behavior may remain outside the domain of systematic investigation for a very long time . . . The limitations of our existing social scientific methodologies ought not provoke us to wish that human behavior were simpler than we know it to be; instead they should provoke us to search for methodologies that are adequate to the task of understanding the exquisite complexity of human development" (Turkheimer and Waldron, 2000, 93).

Cultural and Statistical Complexities

It is already clear that some of the problems encountered in establishing bona fide behavioral genes are related to the failure to take into account the complex world we live in. For example, a widely publicized report of a gene for alcoholism (dopamine receptor D4 gene) was criticized for not considering issues of what statisticians call population stratification (Gelernter et al., 1991; Noble and Blum, 1991). The researchers reported that a particular allele of this gene showed high association with alcoholism. However, critics pointed out that these studies did not control for the possibility that these particular alleles might be more common in some ethnic or "racial" populations than in others. If the allele at issue happened to be more prevalent in a particular population that showed high frequencies of alcoholism, a high correlation would be found, but there would be no necessary causal relationship between that allele and alcoholism. Rather, the high alcoholism rates in that population might have been related to economic issues, to problems of discrimination, or to other historical factors influencing behavior of the group. The problem of population stratification may have also plagued studies that reported an association between a genetic variant of another dopamine receptor gene (D2) and novelty-seeking behavior (Benjamin et al., 1996; Ebstein et al., 1996; Baron, 1998).

These cases involving alleles of dopamine receptor genes illustrate the importance of looking at the world with an appreciation for the complexities of human culture. Accepting genetic complexity alone may not be sufficient.

I will discuss another widely reported study to point out further examples of the complexities in the search for genes associated with behaviors. In 1987, researchers reported the identification of a genetic locus that conferred susceptibility to bipolar manic-depressive illness (Egeland et al., 1987). They chose to examine an extended Amish family from Pennsylvania, because there was a high frequency of the condition among its members. The research group accumulated a large set of chromosomal markers covering all the human chromosomes in each family member. They then asked whether there were any markers that were often present in those members who had bipolar illness and absent in those who did not. They found such markers, and after analysis of their data, they believed that they had found a statistically significant candidate on human chromosome 11 for a region linked to the susceptibility to the illness. However, within two years of the publication of this study, two additional members of this family developed bipolar illness and when their chromosomes were analyzed, they were found not to carry the same chromosomal marker as the others. The statistical significance of the association with the marker on chromosome 11 disappeared. The researchers published a retraction (Robertson, 1989).

There has never been a clear-cut explanation for how the impressive initial positive results could turn out to be so wrong. One possible source of the errors seen in this field, in general, may lie in the details of the calculation used to determine which findings are likely to be significant. These complex details, not surprisingly, are rarely discussed when such reports reach the public. Yet, analysis of them reveals a serious problem with these approaches that mandates extreme conservatism in conclusions until the studies are replicated by others, perhaps even several times (Lander and Krugylak, 1995). The problem is as follows: once researchers have identified regions of the genome where gene mutations predisposing to a trait (e.g., bipolar illness) may lie, they must ask whether the finding is meaningful or is due to chance. Consider that when we flip six coins multiple times, we expect to find them landing with six heads up only very rarely. However, there is always a chance, albeit slim, that on the very first time we flip the coins, six heads will appear. Researchers have developed approaches that allow them to estimate the likelihood that a finding in gene mapping is due to such chance happenings. To do this, they calculate what is known as an LOD (logarithm of the odds) score, a probability value. However, such calculations cannot be made without knowing or, at least, hypothesizing the mechanism of inheritance and expression of the trait in question. For most behavioral traits, little knowledge of these mechanisms is available. So, researchers must consider a variety of models for the pathway from the altered gene to the phenotype. These multiple models are taken into account in sophisticated, statistically oriented computer programs, which can vary a range of parameters and ask whether any particular combinations of values for these parameters give good (high) LOD scores. High LOD scores for a particular chromosomal locus indicate a high probability that it contributes to the manifestation of the trait. The parameters that are varied include the degrees of dominant and recessive behavior of the mutant gene, the degree of penetrance of the condition, the amount of recombination between the chromosomal marker and the actual causative gene, and the age of onset of the condition. Researchers may also vary the diagnostic criteria so that members of a family being studied are switched from the affected (ill) to the unaffected category, or vice versa. From this analysis, a set of LOD scores is calculated that can vary substantially over the range of parameter values that are used for any one chromosomal locus. Researchers look for those genetic loci that over some range of parameters give a "high" LOD score. In the case of human behavior genetics, they have considered an LOD score of 3.0 to indicate that correlation of a particular locus with a behavioral trait is highly likely to be meaningful.

What is crucial to note in such approaches is that each time a numerical value is chosen for parameters in calculating the LOD scores, a different hypothesis is being tested. Researchers are testing multiple hypotheses about how the condition is inherited. Because they are testing not one but many hypotheses, there is an increased likelihood that a high LOD score associated with one set of properties has occurred by chance. That is, as more and more hypotheses are tested, the probability that an association that is found is merely due to chance becomes stronger and stronger. As pointed out above, if we flip six coins enough times, it is likely that eventually six heads will appear in a particular flip. Despite this important qualification to such studies, this approach does provide candidates for relevant chromosomal loci that can then be tested by other researchers. But, given the uncertainty generated by the testing of multiple hypotheses, the finding is not convincing until it is replicated. In light of the fundamental uncertainty resulting from this aspect of the approach, there is no basis for such a finding to be reported as significant either in the scientific report or in the media.

A second problem may be that researchers are missing out, in their statistical programs, on a category of important factors in the manifestation of a disease. For example, it could be that environmental factors play unexpected roles in the development of the condition in a family where genes are clearly important. In the case of the study on bipolar illness, the researchers in their subsequent retraction suggest that the foremost problems are "genetic heterogeneity" and "the presence of phenocopies." Phenocopies, in this instance, are those individuals who suffer from the condition not as a result of genetic influences but because of environmental effects. For example, imagine that many members of a family do have a locus on chromosome 11 that confers susceptibility to bipolar illness. However, in a family that has such a high proportion of its members exhibiting the condition, the environment of the family may be conducive to the development of the illness even in members of the family who don't have the susceptibility genes. Perhaps even the long-term involvement of researchers in the family may heighten the family awareness and concern over bipolar illness and increase the chances that the genetically "unaffected" members of the family will contract the condition. (The suggestion by the researchers of "phenocopies," of course, means that they are considering the possibility of significant environmental sources of manic-depressive illness.)

So, it may even be that the initial finding of a susceptibility gene on chromosome 11 was correct, but confounding complex intrafamilial psychological factors may have turned a significant statistic into an insignificant one. This discussion illustrates the added depth of analysis one might bring to such studies by taking seriously the cultural, social, and psychological factors that may significantly influence study results.

The Consequences

I have suggested that researchers in human behavioral genetics have taken an overly simplistic view of human social behaviors and aptitudes. The failure to consider more complex views of the interactions both between genes and between genes and the environment may explain the absence of any bona fide findings of genes associated with the behaviors they study. Nevertheless, the studies have often been presented by scientists as conclusive, thus attracting considerable media and public attention. Journalists have moved from conclusions based on the simplistic assumptions underlying the studies to present to the public simplistic views of human social problems and human social arrangements. This translation is sometimes encouraged by the scientists themselves, providing journalists with provocative statements for their newspapers and magazines. It is only recently, as the more savvy reporters have recognized the difficulties encountered by geneticists in pinpointing specific genes, that the media coverage has diminished and become more sophisticated.

A relatively recent example of studies on a behavioral problem in a Dutch family illustrates the potential magnification of effects that can take place when scientists do not take care in the presentation of their results and the media picks up on the apparent implications. This particular example is interesting because it may be considered the one case in which a well-characterized gene has been convincingly connected to a behavioral outcome. In 1993, scientists reported that a mutation in the gene for the enzyme monoamine oxidase A in an extended Dutch family was associated with aggressive behavior on the part of males who carried the mutation (Brunner et al., 1993a, 1993b). The mutation completely eliminated the enzyme activity. The data were generally persuasive. One could criticize the reports in that the mapping, biochemistry, and molecular genetics were very carefully done, while the evaluation of the behavior of individual males was sketchy, often relying on reports of other family members. Furthermore, since the "affected" males exhibited some degree of mental retardation, it is not clear what the line of connection is between the mutation and the behaviors. Nevertheless, something real appears to have been found in this study. There is good reason to think that altering MAOA metabolism can have a severe impact on some of the biochemical reactions required for the development and normal functioning of the nervous system. Consequently, it would not be surprising if this mutation did indeed affect mental functioning and even contribute to behavioral abnormalities. But, these findings do not mean that the MAOA gene is a "criminal" or "aggression" gene. Yet, that is what was implied in much of the media coverage that followed (see discussion of media coverage below).

The MAOA gene is not a "criminal" gene for the same reason that the gene altered in the disease phenylketonuria (PKU) is not an intelligence gene. PKU is a rare disease that, if untreated, results in severe mental retardation. However, only a tiny proportion of cases of mental retardation are caused by PKU. No one has suggested that any significant amount of the normal variation in intelligence among people is due to variations in the PKU gene. Analogously, the mutation completely eliminating MAOA activity is extremely rare, and as a result, is responsible for, at most, a tiny fraction of antisocial behavior. Following the finding of the Dutch group, researchers attempting to detect such mutations in other families or in individuals who are unusually aggressive have turned up no other examples. Drawing conclusions about the origins of behavior, in general, from an extreme and rare example is at best unhelpful.

At any rate, there is no such thing as an "aggression" or "criminal" gene. It is certainly true that some of the people who commit violent crimes are more aggressive than the average person and it may even be true that, in some cases, their aggressive behavior is influenced by their genes (along with their environment). However, it does not follow that differences in aggression among people can be explained generally by the presence or absence of mutations in a few identifiable genes. Rather, in view of what we have learned from psychology and sociology about the complexity of aggressive behavior, it is most probable that the discovery of any gene variants associated with aggressive or criminal behavior will make, at best, only a small contribution to explaining or understanding these behaviors.

The conclusions to the two papers from the Dutch research group were relatively limited and careful except that, in each of them, the authors hinted that their findings might have broader implications for the study of aggression in general in the population when they stated, for example, that "should a mutation in the MAOA structural gene be identified in our family, this will have implications for the study of the biological mechanisms underlying disturbed aggression regulation in general" (Brunner et al., 1993b, 1038). This hint was not missed. A reporter for *Science,* in an article entitled "Evidence Found for a Possible 'Aggression Gene,'" suggested "it might be possible to identify people who are prone to violent acts by screening for MAOA gene mutations" (Morell, 1993, 1722). The scientists' conclusions and the more provocative *Science* news article aroused tremendous media interest. A *Newsweek* article entitled "The Genetics of Bad Behavior" included a photograph of a violent confrontation between Palestinians and Israelis, implying a genetic basis for world strife (Cowley and Hall, 1993). A TV news report used films of U.S. street gang violence as a backdrop for a report on the MAOA study (X. Breakefield, personal communication). In a murder trial in Georgia, lawyers' attempts to use genetics as a defense were covered in a *Wall Street Journal* article headlined: "Man's genes made him kill, his lawyers say" (Felsenthal, 1994). Dr. Xandra Breakefield, one of the scientists involved in the study, was called upon by these defense lawyers to testify on the genetic basis of aggressive and violent behavior. Even though the legal appeal to genetics was rejected, this case and the publicity for the Dutch study illustrate the ways in which a relatively minor genetic advance can rapidly be transmitted to the public, misinterpreted, and then incorporated into discussions of social policy. Further, attention to the Brunner study grew with articles in many popular magazines and leading newspapers, which discussed the possible genetic basis of criminal behavior. A *U.S. News and World Report* article on behavior genetics was featured on the front cover with a picture of an infant in prison clothes and the headline "Born Bad?" (Herbert, 1997).

In July 1996, at Woods Hole on Cape Cod, Massachusetts, 35 judges from both federal and state courts met with 20 scientists to discuss the implications of the revolution in genetics for the legal system (Blakeslee, 1996). Judges learned how to sequence DNA in the lab and listened to lectures on the latest developments in DNA fingerprinting. According to the *New York Times,* during round-table discussions of the ethical issues raised by the new genetics, "judges asked what would happen if science demonstrated that genes controlled behavior or that bad early environments conspired with genes to turn some people inevitably into criminals" (C9).

How, then, did we move from this limited study of a rare genetic condition to a court case and judges worrying about whether some people are "inevitably criminals"? I would suggest that a sequence of steps, beginning with the way in which the MAOA researchers presented their work, played a role in stimulating public interest in the social implications of the study. The attempt by the authors of the MAOA study to generalize from their results in the scientific papers is a normal practice in science. Yet, in the case of problematic social questions such as the social and biological origins of aggression, criminality, and the like, scientists should be much more aware of the potential public consequences of such generalization (or overinterpretation). Sensitivity to the long history of these consequences should encourage much greater care in the manner in which results are presented than is usually the case by those scientists engaged in behavioral genetics research. To their credit, the scientists involved in the MAOA study showed concern about the public representations of their reports. Dr. Breakefield was dismayed enough by the publicity to announce that she would no longer work on links between violence and genes (Breakefield, 1994). Dr. Brunner's later statement that "the notion of an 'aggression gene' does not make sense" clearly reflected concern for the ways in which the study was interpreted by the media (Brunner, 1995).

This is one of many such examples that show how preliminary and, in most of the cases, faulty scientific results in the field of human behavioral genetics can be quickly translated into discussions of social implications. Not infrequently, these implications are incorporated into the formulation of social policy. The sequence of events described in the trip from publication of the MAOA study in *Science* to public policy discussions is typical of many instances of misrepresentation of results from the field of behavior genetics to the public. Other examples of overinterpretation of the science include the distorted reports that XYY males were superaggressive, which led to problematic genetic screening programs in the 1960s (Beckwith and King, 1974; Pyeritz et al., 1977). A study from 1980 that hinted at biological factors in the male-female differences in math performance influenced attitudes of parents toward their daughters' school performance and affected the thinking of schoolchildren themselves

(Benbow and Stanley, 1980; Fennema, 1981; Beckwith, 1983). The report of a chromosomal locus associated with male homosexuality in 1993 (Hamer et al., 1993) resulted in a Colorado court agreeing to hear genetic evidence while considering the legality of gay rights legislation (Bayliss, 1993; Beckwith and Alper, 2002). One of the largest projects designed to assess the genetic contributions to human behavior and aptitudes is the study of identical twins led by Dr. Thomas Bouchard at the University of Minnesota (Bouchard et al.,1990). Published reports from this group have suggested that a wide range of such traits are substantially influenced by genetics, with heritability (see chapter 1) estimates hovering around the 50 percent range. These findings have led some of the researchers associated with the project to express prescriptive statements to the public. For instance, referring to their claim that "fearlessness" is subject to strong genetic determinants, team member Dr. Nancy Segal states that "parents can work to make a child less fearful, but they can't make that child brave" (Leo, 1987). Segal's colleague, Dr. David Lykken, speaking of the supposed genetic limits in some individuals that establish a "set point" of happiness recommends: "Find the small things that you know give you a little high . . . In the long run, that will leave you happier than some grand achievement that gives you a big lift for a while" (Goleman, 1996, C1). Both of these prescriptions recognize that genetics does not imply a fixed limit to the expression of a trait. But, by suggesting how people should behave, their authors implicitly claim knowledge of just how flexible the impact of genes is.

Finally, the barrage of news stories suggesting that a wide range of our behavior is genetically controlled conveys a sense of genetic fatalism to the general reader. This extreme interpretation of behavior genetic studies is exemplified by the judges who asked whether the "genetics of bad behavior" has shown that criminal behavior is "inevitable."

Conclusions

Human behavioral genetics has largely passed from the era of nonmolecular studies (twins, families, etc.) to the era of molecular studies (linkage analysis and gene identification). The earlier nonmolecular research has repeatedly suffered from premature conclusions and poorly designed studies. While the new DNA technologies hold promise for putting the field on a more solid footing, the results so far have been disappointing. The problems in defining single genes as strong contributors to a range of behavioral traits have catalyzed a significant reformulation of thinking about the origins of these traits. While most researchers in the field have focused on genetic complexity as explanatory of the difficulties encountered, others have pointed to the long-standing neglect of environmental contributions to behavioral variation as part of the problem. Here, I argue that a major reason for the difficulties in obtaining conclusive results in this field is that researchers have not integrated more fully into their studies the analysis of familial, cultural, and social influences on human behavior and human aptitudes.

Over its nearly 100-year history, the field of human behavior genetics has received widespread public attention, despite the tentative nature of its findings. In some cases, the significance of this work has been so exaggerated by both scientists and the media that it has been used in unwarranted fashion to influence social policy. The problematic history of this field should encourage behavior geneticists to exhibit more care in the presentation of their conclusions and in discussing the social implications of their work.

Recent Developments

Several new studies have appeared that, taken together, represent an approach to genetics of human behavior consistent with many of the changes I have suggested here. This new research offers a more sophisticated examination of the interaction between environment and genes in the manifestation of human behaviors. Taken in conjunction with papers I have referred to earlier (Anthony, 2001; Kendler and Gardner, 2001; Hamer, 2002; Rutter, 2002), the three studies I will mention may reflect a new direction in the field. These are preliminary studies, which can be subject to certain criticisms and to the strong caveat, mentioned throughout this chapter, that such studies require replication before being accepted. In addition, there remains the issue of how emphasis is placed by the authors of the papers and the media on the genes, on the environment, or on both in considering the implications of this work.

Two of these studies were collaborative efforts between the Dunedin Multidisciplinary Health and Development Study of New Zealand and behavioral genetic researchers in Wisconsin and the United Kingdom. In the first study, the researchers studied the behavioral effects of a common genetic polymorphism leading to presumed lowered MAOA levels in humans. They found that, when combined with a childhood of parental abuse, the polymorphism is associated with a significantly higher degree of antisocial behavior than seen with a control group with the more common form of the gene (Caspi et al., 2002). For those individuals with the same polymorphism who have not suffered child abuse, there are no signs of increased antisocial behavior. A gene, which in one environment, has no detectable influence on an individual's social behavior, in another environment seems to have a dramatic effect.

This research appears to provide a striking case of gene-environment interaction, although this conclusion must be considered tentative until the results are replicated by other researchers and until certain methodological questions are answered (Stokstad, 2002). For example, the authors assumed that the individuals with the polymorphism in this study expressed low MAOA levels on the basis of the measurements of those levels in other studies. Nevertheless, the appearance of this report itself represents a striking example of the consideration of environmental factors in genetic studies of behavior. In fact, one of the co-authors, Terrie Moffitt, suggests that environmental factors were a "magic key" in finding the genetic effect and the gene (Stokstad, 2002).

The second study from this collaborative effort reports that the "short version" of the serotonin transporter gene is associated with greater vulnerability to stress. The result for those who have this allele is an increased likelihood of suffering from depression (Caspi et al., 2003). As with people with "low MAOA levels" in the earlier Caspi study, people with the "short version" of the gene in the newer study who did not suffer significant stressful events behaved no differently, in this regard, than those who carried the "long version" of the gene. Again, a genetic variant effects behavior under one condition but not under another.

Finally, Eric Turkheimer and collaborators published a report on the influence of environment on IQ, as it relates to social class (Turkheimer et al., 2003). This study does not deal directly with genes, but rather is a nonmolecular study of families, including many pairs of identical twins. The authors conclude that while genetic factors seem to help explain IQ differences among those coming from high SES backgrounds, environmental factors seem to help explain IQ differences among those coming from low SES backgrounds. Whether or not one considers IQ a good measure of a person's capabilities or considers twin and family studies very definitive, twin studies can be useful in revealing environmental effects.

These three studies may be harbingers of a shift in approach within human behavior genetics. Despite this interesting development, there is still a further step from the research stage to its public presentation, where genes can receive undue emphasis. The concluding sentence of the new MAOA paper, for example, suggests what the authors see as a potential application of their results: "Both attributable risk and predictive sensitivity indicate that these findings could inform the development of future pharmacological treatments" (853). This is a reasonable extension of the author's preliminary findings. It represents an attempt to move from the finding of the gene to a treatment. Yet, there are no similar concluding remarks on "development of future" programs to reduce child abuse, even though the effect of child abuse is as striking as the effect of the polymorphism. For it is not only those children with the particular MAOA polymorphism who have been subjected to abuse that show the increased antisocial behavior. The researchers found, not surprisingly, that those with the more common form of the MAOA gene were also liable to exhibit antisocial behavior if subjected to child abuse. One might have taken the findings of this research as reason to indicate the need for more forceful action on child abuse as well as investigation into possible treatments. Particularly because the path from gene discovery to treatment is nearly always long and arduous, a more balanced discussion of implications is called for. While the authors have presented evidence for a strong gene-environment interaction, their consideration of remedies for the social problem focuses alone on the use of the genetic finding to develop treatments. Contrast this focus with the comment of behavioral geneticist Irving Gottesman, who said that their study on IQ and SES "gets away from the pessimistic conclusion that . . . you're wasting your money on Head Start" (in Weiss, 2003). As behavior geneticists go in this new direction, it will be fundamentally important to remember the history of traveling in quite another.

REFERENCES

Alper, J. S. (2002). "Genetic Complexity in Human Disease and Behavior." In J. S. Alper, C. Ard, A. Asch, J. Beckwith, P. Conrad, and L. N. Geller, eds. *The Double-Edged Helix: Social Implications of Genetics in a Diverse Society.* Baltimore: Johns Hopkins University Press: 17–38.

Anthony, J. C. (2001). "The Promise of Psychiatric Enviromics." *British Journal of Psychiatry* 178(suppl. 40): S8–S11.

Bailey, M., and R. Pillard. (1991). "A Genetic Study of Male Sexual Orientation." *Archives of General Psychiatry* 48: 1089–96.

Bailey, J. M., R. C. Pillard, K. Darwood, et al. (1999). "A Family History Study of Male Sexual Orientation Using Three Independent Samples." *Behavior Genetics* 29: 79–86.

Baron, M. (1998). "Mapping Genes for Personality: Is the Saga Sagging?" *Molecular Psychiatry* 3: 106–8.

Bayliss, H. J., district court judge. (1993). "Findings of Fact, Conclusions of Law and Judgment: Evans vs. Romer." Transcript of Colorado Amendment 2 Trial. Civil action #92, CV7223.

Beckwith, J. (1983). "Gender and Math Performance: Does Biology Have Implications for Educational Policy?" *Journal of Education* (Boston University) 165: 158–74.

Beckwith, J., and J. S. Alper. (2002). "The Genetics of Human Personality: Social and Ethical Implications." In J. Benjamin, R. P. Ebstein, and R. H. Belmaker, eds. *Molecular Genetics and Human Personality.* Washington, D.C.: American Psychiatric Publishing: 315–31.

Beckwith, J., and J. King. (1974). "The XYY Syndrome: A Dangerous Myth." *New Scientist* 64: 474–76.

Benbow, C., and J. Stanley. (1980). "Sex Differences in Mathematical Ability: Fact or Artifact?" *Science* 210: 1262–64.

Benjamin, J., L. Li, C. Patterson, B. D. Greenberg, et al. (1996). "Population and Familial Association between the D4 Dopamine Receptor Gene and Measures of Novelty Seeking." *Nature Genetics* 12: 81–84.

Blakeslee, S. (1996). "Genetic Questions are Wending Judges Back to Classroom." *The New York Times* (July 9): C1, C9.

Bouchard, T. J., Jr., D. T. Lykken, M. McGue, et al. (1990). "Sources of Human Psychological Differences: The Minnesota Study of Twins Reared Apart." *Science* 250: 223–28.

Boyle, M. (1990). *Schizophrenia: A Scientific Delusion?* New York: Routledge.

Breakefield, X. Presentation at Harvard Medical School Conference, "Genes That Make News: News That Makes Genes." December 3, 2004.

Brunner, H. G. (1995). "MAOA Deficiency and Abnormal Behavior: Perspectives on an Association." In M. Rutter, ed. *Genetics of Criminal and Antisocial Behavior* (Ciba Foundation Symposium 194). Chichester: Wiley: 155–64.

Brunner, H. G., M. Nelen, X. O. Breakefield, et al. (1993a). "Abnormal Behavior Associated with a Point Mutation in the Structural Gene for Monoamine Oxidase A." *Science* 262: 578–83.

Brunner, H. G., M. R. Nelen, P. vanZandvoort, et al. (1993b). "X-linked Borderline Mental Retardation with Prominent Behavioral Disturbance: Phenotype, Genetic Localization, and Evidence for Disturbed Monoamine Metabolism." *American Journal of Human Genetics* 52: 1032–39.

Caspi, A., J. McClay, T. E. Moffitt, et al. (2002). "Role of Genotype in the Cycle of Violence in Maltreated Children." *Science* 297: 851–54.

Caspi, A., K. Sugden, T. E. Moffitt, et al. (2003). "Influence of Life Stress on Depression: Moderation by a Polymorphism in the 5-HTT Gene." *Science* 301: 386–89.

Cowley, G., and C. Hall. (1993). "The Genetics of Bad Behavior." *Newsweek* (November 1): 57.

Devlin, B., M. Daniels, and K. Roeder. (1997). "The Heritability of IQ." *Nature* 8: 468–71.

Donat, A., S. McNeil, D. R. Fitzpatrick, et al. (1997). "The Incidence of Cystic Fibrosis Gene Mutations in Patients with Congenital Bilateral Absence of the Vas Deferens in Scotland," *British Journal of Urology* 79: 74–77.

Ebstein, R. P., O. Novick, R. Umansky, et al. (1996). "Dopamine D4 Receptor (D4DR) Exon

III Polymorphism Associated with the Human Personality Trait of Novelty Seeking." *Nature Genetics* 12: 78–80.

Egeland, J. A., D. S. Gerhard, D. L. Pauls, et al. (1987). "Bipolar Affective Disorder Linked to DNA Markers on Chromosome 11." *Nature* 325: 783–87.

Felsenthal, E. (1994). "Man's Genes Made Him Kill, His Lawyers Claim." *Wall Street Journal* (November 1): B1–B5.

Fennema, E. (1981). "Women and Mathematics, Does Research Matter?" *Journal of Research in Mathematics Education* 12: 380–85.

Gelernter, J., S. O'Malley, R. Risch, et al. (1991). "No Association between an Allele at the D_2 Dopamine Receptor Gene (DRD2) and Alcoholism." *Journal of the American Medical Association* 266: 1801–7.

Goleman, D. (1996). "Forget Money; Nothing Can Buy Happiness, Some Researchers Say." *New York Times* (July 6): C1, C9.

Hamer, D. (2002). "Rethinking Behavior Genetics." *Science* 298: 71–72.

Hamer, D. H., S. Hu, V. L. Magnuson, N. Hu, et al. (1993). "A Linkage between DNA Markers on the X Chromosome and Male Sexual Orientation." *Science* 261: 321–27.

Herbert, W. (1997). "How the Nature vs. Nurture Debate Shapes Public Policy—and Our View of Ourselves." *U.S. News & World Report* (April 21): 72–80.

Ingraham, L. J., and S. S. Kety. (2000). "Adoption Studies of Schizophrenia." *American Journal of Medical Genetics* 97: 18–22.

Jackson, D. (1960). "A Critique of the Literature on the Genetics of Schizophrenia." In D. Jackson, ed. *The Etiology of Schizophrenia.* New York: Basic.

Joseph, J. (1998). "The Equal Environment Assumption of the Classical Twin Method: A Critical Analysis." *Journal of Mind and Behavior* 19: 325–58.

Kamin, L. (1974). *The Science and Politics of I.Q.* Potomac, Md.: Erlbaum.

Kendler, K. S., and C. O. Gardner. (2001). "Monozygotic Twins Discordant for Major Depression: A Preliminary Exploration of the Role of Environmental Experiences in the Aetiology and Course of Illness." *Psychological Medicine* 31: 411–23.

Lander, E. S., and L. Kruglyak. (1995). "Genetic Dissection of Complex Traits: Guidelines for Interpreting and Reporting Linkage Results." *Nature Genetics* 3: 241–47.

Lander, E. S., and N. J. Schork. (1994). "Genetic Dissection of Complex Traits." *Science* 265: 2037–48.

Leo, J. (1987). "Exploring the Traits of Twins." *Time* (January 12): 63.

MacKintosh, N. J., ed. (1995). *Cyril Burt: Fraud or Framed?* Oxford: Oxford University Press.

Meschede, D., A. Eigel, J. Horst, et al. (1993). "Compound Heterozygosity for the DeltaF508 and F508C Cystic Fibrosis Transmembrane Regulator (CFTR) Mutations in a Patient with Congenital Bilateral Aplasia of the Vas Deferens," *American Journal of Human Genetics* 53: 292–93.

Morell, V. (1993). "Evidence Found for a Possible 'Aggression Gene.'" *Science* 260: 1722–23.

Noble, E. P., and K. Blum. (1991). "The Dopamine D_2 Receptor Gene and Alcoholism." *Journal of the American Medical Association* 265: 2667.

Osier, M. V., A. J. Pakstis, H. Soodyall, D. Comas, et al. (2002). "A Global Perspective on Genetic Variation at the *ADH* Genes Reveals Unusual Patterns of Linkage Disequilibrium and Diversity." *American Journal of Human Genetics* 71:84–99.

Owen, M. J. (1992). "Will Schizophrenia Become a Graveyard for Molecular Geneticists." *Psychological Medicine* 22: 289–93.

Owen, M. J., A. G. Cardno, and M. C. O'Donovan. (2000). "Psychiatric Genetics: Back to the Future." *Molecular Psychiatry* 5: 22–31.

Paterson, A. D. (1997). "Case-control Association Studies in Complex Traits—the End of an Era?" *Molecular Psychiatry* 2: 277–78.

Pyeritz, R., H. Schreier, C. Madansky, et al. (1977). "The XYY Male: The Making of a Myth." In Ann Arbor Science for the People, ed. *Biology as a Social Weapon*. Minneapolis: Burgess: 85–100.

Risch, N., and D. Botstein. (1996). "A Manic Depressive History." *Nature Genetics* 12: 351–53.

Robertson, M. (1989). "False Start on Manic Depression." *Nature* 342: 222.

Rowe, D. C. (1994). *The Limits of Family Influence: Genes, Experience and Behavior.* New York: Guilford.

Rutter, M. (2002). "Nature, Nurture and Development: From Evangelism through Science toward Policy and Practice." *Child Development* 73: 1–21.

Schaffner, K. F. (2001). "Genetic Explanation of Behavior of Worms, Flies and Men," In D. Wasserman and R. Wachbroit, eds. *Genetics and Criminal Behavior.* Cambridge: Cambridge University Press: 79–116.

Somkuti, S. G., S. S. Wachtel, J. S. Schinfeld, et al. (2000). "46,XY Monozygotic Twins with Discordant Sex Phenotype." *Fertility and Sterility* 74: 1254–56.

Spitz, E., and M. Carlier. (1996). "La méthode des jumeaux de 1875 à nos jours." *Psychiatrie de l'enfant* 39: 137–59.

Steele, C. M., and J. Aronson. (1995). "Stereotype Threat and the Intellectual Test Performance of African Americans." *Journal of Personality and Social Psychology* 69: 797–811.

Stokstad, E. (2002). "Violence Effects of Abuse Tied to Genes." *Science* 297: 752.

Tsuang, M. T., and S. V. Faraone. (2000). "The Frustrating Search for Schizophrenia Genes." *American Journal of Medical Genetics* 97: 1–3.

Turkheimer, E., A. Haley, M. Waldron, et al. (2003). "Socioeconomic Status Modifies Heritability of IQ in Young Children." *Psychological Science* 14: 623–68.

Turkheimer, E., and M. Waldron. (2000). "Nonshared Environment: A Theoretical, Methodological, and Quantitative Review." *Psychological Bulletin* 126: 78–108.

Wachtel, S. S., S. G. Somkuti, J. S. Schinfeld, et al. (2000). "Monozygotic Twins of Opposite Sex." *Cytogenetics and Cell Genetics* 91: 293–95.

Weiss, R. (2003). "Genes' Sway over IQ May Vary with Class Study: Poor More Affected by the Environment." *Washington Post* (September 2): A1.

CHAPTER FOUR

Mobiles

A Gloomy View of Research into Complex Human Traits

Eric Turkheimer, Ph.D.

My colleagues and I (Turkheimer et al., 2003) published a journal article showing that for our sample of relatively poor 7-year-old twins, family environment was far more important than genes in the determination of individual differences in IQ. (For that portion of the sample raised in at least middle-class environments, genes predominated, as they usually have in earlier twin studies.) We were fortunate enough to get the attention of Rick Weiss, the science reporter for the *Washington Post*, who wrote a story describing our results. As a result, I had the opportunity to answer a great many questions about our findings from the lay public, interested government agencies, and other social scientists. By far the most common was this: Now that we can show that impoverished environments make a difference, what can be said about what the important environmental ingredients are?

This is a serious and well-intentioned question, and it was certainly tempting to speculate about schools, parenting, nutrition, peer groups, or perinatal care. But I didn't, and not only for reasons of scientific reticence in the absence of good data. The honest answer to the question is that I don't think there *is* anything in particular about the environment that is responsible for the effects of poverty, nothing that will set a fruitful course for future research, nothing that would make a particularly good intervention in impoverished homes, none of the things that one would like to be able to say. I don't think there is any single thing in an impoverished environment that is responsible for the deleterious effects of poverty. I don't think there is one element of impoverished environments that will be especially fruitful to study in the future or that there is any precisely targeted intervention one might make in those home environments. Yet I do believe in our finding: differences in family environment are responsible for the majority of IQ differences among impoverished twins. The difficulty arises in the contrast between the idea of "environment" as it represented in twin studies, and the ways in which actual environments cause actual outcomes in actual children. As I explore these relationships in this chapter, I hope to illuminate what we can and can't learn about environmental effects on behavior, and by way of analogy say something about genetic effects on behavior as well.

I hope readers of this volume have by now a basic understanding of the goal of twin studies, which is first to distinguish between the magnitude of the genetic and environmental influences on a trait. Once researchers have determined how much of the phenotypic variation is due to genetic variation and how much is due to environmental variation, then, using the simple model and equation explained in chapter 1, they calculate how much of that environmental variation is due to what they call the "shared environment" and how much is due to the "nonshared environment." By definition, the shared environment is composed of those factors that make siblings in the same family *similar* and the nonshared environment is composed of those factors that make siblings in the same family *different*.

Part of the appeal of basic twin studies is that once you have found the twins, twin studies are very easy to conduct. In fact, it is quite possible to conduct a twin study and obtain estimates of the effects of genes and environment without measuring anything about the environment at all. For that matter, it isn't necessary to measure anything about the genes either. All you need is a good measure of the trait of interest. Then, all you do is measure a trait in twin pairs, and compute the twin correlation (a measure of how similar twins are to each other on the trait, varying from zero, when twins are no more similar than two individuals chosen at random, to 1.0, when twins are exactly the same) separately for identical (MZ) and fraternal (DZ) twins. Since the twin correlations are a measure of how similar twins are for the trait, a comparison of the correlations for genetically identical MZ twins and the correlations for 50 percent genetically identical DZ twins indexes the contribution of genes to differences in the trait: double the difference between the correlations, and you get the genetic proportion of variance; double the DZ correlation and subtract the MZ, and you get the estimate for the "shared" environment; subtract the sum of these estimates from 1.0, and you get the "nonshared" environmental portion. (For more on twin studies, see chapter 1.)

The tendency of behavioral geneticists to reach conclusions about the environment without taking the trouble to measure anything about it has always rankled environmentally oriented researchers (Wachs, 1983). Even when the environment was actually measured in traditional twin studies, it was not specified in any detail, consisting (as was the case in our IQ study) of broad sociological measures of parental education, income, and occupational ratings, hardly the stuff of good environmental analysis. But once more finely grained environmental measures were finally included in behavior genetic research, the payoff was significantly less than might have been hoped. Detailed measures of the shared environment turn out to be substantially heritable themselves, in the sense that when they become parents themselves, identical twins are more similar to each other in their parenting behaviors than are fraternal twins (Plomin and Bergeman, 1991; McGuire, 2003). When relations between particular environmental variables and child outcomes are studied in contexts that allow researchers to estimate the specific environmental effects of one variable on another, there often seems to be nothing there (Reiss et al., 2000).

In the kind of study I am describing, a researcher might record the number of negative communications between a mother and each of her twin children, and the number of delinquent acts in which each of the children engage. The goal of such research is to show that the twin who is the target of more negative communications is also the twin who engages in more delinquent acts. If such research showed that the twin who received more negative communications also engaged in more delinquent acts, then the communications would be demonstrated to be an active ingredient of the nonshared environment (the part of the family environment that makes sibs different). Mary Waldron and I have conducted a meta-analysis that summarized the effects of all studies then available that used this design (Turkheimer and Waldron, 2000). Although it is true that about 50 percent of the total variation in behavioral outcomes can indeed be attributed to the nonshared environment, our meta-analysis found that researchers who used designs like the one I just described could hardly ever specify *which* elements of the environment made children in the same family different. In the 43 studies we analyzed, only about 2 percent of the total variation in behavioral outcomes could be shown to depend on identified factors in the nonshared environment. In other words, we can infer the *total* effect of the factors that make children in the same family different, but we can't seem to specify *which* factors make them different.

So following our example of adolescent delinquency, twin studies show that much of the variability in delinquency is environmental, especially the nonshared variety that makes children raised in the same family different from each other. But what is it about the environment? Parents who make more negative comments to one sibling than the other? Peer groups? Schools? Again, our meta-analysis showed that studies of the relation between any of these particular measures and outcomes in children yielded very little. After almost two decades of research we know little more about the ingredients of the nonshared environment than we did when we started.

What is going on here? Finding a way out of the apparent contradiction between the predominance of the environment when it is studied broadly, and the subsequent disappearance of those same effects when they are studied specifically, requires a realistic account of how environment might affect behavior. Fortunately, such a model is thoroughly intuitive and immediately at hand. I will prime your intuitions about the details of such a model by working through some others that turn out to be too simple for the task.

The simplest model of how the environment in general might affect behavior is predicated on individual environmental events with large, systematic effects on behavior. This model, illustrated in Figure 4.1, which might be called the one-environment-one-effect (OEOE) model, often arises in the early, irrationally exuberant phases of psychological theory development. Early versions of psychoanalysis are an example, in which it once seemed plausible to propose that particular forms of parent-child interaction led to particular patterns and pathologies in development later on. The occasional waves of enthusiasm for birth order as a potent explanation of behavior are another example.

Needless to say, OEOE explanations, psychoanalytic or otherwise, have not fared very well as scientific explanations of behavior. Recognizing that it is probably futile to expect an OEOE model to describe the environmental causes of actual behavioral outcomes, most social scientists turned to a model in which each of many environmental causes is posited to have a small effect on behavior, which can then be added up over many causes to achieve a reason-

Toilet training ———► Personality

Fig. 4.1. A "one-environment, one-effect" model.

able level of explanation: that model, illustrated in Figure 4.2, might be called a quantitative environmental effect (QEE) model. QEE models are best characterized by the statistical procedure that is commonly used to investigate them: multiple regression, in which each of several correlated predictors is allowed to have an independent, (usually) small, and (usually) additive effect on outcome. So, for example, a researcher who is interested in why some children engage in more delinquent acts than others might obtain a variety of information about parental education and childrearing practices, school quality, neighborhood and peer-group characteristics, and the like, and then use multiple regression to find out how the several variables can be optimally weighted to predict delinquency scores.

Social scientists have become so accustomed to this kind of statistical analysis and its various routine justifications that it has become difficult to bear in mind that such analyses might actually be intended to explain the causes of a real phenomenon. Instead, researchers either talk of "predicting" an outcome, although it is the rare application that is actually designed for the purpose of predicting anything, or disguise their causal intentions in circumspect language about outcomes that are "linked to" or "influenced by" the predictors. But if taken seriously, regression-based data analysis procedures specifically imply a QEE causal model. The causal implications of statistical prediction models are routinely ignored precisely because models of this kind never actually end up explaining anything, beyond enumerating lists of variables that appear to have nonzero associations with outcome while controlling for an incomplete and arbitrary list of other variables.

Social scientists don't like to say it, but the reason the QEE model has been a failure in terms of causal explanation is glaringly obvious: no complex behaviors in free-ranging humans are caused by a linear and additive set of causes. Any important outcome, like adolescent delinquent behavior, has a myriad of interrelated causes, and each of these causes has a myriad of potential effects, inducing a squared-myriad of environmental complexity even before one gets to the certainty that the environmental effects co-determine each other, or that the whole package interacts with the just-as-myriad effects of genes (Figure 4.3). Following Plomin and Daniels (1987), I have referred to this

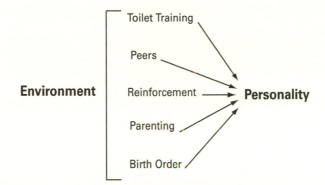

Fig. 4.2. A quantitative-environmental-effect model.

situation, with its discouraging implications for successful social science, as the gloomy prospect. (I recently attended a talk by Steven Hyman, former head of the National Institute of Mental Health and author of chapter 5 in this volume, in which he referred to a "nightmare," in which the causes of mental illness are broken up into so many tiny nonlinear pieces that scientists can never get a handle on them. Plomin's gloomy prospect might also be known as Hyman's nightmare. For Hyman's more optimistic vision of the future of such research, see chapter 5.)

As a social scientist, one can respond to the gloomy prospect in any number of ways. Plomin always returns to the conclusion that the failure to find something is not evidence that it isn't there; instead, it is evidence that we need to look harder (Plomin et al., 2001). Although I can't hide my skepticism about these ongoing efforts, neither do I object to them: that's the way science works, and the day someone finds a specific within-family environmental variable or an individual genetic locus with a substantial, noncontingent, and reproducible causal effect on a psychological outcome (not just a significant correlation or linkage, which obviously exist!) she will be right and I will be wrong. Alternatively, one could shrug at all the overwhelming complexity of environmental causation and contemplate abandoning the effort, as I may have sometimes been guilty of doing myself. Far better, of course, is to get serious about the prospects of doing the best one can at understanding complex behavioral phenomena, at least around the edges. Rutter and colleagues (2001) produced a formidable catalogue of methods to this end.

One example of doing the best one can is the point of this chapter. Faced

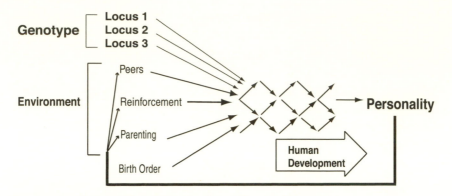

Fig. 4.3. A gloomy model of genetic and environmental effects.

with the squared-myriad of ways that an impoverished environment might inhibit intellectual ability, one imperfect but potentially useful technique is to find a way to add them all together, willy-nilly. Bad schools, inferior nutrition, indifferent parenting, dangerous neighborhoods, antisocial peers, childhood diseases, environmental toxins, you name it, all rolled together into one variable called "socioeconomic status." Socioeconomic status is a coarse, normative, ceteris paribus type of variable, and it has been much vilified by environmentalists put on the defensive by behavioral genetics. But the very coarseness of socioeconomic status can make it a blunt instrument for the detection of environmental effects that on their own are too small, uncontrolled, and nonlinear to be detected reliably, which is the role it played in our study of the genetics of intelligence.

So while I don't doubt that the socioeconomic interaction we reported must be composed of *something,* I fear that any effort to specify its composition will only lead to gloomily unsatisfying social science. Fortunately, the finding still has real consequences. Improving individual aspects of the conditions of impoverished children will probably have small positive effects, none reliably larger than the others. Removing children from poverty entirely will probably have large positive effects, a prediction that has content even without specifying exactly what "poverty" entails. Start by improving the constituents of the socioeconomic index—family income and the education and occupations of parents—and most of the rest will follow along.

I promised to conclude with an extension of my argument to the genetics of behavior. It might seem as though nothing could be farther from the gloomy muddle of environmental behavioral science than the gleaming modern science of genetics. Genetics, especially molecular genetics and its technological cousin neuroscience, are the latest in a long line of scientific white knights that have come to wake social science from its gloomy nightmare.

When I traced models of environmental causation from the simplicity of OEOE, through the regression-based QEE model, to the gloom of Hyman's nightmare, I deliberately followed a course set by the geneticists themselves. Corresponding to the OEOE model is what Plomin (1995) has called the one-gene-one-disorder (OGOD) model, useful enough for traditional medical genetics, but now universally recognized as inadequate for medical disorders as complex as diabetes or heart disease, to say nothing of schizophrenia or delinquency. In place of the OGOD model, Plomin proposes the QTL (quantitative trait locus) model on which so much of modern molecular behavioral genetics has pinned its hopes. In the QTL model, each of a great many environmental loci makes a small, but reliable, independent, and additive contribution to an outcome.

The QTL model corresponds to the regression-based QEE model of environmental effects, except that genetic models are rarely so multivariate as to contemplate anything as sophisticated as multiple regression, the search for "genes for" schizophrenia or intelligence or delinquency generally proceeding one at a time. Yet somehow, what has come to seem almost pathetically futile in environmental social science—observing that parents who place mobiles over their children's cribs have children who do better in third grade, and concluding that early visual stimulation plays an important causal role in school success—acquires a crisply technological, optimistically modern ring when exactly the same mistake is made in a genetic context. If a particular genetic locus occurs more frequently in a sample of very bright children than in a sample of borderline retarded children, it means either that the locus is a specific link in a direct causal chain leading from genes to neurons to brain function to intelligence, or it means that the locus is a mobile hanging in the vast, interactive, uncontrolled causal network that eventuates in some children performing better on IQ tests than others.

Which of these causal models you choose to believe in depends on the particular balance of scientific optimism versus realism you prefer. There is no proving that it is impossible to identify the additive set of QTLs that are jointly responsible for intelligence, which is why I do not object to the widespread efforts to sort it all out. Like mobiles over cribs, genes correlated with intelligence may not be causal in any straightforward sense, but neither are they irrelevant;

and for now, the daunting network of correlations is all we have to go on. So as I have already said, the correct response is not to give up, but rather to change our scientific expectations in a direction that is potentially gloomy but refreshingly humanistic. The reductionist and antipsychological expectation that we are going to identify a potent environmental ingredient that explains the effects of poverty on IQ, or explains schizophrenia or delinquency via the genome project or the Decade of the Brain or whatever technological marvel comes next, will never be fulfilled. As scientists or consumers of science, we need to recognize that when technology from the natural sciences meets problems from the social sciences, the result is not social science exposed at last to the bright light of natural science, but rather technology that has become entangled in the prevailing social scientific gloom. Once we can accept this state of affairs, we will be ready to proceed with a humbler program of genetically and neurologically informed social science that may allow us to understand complex behavior a little better while we wait for the millennium of scientific psychology to arrive.

REFERENCES

McGuire, S. (2003). "The Heritability of Parenting." *Parenting: Science and Practice* 3: 73–94.

Plomin, R. (1995). "Molecular Genetics and Psychology." *Current Directions in Psychological Science* 4: 114–17.

Plomin, R., K. Asbury, and J. Dunn. (2001). "Why Are Children in the Same Family So Different? Nonshared Environment a Decade Later." *Canadian Journal of Psychiatry* 46: 225–33.

Plomin, R., and C. S. Bergeman. (1991). "The Nature of Nurture: Genetic Influence on 'Environmental' Measures." *Behavioral and Brain Sciences* 14: 373–427.

Plomin, R., and D. Daniels. (1987). "Why are Children in the Same Family so Different from One Another?" *Behavioral and Brain Sciences* 10: 1–16.

Reiss, D., J. M. Neiderhiser, E. M. Hetherington, et al. (2000). *The Relationship Code: Deciphering Genetic and Social Influences on Adolescent Development.* Cambridge, Mass.: Harvard University Press.

Rutter, M., A. Pickles, R. Murray, et al. (2001). "Testing Hypotheses on Specific Environmental Causal Effects on Behavior." *Psychological Bulletin* 127: 291–324.

Turkheimer, E., A. Haley, M. Waldron, et al. (2003). "Socioeconomic Status Modifies Heritability of IQ in Young Children." *Psychological Science* 14: 623–28.

Turkheimer, E., and M. Waldron. (2000). "Nonshared Environment: A Theoretical, Methodological, and Quantitative Review." *Psychological Bulletin,* 126: 78–108.

Wachs, T. D. (1983). "The Use and Abuse of Environment in Behavior-Genetic Research." *Child Development* 54: 396–407.

CHAPTER FIVE

Using Genetics to Understand Human Behavior

Promises and Risks

Steven E. Hyman, M.D., Ph.D.

The genetics of behavior is seen by some as the key to unlocking the secrets of dread diseases such as autism, schizophrenia, and bipolar disorder. It is seen by others as a tool of stigmatization and discrimination. I believe that virtually all scientists in a position to apply modern genetic and genomic tools to behavior are motivated by a concern for the public health. Yet it is also true that for many phenotypes (traits), there is no bright line between normal behavioral variation and disease. Moreover, the technologies and scientific approaches that might permit us to understand the genetic risk factors for mental illness will almost certainly be applicable to dissect normal traits such as intelligence. Such issues were a major concern for me during my tenure as director of the National Institute of Mental Health (NIMH), which is the world's largest funder of genetic studies of behavior.

During my time as director, the NIMH investment in human genetics grants increased from approximately $30 million a year to approximately $50 million a year, while substantial funds from the intramural research program in Bethesda were reprogrammed for human genetics as well. At the same time funding for genetic studies in animal models was markedly increased, with substantial new investments in such areas as transgenic and gene knockout mouse models, large-scale mouse mutagenesis projects, and other genetic approaches to neurobiology and behavior. Overall this was a period of great excitement about genomics and genetics at NIH broadly, as the Human Genome Project moved toward completion, along with the sequencing of the mouse and other model organisms. Together these efforts promised greatly improved infrastructure and tool sets for research in human genetics.

For NIMH, with its mission of eliminating the burden of disease attributable to mental illness, genetics seemed particularly important as a possible shortcut to understanding the staggering complexity of the brain and its ills, setting better-grounded diagnostic criteria for disorders, and finding much needed new treatments. The brain is the most complex object of human scientific inquiry, with thousands of distinct cell types among its approximately 100 billion cells, and perhaps 100 to 1000 trillion synaptic connections that are organized into myriad precise, yet plastic circuits and modulatory systems that communicate via more than 100 different chemical neurotransmitters and a far larger number of receptors. In response to environmental inputs, physiological signals, and even thoughts, neurotransmitters activate complex signaling pathways within cells that lead to short-term cognitive, emotional, behavioral, physiologic, and hormonal responses, and at the same time initiate cascades leading to memory formation and adaptation to the environment. For families concerned with mental illness, basic investigations of the brain seemed to be moving not much faster than the tectonic plates that carry the earth's continents. We needed more clues about the challenging illnesses that had as their symptoms alterations in higher cognitive function, emotion, and behavioral control. Genetics promised to provide them. In fact, it was not to prove so easy.

Indeed, despite the real promise of genetics, at the time that I became NIMH director in 1996, the study of genetics at the institute could only be described as troubled. Genetic studies of mental illness had not proven productive. Early announcements of linkages of mental illness to genetic markers had gone unreplicated or had been retracted (e.g., Egeland et al., 1987; Kelsoe et al., 1989). The institute was funding many studies that were too small to achieve the statistical power to succeed or were otherwise methodologically too weak to have much promise of identifying alleles that increased risk of mental illness. (Alleles are the variant forms of any given gene within the human population.) Moreover, the institute's early attempts to produce larger coalitions of investigators and therefore increase the statistical power of studies were rife with dis-agreements born, at least in part, from competition among teams of investi-gators. Except for notable successes in Alzheimer disease, a condition that, unlike schizophrenia or mood disorders, had clearly identifiable pathologic le-sions and, more important, rare Mendelian forms (i.e., forms of the disease re-sulting from the effects of a single genetic mutation acting in deterministic fashion), molecular approaches to behavioral genetics had little to show for their efforts (Cowan et al., 2002; Merikangas et al., 2002). Critics began to ar-gue that scientific efforts to find genes for mental illnesses were either ill con-ceived or even impossible.

Alongside these scientific challenges, NIMH was also emerging from a tur-bulent period in which concerns about genetic and other biological studies of behavior, most notably studies of violence and criminal behavior, had led to protests about the goals of the institute, criticism of its leadership (Hilts, 1992a), and a widely publicized cancellation of a conference on genes and vi-olence (Hilts, 1992b). Critics expressed concerns about a possible resurgence of genetic determinism as a malign social force, about misuse and misinter-pretation of genetic data, and about the potential stigmatization of minority groups by this research. The last permanent NIMH director before my arrival had been forced to resign over remarks on the biological underpinnings of vi-olence that had been interpreted as racially insensitive. Between the scientific difficulties and such criticisms of behavioral genetics, it seemed possible that genetic studies at NIMH might become a scientific backwater mired in rapidly outdated strategies and lacking in public support, just when genomics, and with it, human genetics was about to take a quantum leap forward.

Paradoxically, the same fundamental observation that could have given comfort to those who feared a deterministic genetics of behavior would also frustrate those who hoped that genetics would speed cures for terrible illnesses: the genetic underpinnings of behavior are highly complex. By the mid-1990s, it was quite clear, although not widely appreciated, that simple determinist models of the sort holding that "one mutant gene gives rise to one defective protein, which gives rise to a deviant behavioral trait" had no relevance to common behavioral phenotypes (if, indeed, the boundaries of such putative phenotypes could readily be drawn) or, for that matter, to any common form of mental illness. Single-gene disorders of behavior tend to be relatively rare and to result in severe phenotypes, such as Huntington disease. Those that ap-pear early in life, such as Rett syndrome, often exhibit multiple neural abnormalities, including mental retardation. An interesting exception to such generalizations is provided by a point mutation in the *FOXP2* gene, a gene that encodes a transcription factor (a protein that controls the expression of other genes). This mutation was found in those members of a family who exhibited severe abnormalities in language articulation and grammar, but not in other aspects of cognition. Although this is a very rare disorder, the *FOXP2* mutation is an example of a single-gene disorder limited to one aspect of higher cognition (language) rather than a multisystem neuropsychiatric disease. Notwithstanding this example, it appears that common phenotypes related to higher cognitive function, emotion, and behavioral control are genetically complex; at present they are hypothesized to result from nonlinear interactions of multiple, often heterogeneous genetic loci (i.e., different in different families), environmental factors, and chance. In short, there is no "violence gene," no "anxiety gene," no "intelligence gene," and no "gene for schizophrenia." For such phenotypes, genes remain important in aggregate, but their contributions must be understood in terms of probabilities and risk, not in terms of certainties or simple causality.

This emerging scientific picture of complexity was not, and perhaps is still not fully grasped by the broad public—or for that matter by some social scientists and policy makers. Historically, few areas of biology have been so misconstrued and misused to cause so much mischief in society. The hereditary influence on behavior was a major focus of the eugenics movement that led to sterilization of people considered "unfit" in many countries, including the United States, and contributed to mass murder in Nazi Germany. Of course, the scientific truth that behavioral disorders are genetically complex makes behavioral eugenics scientifically as deluded as it was morally repugnant. No one is a perfect genetic specimen. All human beings carry risk alleles for common medical conditions, including mental disorders. The variants that might contribute to illness might actually be beneficial in some combinations (explaining why they are widespread) and neutral in others. Only in certain infelicitous combinations do they create risk (although still not the certainty) of disease.

Controversy flared in the United States in the mid-1990s as a result of attempts to explain racial and ethnic differences in IQ test scores on the basis of genetics, and to claim, therefore, that these differences are relatively fixed (Herrnstein and Murray, 1994). A large number of twin studies have established that among individuals raised in an adequate environment, genetic differences help to explain why people score differently on IQ tests and thus are said to have different levels of general intelligence, or g (Plomin, 1999). (This is not the place to debate the validity of IQ as a phenotype or its uses in our society.) Herrnstein and Murray (1994) argued that widely observed differences between groups on average performance on IQ tests reflected group genetic differences, which, they argued, would make them resistant to environmental intervention. Even a decade later, no one knows how many genes might be involved in general intelligence, or how the relevant variants of those genes might be distributed in populations. What we are learning about the genetic complexity of behavioral traits and about genetic variation in human populations—whereas within-group differences account for more than 90 percent of human genetic variation, differences among major groups account for no more than 5 percent (Rosenberg et al., 2002)—makes Herrnstein and Murray's work seem, at best, speculative and certainly not a platform from which to recommend public policy. Even in areas less charged than racial group differences, media reports often reinforce the scientifically untenable idea that a variety of common behavioral traits might result from the action of one gene (or perhaps a few genes) acting deterministically.

For the NIMH, a research agency with the goal of defeating mental illness, the challenge in 1996 was to better address ethical and social concerns while at the same time refocusing the science to give it a chance to succeed despite extraordinary difficulties posed by murky behavioral phenotypes and genetic complexity. Beginning in 1996, I worked with research and advocacy communities to develop policies for genetics research for the NIMH, so that the tools of genetics could eventually benefit people with mental illness.

Genes and Mental Illness

For both ethical and practical reasons, human genetics is an observational, not an experimental, science. Thus, the practice of human genetics differs markedly from study of other organisms in which breeding and environmental factors can be rigidly controlled, mutagenesis can be performed, and, in some cases, genes can be directly inserted or deleted. Before the advent of molecular genetics, human behavioral genetics was limited largely to analyses that attempted to quantify genetic versus nongenetic influences on behavioral phenotypes and to determine the modes of inheritance in cases in which genes proved relevant. Quantitative (or classical) genetic studies of behavior depended on observational designs in which genetic and environmental influences might be teased apart or in which patterns of segregation of genes might be inferred. These designs included multigenerational family studies, twin studies, and adoption studies. Multigenerational family designs permit the analysis of modes of inheritance across generations. Based on their relative convenience and analytic power, many behavioral genetic studies investigated phenotype concordance in twins, comparing identical twins versus fraternal twins raised together. That is, they investigated how similar identical twins raised together were with respect to some trait (e.g., height or schizophrenia or "IQ") and compared those observations with observations regarding how similar fraternal twins raised together were with respect to the same trait. On the assumption that identical twins are raised in the same environment and that fraternal twins are too, and given the fact that identical twins share 100 percent of their DNA and fraternal twins share on average only 50 percent of theirs, researchers make inferences about the magnitude of the role of genes in the emergence of a particular trait. (See chapter 1 in this volume for a lengthier introduction to the logic of such investigations.) To be sure, the methodology of twin studies has the weakness that the 100 percent shared-DNA condition (identical twins) cannot truly be balanced by a 100 percent shared-environment condition in humans. Indeed, creating truly identical conditions even for lab rats has proved to be very difficult (Crabbe et al., 1999).

Studies of individuals who had been adopted away from their biological families early in life better distinguished the influences of heredity and environment, and studies of twins separated early in life provided an even more powerful design. But adoption studies are difficult to perform, since they depend on societies making both records and people available for examination and interview. Moreover, the selection of adoptive families by social service agencies and the phenomenon of gene-environment covariation (whereby the individual helps select or create his or her own experiential environment) have moved some observers to question the validity of the investigators' assumption that the environments of the adoptees are really so different. (For a lengthier critique of the assumptions at work in twin and adoption studies, see chapter 3 in this volume.)

Measures frequently used in thinking about disease phenotypes and other traits that can be derived from both twin and family studies are recurrence risk ratios (λ), which quantify the likelihood of sharing a phenotype with another person as a function of relatedness and therefore as a function of the percent-

Table 5.1. Recurrence Risk Ratios (λ) for Selected Psychiatric Disorders

Disorder	Siblings (λ)	Identical Twins (λmz)
Autism	60	>1000
Schizophrenia	9	48
Bipolar disorder	7	60
Alcohol dependence	7	
Major depression	2–3	16
Panic disorder	3–7	

Sources: Data from National Institute of Mental Health, 1998; Merikangas and Risch, 2003.

Note: For comparison λ for breast cancer is 1.8 and for type II diabetes is 4.3 for siblings.

age of DNA shared. As I will discuss at greater length later, recurrence risk ratios, like heritability estimates (which are discussed at length in chapter 1) can serve as a rough and ready measure to prioritize disease phenotypes for molecular genetic investigation based on the notion that the greater the contribution of genes to a phenotype, the higher the likelihood of identifying the genetic loci that contribute risk. Both heritabilities and recurrence risk ratios are measures of the *aggregate* genetic contribution to a phenotype no matter how complex the genetic contribution; thus, a high recurrence risk ratio is not a guarantee of success in identifying *actual loci* contributing to a phenotype.

Extensive family and twin studies (McGuffin et al., 1996; Sullivan et al., 2000; Kendler, 2001) and a smaller number of adoption studies (e.g., Kety et al., 1968; Kendler et al., 1994; Sigvardsson et al., 1996) have led to the conclusion that genes contribute significantly to risk of autism, schizophrenia, bipolar disorder, major depression, anxiety disorders, alcoholism, and other disorders of brain and behavior. Recurrence risk ratios derived from many studies (Table 5.1) are consistent with a major role for genes in risk of mental illness. With the development of modern genomic and other molecular tools, we can now begin to address the extraordinary challenge of how genetic differences influence biochemical and cellular networks that affect the emergence of complex traits; thus, the traditional quantitative genetic analyses are no longer a goal in themselves, but a tool.

The goal of behavioral genetics in the twenty-first century is to identify the precise genetic variants that contribute to behavioral phenotypes. These discoveries, in turn, become tools of inquiry for neuroscience and for the neurobiology of disease. To provide just one kind of example of how gene identification provides tools for neuroscience, genes found to be associated with Alzheimer disease, Parkinson disease, or Rett syndrome in humans have been inserted into mice or used to replace the endogenous mouse gene, thus producing potential animal models for research and treatment development (Dodart et al., 2002; Shahbazian et al., 2002). Clearly, mouse models will never provide perfect replicas of human cognitive and behavioral disorders, such as schizophrenia, but they can prove very useful as partial models (Watase and Zoghbi, 2003). For example, a knock-in mouse (i.e., a mouse in which the endogenous gene was replaced by a gene of the investigator's choosing) made to express a human Rett disease mutation in the causative *MEPC2* gene shows abnormalities in social behavior (Shahbazian et al., 2002). This experiment was possible because Rett is a Mendelian (single-gene) disorder; what might not have been predicted is that human social deficits could be even partially modeled in a mouse. Overall there is growing evidence that useful, if imperfect mouse models can be constructed by inserting genes that confer disease risk in humans.

In sum, the importance of quantitative or classical genetic analyses of behavior now lies in helping to define phenotypes, suggesting paths of gene-environment interaction, and setting priorities for molecular analyses. The scientific future for behavioral genetics lies in providing tools to understand the brain in health and disease, and to point the way toward new therapies for brain disorders.

Mendelian and Non-Mendelian Disorders

During the past 15 years, approximately 1200 genes that cause human disease have been identified through positional cloning (Botstein and Risch, 2003). These discoveries have facilitated studies of the mechanisms of disease and attempts to develop new therapies. In essentially all cases, however, these successes have involved genes that act in Mendelian fashion, the situation in which a mutation in a single gene is responsible for the disease phenotype such as cystic fibrosis, Huntington disease, or Rett syndrome. In some cases a disease may actually represent multiple Mendelian disorders, such as familial Alzheimer disease (Selkoe and Podlisny, 2002) or retinitis pigmentosa (Rivolta et al., 2002) in which many different mutations in different genes produce the disorder, but within each pedigree, this is still a single-gene disorder. The deleterious nature of the mutations that cause Mendelian disorders tends to make these diseases relatively rare by decreasing reproductive fitness. Most common diseases and normal variant phenotypes are genetically complex (Kennedy et al., 2003).

Despite extraordinary success in identifying genes for Mendelian disorders, the tools of the recent past were not powerful enough to permit much success in identifying the complex genetic underpinnings of common human phenotypes. Where genes that contribute to complex disorders have been identified, such as the APOE locus in the common, late-onset forms of Alzheimer disease (Selkoe and Podlisny, 2002), they exert relatively large, and therefore more readily detectable, effects.

The genetic investigation of common behavioral phenotypes has been particularly frustrating, although some compelling candidate genes for schizophrenia have recently been identified (Chumakov et al., 2002; Stefansson et al., 2002). For the best-studied behavioral phenotypes, which are mental illnesses, comparison of concordance ratios between identical and fraternal twin pairs (which deviate markedly from expected Mendelian ratios), segregation analyses of multigenerational pedigrees, and attempts to establish linkage to genetic markers (Risch et al., 1999) have converged on the conclusion, already described above, that the common forms of psychiatric disorders are genetically complex. This means that psychiatric disorders do not arise from the action of single genes acting causally, but from the interplay of multiple genes and nongenetic factors, environmental, stochastic (chance occurrences during brain development, "dust in the machine") and chaotic (issues that arise in wiring up 100 to 1000 trillion synapses) each contributing a relatively small effect. In addition, because gene-gene and gene-environment interactions operate hierarchically during brain development (i.e., later effects are dependent upon earlier developmental events), epistatic rather than additive interactions are likely to be the rule. This means that some genes that exert an effect later in brain development might confer disease risk only if certain genetic (or environmental) effects had occurred earlier. In this scenario, the effects of the later-acting gene are not additive with the earlier events, but conditional on them. One interesting observation that has been made repeatedly in transgenic mice is that the insertion of a gene that is expected to exert a major effect may, in fact, have widely varying effects depending on the mouse strain into which it is inserted. In such cases, the genetic differences that characterize different strains modify the effect of the new gene or of the gene knockout (Holmes et al., 2003). It has become clear that gene products (proteins) perform their biological functions within interacting molecular networks, making it difficult, and sometimes impossible, to state meaningfully the function of a single gene in isolation.

Certainly it makes no sense to oppose nature and nurture. The evidence we have suggests that genetic and nongenetic factors are not simply additive, but, to a large extent, interactive during brain development. Genes affect a child's experience of the environment both by influencing the perceived salience of diverse stimuli and by influencing the environments that a person may approach or avoid. Genes may even alter the environment itself; for example, a child's temperament, which is partly genetically influenced, may elicit widely divergent behaviors on the part of parents, teachers, and peers. In turn, the environment (e.g., lived experience, drugs, illness) influences gene expression throughout life and therefore helps shape the synapses and circuits that ultimately control behavior. In the end, the brain is the great integrator, shaping neural circuits and their responsiveness and remodeling them over time based on genetic factors, a wide diversity of environmental influences, and stochastic and chaotic factors that play at least some role in gene expression within neurons, and the synaptic connections between neurons.

As mentioned in the introduction to this volume, one not-yet-replicated but very interesting study suggests how important gene-environment interactions are in the emergence of a phenotype. A longitudinal study followed a birth cohort with regular examinations of the subjects into their mid-20s. In a genetic association study that used this cohort, a polymorphism in the promoter of the gene encoding the serotonin transporter was found to moderate the influence of stressful life events on depression. Individuals with a shorter version of this promoter (that confers lower levels of expression on the gene), who also experienced stressful life events, had an elevated risk of depression. Neither the short polymorphism alone nor stressful experience in the absence of the short polymorphism elevated risk (Caspi et al., 2003).

Based on such considerations few modern scientists would disagree with the proposition that nature and nurture are inextricably intertwined as they influence brain and behavior. Indeed, the nature-nurture debate is often declared to be at an end. Unfortunately, it is not entirely clear that the evaporation of the nature-nurture dichotomy at a scientific level has as yet deeply influenced the broad social understanding of behavior. When the nature-nurture dichotomy is seen through the additional distorting lens of Cartesianism (that sees mind and body as categorically separate), distorted treatments for mental illnesses and poor policy interventions for human behaviors are the result. If an unwanted behavior or poor performance is genetically influenced (as most complex human behaviors surely are), then it does not follow that improving that behavior must be accomplished through biological means such as pharmacology. Phenylketonuria results from mutations in a single gene, but the most effective clinical response is environmental: reducing the amount of phenylalanine in the affected individual's diet. Of course, there are limits set by our genes—as is often pointed out, we cannot learn to fly—yet, on the other hand, many genetically influenced traits are in highly susceptible to significant modification.

The Genotype Problem Is Matched by a Phenotype Problem

Genetic complexity is one clear obstacle to success in identifying disease risk genes; another is the difficulty of defining behavioral phenotypes. To appreciate the difficulty of "carving nature at the joints" when it comes to behavioral traits, it helps to consider the difficulties that researchers have encountered as they have tried to set boundaries around psychiatric disorders to permit accurate diagnosis, neurobiological investigation, and treatment research. The late-twentieth-century approach to psychiatric diagnosis was shaped by the plausible approach outlined by Robins and Guze (1970). They argued that reliable and valid diagnoses of psychiatric disorders would follow from careful clinical description, laboratory studies, clear delineation of one disorder from another, family history, and the stability of diagnosis over the lifetime. This approach, which continues to provide the intellectual underpinnings for the *Diagnostic and Statistical Manual of Mental Disorders,* 4th edition (DSM-IV, American Psychiatric Association, 1994) and the International Classification of Disease, 10th edition (ICD-10, World Health Organization, 1992) classifications of mental illness, has undoubtedly met with some success. The high values for recurrence risk ratios (λ) shown in Table 5.1 demonstrate that current diagnostic categories are not simply "noise," but are picking out symptom complexes with substantial heritability. Yet, when one looks carefully, the Robins and Guze criteria do not actually converge on valid diagnoses. For example, selecting for stability of diagnosis in schizophrenia is best accomplished by choosing as cases those individuals who have a chronic illness, but if we do this, we find that this characteristic does not necessarily segregate in families. Indeed, bipolar patients are found in pedigrees with schizophrenia (Berretini, 2002). In addition, major depression and generalized anxiety disorder, discreet in the DSM classification, may share genetic risk factors and very frequently co-occur (Kendler, 1996). For personality disorders, as classified in the DSM-IV (American Psychiatric Association, 1994), it is rare that a patient receives only one diagnosis; the rule is to meet criteria for multiple personality disorders, and often a mood and substance use disorder as well (Skodol et al., 2002). Such findings might have been difficult to understand prior to our current hypothesis that risk for mental disorders is genetically complex. The high frequency of co-occurring psychiatric disorders in clinical populations likely has many origins, including shared (or blurred) risk at the genetic and environmental levels, as well as scenarios in which one disorder is a risk factor for another.

How can the boundaries of mental illnesses and other behavioral phenotypes be better articulated? First, it is not likely that sharp syndromal boundaries can be specified for most common, genetically complex disorders, behavioral or otherwise. "Specific" mental illnesses likely represent a cluster of pathophysiologically closely related entities with some differences in onset, underlying biology, course, treatment response, and outcome, depending on the precise risk factors that exist within the affected person. Second, even if circular reasoning is scientifically inelegant, the determination of phenotypes is likely to be iterative. The discovery of the mutations that cause spinocerebellar ataxias, for example, have clarified the phenotypes, and even the number of distinct disorders even in a relatively simple group of Mendelian illnesses. Third, it is likely that clinical neurobiology, such as the combination of neuro-imaging techniques with better cognitive and emotional stimuli than are now generally employed, will improve the objectivity of diagnosis over the current checklist approach. Nonetheless, "carving nature at the joints" will prove to be quite difficult for behavioral phenotypes, and, as we are finding, in some cases there may be no clear joints. (See chapter 6 for more extended reflections on the problems surrounding the definition of phenotypes.)

Setting Priorities

The scientific challenges to finding risk genes for mental illnesses are daunting, and yet the new informational infrastructure and technologic approaches to genetics make it possible that such loci will be found. Advances include the sequencing of the human genome (Genome International Sequencing Consortium, 2001; Venter et al., 2001) and the genomes of several model organisms, the identification of several million single nucleotide polymorphisms (SNPs), the most common form of variation in the human genome (Sachidanandam et al., 2001; Venter et al., 2001), the systematic identification of haplotype blocks in which SNPs are correlated with each other (Gabriel et al., 2002), the development of new sequencing technologies, and improved statistical methods. Although there is not yet clear agreement as to the best approaches to take (Botstein and Risch, 2003), it is likely that some complex disorders will be analyzable with modern approaches (Collins and McKusick, 2001). Ultimately, the application of genetic results to neurobiology will require the development of systems biology approaches that recognize the interaction of multiple components in the function of intracellular signaling networks and of multiple cells and synapses in the function of circuits.

Although the ultimate shape of the genomics/genetics tool kit was far from clear when I arrived at NIMH in 1996, what was clear was that it was time to readdress thoroughly the NIMH approach to genetics. This was undertaken through a broad process of consultation and reflection. The central component of this process was a Genetics Working Group of the National Advisory Mental Health Council that issued its report in 1998 (National Institute of Mental Health, Genetics Workgroup, 1998). This report recommended that the NIMH focus its resources and efforts on its public health mission, and therefore give priority to genetics research concerned with illnesses, rather than nondisease phenotypes like aggression or IQ. Furthermore, the work group recommended that highest priority be given to illnesses that had substantial public health significance but that were also known to have a major genetic component of risk (as determined by such values as recurrence risk ratios). With additional consultation, I made the decision to focus the lion's share of our genetics efforts on schizophrenia, bipolar disorder, early-onset major depression, and autism. Major depression, schizophrenia, and bipolar disorder qualify in part because of their very large contributions to worldwide disease burden as measured by Disability-Adjusted Life Years (DALYs), that is, healthy years of life lost to disability or premature mortality (Murray and Lopez, 1996). Autism qualified, as did schizophrenia, and bipolar disorder because of their very high recurrence risk ratios. The priority in the investigation of major depression was set on those pedigrees with many affected individuals and relatively early onsets (Weissman et al., 1984) because the genetic contribution to risk appeared to be greatest in this subgroup. With this policy, other phenotypes would be studied with NIMH funds, but these four disorders would get the most attention and resources.

My colleagues and I were not unique in thinking such an approach was wise; a 2003 opinion piece in *Science* on prioritizing complex diseases for analysis also argues for giving priority to diseases that produce a large public health impact and have a substantial contribution to risk from genes (Merikangas and Risch, 2003). Of course, the limitation to this approach is that aggregate measures such as recurrence ratios (λ) do not illuminate the underlying complexity of risk. It is possible that a disorder that ranks high in terms of both public health significance and λ might turn out to be extremely difficult to analyze because a large number of genes must interact to produce the heritable component of risk. (Or, as the editors say in their introduction, it is important to remember that our understanding of the genetic influence might remain weak even in the many cases where the genetic influence itself is strong.)

Policies were also developed to address the statistical weaknesses of older study designs given the small contribution to risk likely to be derived from any single genetic locus or environmental factor. In particular, it seemed important to facilitate the collection of large samples and extended phenotype information for each disorder and to ensure that as new technologies and scientific hypotheses emerged, samples did not have to be collected again de novo. NIMH therefore set as a policy that DNA samples and phenotype data collected with public monies (NIMH grants) should be made available to all qualified scientists. We would pay the costs of banking DNA samples or producing and storing cell lines and of maintaining databases. We therefore required investigators applying for human genetics grants to include a "sharing plan" as part of their application. This would become a matter for peer review, and if the grant were awarded would become part of the terms and conditions of the grant. This mandated sharing approach was initially seen as intrusive and burdensome by many investigators, but welcomed by most disease advocates. A group of families with autistic children, led by the voluntary group, Cure Autism Now (CAN), founded their own DNA repository, Autism Genetic Resource Exchange (AGRE), which was subsequently funded by NIMH. The sharing policy is now well accepted by NIMH investigators, but only a minority of NIH institutes have adopted similar approaches to complex disorders despite the relatively positive NIMH experience. This policy also required new attention to human subject protections, especially privacy and informed consent, since samples might eventually be used by scientists other than those who had obtained the consent.

Given the continuing emergence of new tools and the ongoing difficulties of investigating complex disorders, planning processes for genetics have continued at NIMH. A genetics work group met in 2001 as part of a broad reevaluation of research on mood disorders. This group recommended that the NIMH support continued efforts to identify the most heritable subtypes of major depression and make an effort to find underlying neural phenotypes (or endophenotypes) that could be measured with greater precision than the descriptive phenotype that would yield a DSM-IV diagnosis.

The clear focus on disease, rather than on aggression, IQ, or other interindividual differences along a normal continuum, was useful for the NIMH in three ways. First, funds were brought more clearly to bear on our public health mission, increasing the confidence of our advocacy groups and of the Congress that we had not lost our way. Second, the ultimate goals of genetic research on disease, better diagnoses and better treatments, are broadly and appropriately seen as "goods." In contrast, even though youth violence should be construed as a public health problem as well as a criminal justice issue, the attempt to find medical solutions to youth violence (except in children with diagnosable disorders) raises enormously difficult issues concerning personal responsibility, stigmatization by early identification of those deemed to be "at risk," and in some cases civil liberties. These are important issues that society must debate, and I do not believe that any honest search for knowledge should be suppressed. But for the NIMH at the turn of the twenty-first century, these were divisive distractions from the core mission. Finally, with a new focus of genetics research on disease, open discussion of the enormous challenges of genetics research, and public discussion of ethical and informed consent issues, the political problems of NIMH literally melted away. The questions to me from the Congress were about how the NIMH would use the tools of the genome project, and about whether minority groups would benefit enough from our research (given the increasingly well-documented outcome disparities for African American and Hispanic minorities)—they were not about whether our research would worsen discrimination against minorities.

Of course, this approach put off some of the difficult issues that must still be addressed. For example, as the introduction to this volume emphasizes, recent research suggests that in the main, mental illnesses are not categorically discontinuous from normal variation. While the current diagnostic classifications, the ICD-10 (World Health Organization, 1992) and DSM-IV (American Psychiatric Association, 1994), treat such disorders as attention deficit hyperactivity disorder (ADHD), major depression, and autism as categorical, there is substantial evidence that they represent complex dimensional disorders that shade into the normal (Kendler and Gardner, 1998; Spiker et al., 2002). Before long, the analysis of normal variation by genetic methods will have to be addressed in more depth than the Hastings Center–American Association for the Advancement of Science (AAAS) project has already attempted.

Conclusions

Despite the genome project's great success in sequencing human genes, one must remain sober about the prospect of solving the genetics of complex behavioral disorders. It is quite possible that gene-gene and gene-environment interactions will be so complex that we will remain limited in our capacity to build adequate models or to find better diagnostics and treatments for mental illness. We will see. As NIMH director I made major investments in genetics, both because the alternatives seemed far less promising, and because, with new tools and large enough samples, the probability of at least some successes with public health implications seemed high enough to invest public funds. And despite the controversies and contentious history, behavioral genetics is a critical part of our scientific future and is likely to be one of the cornerstones in improving life for people with mental illness. If the goals of early behavioral genetics were once to quantify the degree of heritability of a particular behavioral variant, the goals are now very different. Ultimately, the information from behavioral genetics will provide a critical set of tools to understand the brain and the neural underpinnings of behavior. I would argue that the main thrust of behavioral genetics in the near term must be toward an understanding of illness—patterns of behavior that produce distress, disability, and even death. However, the human quest for self-understanding and for improving our ability to function will also shed light on the mechanisms underlying normal behavior. By moving beyond the notion of heritability to the mechanisms by which gene-environment interactions shape the brain, we are less likely to succumb to simple deterministic models that have led in the past to harmful social policies.

Ultimately, of course, it is our brains and not our genes that control behavior. Although genes are critically important, they do not by themselves cause the brain to be built and therefore do not, except in the case of rare, highly penetrant Mendelian disorders, provide us with a causal description of what might happen or has happened to any individual. At the same time, given the complexity of the brain, it is hard to imagine that we will understand it well without important insights from genetics.

REFERENCES

American Psychiatric Association. (1994). *Diagnostic and Statistical Manual of Mental Disorders.* 4th ed. Washington, D.C.: American Psychiatric Association.

Amir, R. E., V. Veyver, B. Wan, et al. (1999). "Rett Syndrome is Caused by Mutations in X-linked MECP2, Encoding Methyl-CpG-binding Protein 2." *Nature Genetics* 23: 185–88.

Bailey, A., A. Le Couteur, I. Gottesman, et al. (1995). "Autism as a Strongly Genetic Disorder: Evidence from a British Twin Study." *Psychological Medicine* 25: 63–77.

Berrettini, W. H. (2002). "Are Schizophrenic and Bipolar Disorders Related? A Review of Family and Molecular Studies." *Biological Psychiatry* 48: 531–38.

Botstein, D., and N. Risch. (2003). "Discovering Genotypes Underlying Human Phenotypes: Past Successes for Mendelian Disease, Future Approaches for Complex Disease." *Nature Genetics* (suppl. 33): S228–S237.

Caspi, A., K. Sugden, E. Miffitt, et al. (2003). "Influence of Life Stress on Depression: Moderation by a Polymorphism in the 5-HTT Gene." *Science* 301: 386–89.

Chumakov, I., M. Blumenfeld, O. Guerassimenko, et al. (2002). "Genetic and Physiological Data Implicating the New Human Gene G72 and the Gene for D-amino Acid Oxidase in Schizophrenia." *Proceedings of the Natural Academy of Sciences* USA 99(21): 13675–80.

Collins, F. S., and V. A. McKusick. (2001). "Implications of the Human Genome Project for Medical Science." *Journal of the American Medical Association* 285: 540.

Cowan, W. M., K. L. Kopnisky, and S. E. Hyman. (2002). "The Human Genome Project and Its Impact on Psychiatry." *Annual Reviews in Neuroscience* 25: 1–50.

Crabbe, J. C., D. Wahlseten, and B. C. Dudek. (1999). "Genetics of Mouse Behavior: Interactions with Laboratory Environment." *Science* 284: 1670–72.

Dodart, J. C., C. Mathis, K. R. Bales, et al. (2002). "Does My Mouse Have Alzheimer's Disease?" *Genes, Brain, Behavior*1(3): 142–55.

Egeland, J. A., D. S. Gerhard, D. L. Pauls, et al. (1987). "Bipolar Affective Disorders Linked to DNA Markers on Chromosome 11." *Nature* 325(6107): 783–87.

Elowitz, M. B., A. J. Levine, E. D. Siggla, et al. (2002). "Stochastic Gene Expression in a Single Cell." *Science* 297: 1183–86.

Enard, W., M. Przeworski, S. E. Fisher, et al. (2002). "Molecular Evolution of FOXP2, A Gene Involved in Speech and Language." *Nature* 418: 869–72.

Gabriel, S. B., S. F. Schaffner, J. Nguyen, et al. (2002). "The Structure of Hapolotype Blocks in the Human Genome." *Science* 296: 2225–29.

Genome International Sequencing Consortium. (2001). "Initial Sequencing and Analysis of the Human Genome." *Nature* 409: 860–921.

Herrnstein, R. J., and C. Murray. (1994). *The Bell Curve: Intelligence and Class Structure in American Life.* New York: The Free Press.

Hilts, P. J. (1992a). "Federal Official Apologizes for Remarks on Inner Cities." *New York Times* (February 22).

Hilts, P. J. (1992b). "U.S. Puts a Halt to Talks Tying Genes to Crime." *New York Times* (September 5).

Holmes, A., Q. Lit, D. L. Murphy, E. Gold, and J. N. Crawley. (2003). "Abnormal Anxiety-related Behavior in Serotonin Transporter Null Mutant Mice: The Influence of Genetic Background." *Genes, Brain, Behavior* 2(6): 365–80.

Jaenisch, R., and A. Bird. (2003). "Epigenetic Regulation of Gene Expression: How the Genome Integrates Intrinsic and Environmental Signals." *Nature Genetics* (suppl. 33): S245–S253.

Kelsoe, J. R., E. I. Ginns, J. A. Egeland, et al. (1989). "Re-evaluation of the Linkage Relationship between Chromosome 11p Loci and the Gene for Bipolar Affective Disorder in the Old Order Amish." *Nature* 342(6247): 238–43.

Kendler, K. S. (1996). "Major Depression and Generalised Anxiety Disorder. Same Genes, (Partly) Different Environments—Revisited." *British Journal of Psychiatry* (suppl. 30): S68–S75.

Kendler, K. S. (2001). "Twin Studies in Psychiatric Illness" *Archives of General Psychiatry* 58: 1005–14.

Kendler, K. S., and C. O. Gardner. (1998). "Boundaries of Major Depression: An Evaluation of DSM-IV Criteria." *American Journal of Psychiatry* 155: 172–77.

Kendler K. S., A. M. Gruenberg, D. K. Kinney, et al. (1994). "Independent Diagnoses of Adoptees and Relatives as Defined by DSM-III in the Provincial and National Samples of the Danish Adoption Study of Schizophrenia." *Archives of General Psychiatry* 51: 456–68.

Kennedy, J. L., L. A. Farrer, N. C. Andreasen, et al. (2003). "Genetics of Adult-onset Neuropsychiatric Disease: Complexities and Conundra?" *Science* 302(5646): 822–26.

Kety, S., .S. D. Rosenthal, P. H. Wender, et al. (1968). " The Types and Prevalence of Mental Illness in the Biological and Adoptive Families of Adopted Schizophrenics." *Journal of Psychiatric Research* 6: 345–62.

McGuffin, P., R. Katz, S. Watkins, et al. (1996). "A Hospital-based Twin Register of the Heritability of DSM-IV Unipolar Depression." *Archives of General Psychiatry* 53: 129–36.

Merikangas, K. R., A. Chakravarti, S. O. Moldin, et al. (2002). "Future of Genetics of Mood Disorders Research." *Biological Psychiatry* 52(6): 457–77.

Merikangas, K. R., and N. Risch. (2003) "Genomic Priorities and Public Health." *Science* 302(5645): 599–601.

Murray, C. J, and A. D. Lopez. (1996). "The Global Burden of Disease." In *World Health Organization. Global Burden of Disease and Injury Series*, vol. I. Geneva: Harvard School of Public Health, World Bank, and World Health Organization.

National Institute of Mental Health Genetics Workgroup. (1998). "Genetics and Mental Disorders." Bethesda, Md., NIH Publication No. 98–4268. www.nimh.nih.gov/research/genetics.htm.

Plomin, R. (1999). "Genetics and General Cognitive Ability." *Nature* (suppl. 402): S25–S29.

Risch, N. D., L. Spiker, D. Lotspeich, et al. (1999). "A Genomic Screen of Autism: Evidence for a Multilocus Etiology." *American Journal of Human Genetics* 65: 493–507.

Rivolta, C., D. Sharon, M. M. DeAngelis, and T. P. Dryja. (2002). Retinitis Pigmentosa and

Allied Diseases: Numerous Diseases, Genes, and Inheritance Patterns. *Human Molecular Genetics* 11(10): 1219–27.

Robins, E., and S. B. Guze. (1970). "Establishment of Diagnostic Validity in Psychiatric Illness: Its Application to Schizophrenia." *American Journal of Psychiatry* 126: 983–87.

Sachidanandam, R., D. Weissman, S. C. Schmidt, et al. (2001). "A Map of Human Genome Sequence Variation Containing 1.42 Million Single Nucleotide Polymorphisms." *Nature* 409: 928–33.

Selkoe, D. J., and M. B. Podlisny. (2002). "Deciphering the Genetic Basis of Alzheimer's Disease." *Annual Review of Genomics and Human Genetics* 3: 67–99.

Shahbazian, M., J. Young, L. Yuva-Paylor, et al. (2002). "Mice with Truncated MeCP2 Recapitulate Many Rett Syndrome Features and Display Hyperacetylation of Histone H3." *Neuron* 35: 243–54.

Sigvardsson, S., M. Bohman, and C. R. Cloninger. (1996). "Replication of the Stockholm Adoption Study of Alcoholism: Confirmatory Cross-fostering Analysis." *Archives of General Psychiatry* 53: 681–87.

Skodol, A. E., J. G. Gunderson, B. Pfohl, et al. (2002). "The Borderline Diagnosis I: Psychopathology, Comorbidity, and Personality Structure." *Biological Psychiatry* 51(12): 936–50.

Spiker, D., L. J. Lotspeich, S. Dimiceli, et al. (2002). "Behavioral Phenotypic Variation in Autism Multiplex Families: Evidence for a Continuous Severity Gradient." *American Journal of Medical Genetics* 114(12): 129–36.

Stefansson, H., E. Sigurdsson, V. Steinthorsdottir, et al. (2002). "Neuregulin 1 and Susceptibility to Schizophrenia." *American Journal of Human Genetics* 71(4): 877–92.

Sullivan, P. F., M. C. Neale, and K. S. Kendler. (2000). "Genetic Epidemiology of Major Depression: Review and Meta-analysis." *American Journal of Psychiatry* 157(10): 1552–62.

Thompson, P. M., T. D. Cannon, K. L. Narr, et al. (2001). "Genetic Influences on Brain Structure." *Nature Neuroscience* 4: 1253–58.

Venter, J. C., M. D. Adams, E. W. Myers, et al. (2001). "The Sequence of the Human Genome." *Science* 291: 1304–51.

Watase, K, and H. Y. Zoghbi. (2003). "Modelling Brain Diseases in Mice: The Challenges of Design and Analysis," *Nature Reviews Genetics* 4(4): 296–307.

Weissman, M. M., P. Wickramaratne, K. R. Merikangas, et al. (1984). "Onset of Major Depression in Early Adulthood.: Increased Familial Loading and Specificity." *Archives of General Psychiatry* 41(2): 1136–43.

World Health Organization. (1992) "The ICD-10 Classification of Mental and Behavioral Disorders: Clinical Descriptions and Diagnostic Guidelines." *Geneva, World Health Organization.*

II / Basic Ethical and Social Concepts and Problems

CHAPTER SIX

Social Construction and Medicalization

Behavioral Genetics in Context

Nancy Press, Ph.D.

The concepts of *social constructionism* and *medicalization* can help explain how certain behaviors become available for a search for their genetic underpinnings, why those searches have had only limited success, and what the social consequences, for scientists and for the broader society, are of the failures as well as the continued attempts.

Social Constructionism

Social constructionism refers to a set of social science concepts and methods that are currently highly visible and highly contentious. Social constructionism has been at the center of "science wars" (Labinger and Collins, 2001), media hoaxes (Sokal, 1996a, 1996b), and a small industry in edited volumes (e.g., Stein, 1992; Wiebe et al., 1987). One of the clearest and most complete discussions of the concepts and their controversies is found in Ian Hacking's *The Social Construction of What?* (2000). Hacking provides a taxonomy of social constructionist formulations and the premises underlying them. He states that all types of social constructionist arguments depend on "the constructionist precondition, an axiom that posits, 'In the present state of affairs, X is taken for granted; X appears to be inevitable'" (12). That is, X appears to be a fact in the world. Hacking sees this axiom as a necessary precondition that puts one in the right place for any further moves in the argument. It essentially brackets the concept of X, thus making it possible and logical to move on to the basic constructionist proposition which is: X (the concept or idea) need not be as it seems to be at the current time; X is not determined by the nature of things and is not inevitable; and it is possible that X need not have existed at all.

A particularly clarifying aspect of Hacking's discussion comprises a list of things about which no one has taken a social constructionist position. Interestingly, what these concepts have in common is not that they so patently are real, but rather that they so patently are not. The list includes such things as the British monarchy, legal contracts, and money (12). Hacking points out that since there is no argument with the idea that these are all completely products of human invention, there is no need to bring the social constructionist lens to bear in examining them.

Then what things do become the object of social constructionist inquiry? Hacking provides an astonishing number of concepts about which social constructionist arguments have been published, literally from A (authorship) to Z (Zulu nationalism), with S (serial homicide) and W (women refugees) in between. A look at Hacking's discussion of the social construction of women refugees, based on the work of Moussa (1992), is instructive in making clear the underlying logic of these arguments as well as the essential modesty of what seems at first an outrageous claim. The claim seems far-fetched only if it is taken to mean that there are no actual women who flee from their home countries. But no one makes such a claim. Rather, what is seen as socially constructed is a rubric that then supports the creation of legislation, bureaucracies, newspaper articles, and scholarly studies and, in so doing, actually obscures the individual women, their individual stories and circumstances—and, often the pain and outrage of these stories—within the compound phrase *women refugees*. This is important because this process of social construction makes these women appear as a distinct species of being, an object of legislation and statistical and bureaucratic management, but also eventually blunts their unique and painful stories inside this distancing phrase. Once this new category of *women refugees* is created, it allows a kind of slippage from a focus on the intolerable conditions and circumstances that motivate a particular woman to flee, to a focus on the characteristics that comprise a particular kind of woman—the *woman refugee*. Thus something specific and linked to a particular time and place now appears general, universal, and inevitable. If one imagines that this social construction might occur in regard to a *behavioral trait* rather than about a set of individuals in a particular social circumstance, one begins to see the connection to behavioral genetics, which I examine below.

Social constructionism, however, represents not only a critique but also a method. Once an idea or concept has been bracketed by a claim that it is socially constructed, that it is a contingent, social fact rather than an inevitable product of nature, it is possible to undertake a biographical investigation of that concept: When was it "born"? What were the circumstances that made this birth possible? What sort of life did it have? What has been its effect on the world? And, finally, sometimes, how and when and of what causes did it cease to exist?

Elianne Riska uses just this trope of biography in an article entitled "The Rise and Fall of the Type A Man" (2000). Riska sets as her task the tracing of the social construction of Type A man in the scientific medical literature in the 1950s and 1960s. Sometimes referred to as Type A personality, the phrase *Type A Man* makes particularly clear the creation of a category similar to that of *women refugees*. However, in this case, the constructed aspect is clearer, as there is no particular action (such as fleeing one's home) that separated the Type A man from other men, but rather a set of psychological and behavioral characteristics, which included competitiveness, a drive toward hard and intense work, a general impatience and even hostility in relations with others, along with a decisive leadership style. These traits appeared not only to cluster together, but also to correlate with a greatly increased risk for heart disease. Beginning in the mid-1950s, this concept gained rapidly in popularity and seemed to define a whole set of men who were at risk of death from their own personality. By the mid-1990s, research in this area had virtually ceased and, although the phrase is still occasionally heard, Type A man and Type A personality have become something of a footnote in personality theory. For a while, though, Type A man seemed discovered rather than created, a real and powerful factor in both personality and health. Riska and others provide a variety of explanations for what happened to Type A. These include, but are far from limited to, the rapidly changing roles of men and women in the 1970s, and changes in knowledge about the place of lifestyle (e.g., diet and exercise) in the etiology of heart disease, along with the concomitant drop in heart disease rates during those decades. In fact it seems likely that the complete biography of the concept of Type A man is still to be written. But its short lifespan makes it a powerful example of how a concept can be socially constructed. It seems more than likely that if advances in genetics had happened earlier, the concept of Type A would have been ripe for a genetics search.

Social constructionism thus provides a rich mode of working for historians, anthropologists, and social philosophers. It tells us interesting things about our world that might otherwise be largely invisible. Like any investigation in social history, it is likely to be more specific than general, highly detailed, attuned to "local" conditions, aware of the interactions among factors, and, in general, holistic. It is, in all of this, quite the opposite of the way science must work. Science, with its search for general principles, must "flatten out" the world in its search for connections between a class of phenomena called A and another class called B. Thus, it might appear that there is little point of contact—or criticism—between a social constructionist view of the world and that of science. But I would contend that in behavioral genetics, the view of social constructionists is highly germane, and suggests a particular vulnerability of behavioral genetics: behavioral genetics depends for the subject of its inquiries on traits, concepts, or phenotypes that are often not the product of nature but rather socially constructed, and thus inconstant, phenomena. To the degree that this is the case in any given situation, these phenomena, while often having deep reality in the social world, lack the "construct validity" needed for a natural science inquiry; thus, they may lead behavioral genetics astray.

Construct Validity

To take a very broad example, if a contemporary scientist were to suggest a search for a gene predisposing to the likelihood of being a witch, or even a vulnerability to being affected by witchcraft or demonic possession, no one within the scientific community would expect the endeavor to be successful because no one within that community believes in witchcraft or demonic possession as real things in the world. It is true that a scientist might get support for a search for a genetic predisposition to *believing* that one is subject to demonic possession, but that would be quite different from a search for a gene predisposing to actual demonic possession. That is, whether consciously or not, scientists take a social constructionist view of "witchcraft"—they know that as a social phenomenon witchcraft certainly has had a powerful impact on the world, but they do not believe in witchcraft as a thing-in-itself, with an existence independent of its name, out in the world.

One might then, in parallel to Hacking's basic proposition of social constructionism, posit a basic proposition for behavioral genetics: that the behavior/trait X is determined by the biological nature of things and while possibly affected by the culture in which the person with the trait lives, the underlying form of the trait is invariant and inevitable. Simply stated, the success of any search for the genetic contributions to behavior X, a phenotype, depends on the construct validity of behavior X.

Certainly behavioral geneticists are well aware of the problem of phenotype definition and have striven in recent years to make their definitions ever more rigorous (see Hyman, chapter 5 of this volume). Nevertheless, behavioral geneticists are still beholden to psychology, psychiatry, and, to a certain extent, contemporary public discourse, to present them with the constructs for which genetic underpinnings are sought. It is here, I believe, that they remain vulnerable to the construct validity problem; that is, the fact that the phenotypes they study are socially constructed.

The realm of psychology appears to be in a particularly reductionist moment in which it is averred that all personality variation can be explained as a mix of the "Big Five" factors (openness, conscientiousness, extraversion, disagreeableness, and neuroticism) (Costa and McCrae, 1986). It is, of course, possible that time will prove that, indeed, these five traits form the substrate of all human personality in all societies. However, the history of psychology is littered with other such unifying personality theories, and it may turn out that the Big Five is neither as explanatory nor as universal as currently thought. If this is the case, it would seem to predict the nonreplicability of findings of geneticists who are already using the Big Five as a guide to phenotype-genotype studies (Jang et al., 1996).

One interesting example of such work is that of Johnson and colleagues (2004). These researchers set themselves the task of examining "the extent to which [the Big Five] factors of personality are predictive of leadership dimensions and the extent to which unique genetic contributions to the relationship between personality and leadership style may be identified" (27). Their sample comprised adult pairs of monozygotic (MZ) and dizygotic (DZ) twins. Although the article does not specifically mention it, all participants appear to have been recruited from the same geographic area ("through newspaper advertisements and by word of mouth through local multiple birth associations" [28]). Using pen-and-pencil measurement instruments to assess leadership (the Multifactor Leadership Questionnaire) and personality dimensions (the Personality Research Form), comparing the MZ and DZ twin pairs, the results supported the authors' hypothesis that there is a significant genetic contribution to leadership and that it correlates with certain aspects of the Big Five personality factors.

A perusal of some of the factors in the leadership questionnaire is instructive. They include, for example, attributed charisma, inspirational motivation, individualized consideration, and idealized influence. While there are clearly specific, technical, and carefully thought out definitions of each of these dimensions, the names themselves suggest an important fact: leadership as a behavior—what constitutes it and how valued it is—is tremendously variable from culture to culture and through time.

A telling, recent, example is presented by the fate of several Japanese nationals taken hostage in 2004 in Iraq during the U.S.-British led war. After days of horrific pictures of these hostages being threatened with execution, they were finally released back to Japan, where they were greeted with nothing but opprobrium. A Japanese psychiatrist, interviewed by the *New York Times* (Onishi, 2004), felt that the stress of the hostages' return to Japan was greater than what they had suffered in Iraq, where death by immolation had been threatened. Criticism of them in Japan centered on the fact that they were seen as putting themselves—and thus the country—in a position to be held hostage and humiliated. Although such a public response is clearly within the range of emotions that would have formed some part of a reaction to U.S. hostages upon their safe return to the United States, the difference in overall reaction is, clearly, immense. Perhaps most interesting is that two of the female hostages had gone to Iraq to do aid work with Iraqi street children. Such an act, which would most likely have made these women seem heroic in their altruism in the United States—and slated for media coverage that would, no doubt, have stressed their inspirational motivation—was seen as an act of particular selfishness in Japan. What in the United States would have seemed to be showing leadership through taking charge and setting an example—a kind of entrepreneurial spirit—was in no way congruent with proper leadership style in Japan, where leaders emerge slowly and lead quietly, by indirection, and not by getting themselves noticed.

Clearly such contrasts are merely suggestive until Johnson's study results were to be replicated in Japan (or at least until the exercise were done of trying to achieve construct validity for the leadership scale in that country). But even performing this thought experiment about the construct of *leadership* suggests the dependence of behavioral genetics on, usually locally based, concepts from psychology to form the bedrock of behavioral genetics investigations and the attendant vulnerability to errors regarding construct validity that this dependence yields.

Even if one accepts that this problem exists in regard to the psychology of normal personality, one might still suppose it would be far less problematic when one shifts to the realm of psychiatric disease. Here one is dealing with traits and conditions that are clearly further from species-typical functioning and perhaps, like malaria or cancer, will be the same wherever they are found.

However, that is not the view taken by a group of medical anthropologists and transcultural psychiatrists who formed the National Task Force on Culture and Psychiatric Diagnosis (Mezzich et al., 1999), charged with providing advice on a major revision of the *Diagnostic and Statistical Manual* (1994). In reports written after the completion of the DSM-IV, this group found significant problems with the way culture was incorporated into the diagnostic categories. While commending the more integrated inclusion of culture in this revision than in previous ones, the group felt that an ironic point had been reached where the acceptance of some of the elements of a transcultural anthropologic approach—specifically the distinction between disease and illness—had actually worked in a conservative direction. Disease, as it is understood by medical anthropologists, refers to abnormalities in the structure and function of organ systems; it is the experience from the point of view of science or the practitioner who diagnoses and treats clinical pathology. Illness refers to the lived experience of these problems. As Arthur Kleinman, states, "illness refers to how the sick person and the members of the family or wider social network perceive, live with, and respond to symptoms and disability" (Kleinman, 1988, 3). According to the medical anthropologists and transcultural psychiatrists who formed this task force, the reframers of the DSM-IV discovered in this distinction a way to explain the differences found among psychiatric illness from one culture to the next by situating these differences in the realm of illness—the patient's different, culturally influenced presentation of the condition. However, by doing so, the view that the disease is invariant, representing a natural category in the world, was actually bolstered.

Thus, both psychology and psychiatry seem currently to affirm the sensibleness of searching for the genetic underpinnings of normal personality traits and psychiatric disorders. And one has only to do the briefest examination to see that, indeed, such a search is going on at an amazing clip. For example, a Google search conducted on May 6, 2004, on the phrase "gene found for AND behavior" yielded 9410 hits. The array of traits found in this quick search comprised an extraordinary range of behaviors or conditions, the genetic underpinnings for which some scientist's lab was searching. These included manic depression; depression; obsessive compulsive disorder; alcoholism; obesity; impulsivity; impulsivity linked to violence; anxiety, including reports of a "scaredy cat" gene; anxiety linked to aggression; gambling behavior; novelty seeking; risk taking; a gene predisposing to post-traumatic stress disorder; shyness; spirituality; addictive behaviors in general; and a "sweet-tooth gene."

Medicalization

Yet the fact of a busy industry in "gene searching" for traits that may at least in part be socially constructed does not tell the whole story of what is occurring and what risks it may present to society. For that one needs to add to the mix the concept of *medicalization*.

Medicalization is a term first coined by anthropologist Irving Zola (1972) to refer to a process through which an increasing number of aspects of life were being brought under the purview of medicine. According to those who work within this framework (Ginzburg and Rapp, 1991; Verweij, 1999; Conrad, 1992), medicine, with the patently admirable aim of reducing morbidity and mortality, has become culturally authorized to scrutinize what individuals eat, drink, and inhale; how they spend their leisure time; whether they choose to take the stairs or the elevator; whether they wish to think about breast cancer while taking a shower. Preservation of the best possible health status has become a personal and social responsibility and good health has come to seem not one advantage of socioeconomic success but a marker of the kind of responsible action that led one to become successful in the first place. Social philosopher Michel Foucault (1994) coined the phrase *the medical gaze* to talk about medicine as a type of surveillance in which individuals and their behavior are increasingly brought within a disciplinary focus.

Implicit in this is that medicalization pathologizes what might otherwise be considered simply variations in normal human functioning. Concomitant with this is the idea that this pathologizing, at the same time, reifies behaviors thought to be problematic or pathological, thus creating conceptually distinct phenomena out of what otherwise might not be separated from the flow of daily life, reactions, or sensations. These linked processes of pathologizing and reifying are key to the availability of such behaviors, traits, and conditions for "gene searches."

Abby Lippman (1991), a feminist biologist, coined the term *geneticization* to describe the extension of medicalization to the genetic realm. She believes that the explosion of interest in genetics, especially since the inception of the Human Genome Project, has encouraged the logic of medicalization to expand into the arena of genetics and makes it easy to predict that the number Google hits in the search mentioned above would be large and daily growing larger.

Some Examples

We now have several, related concepts—*social construction,* which suggests that various behaviors and traits examined under the behavioral genetics rubric may lack *construct validity,* and the idea that *medicalization,* with its subcategory of *geneticization,* may represent a force that helps construct and reify the behaviors with which behavioral geneticists are currently engaged. I would like now to explore this schema through some examples, taken from the Google search mentioned above, of a current, although not particularly serious nature.

The first involves the "sweet-tooth gene." Scientific interest in the physiology of taste is longstanding and inquiry is ongoing into the genetic underpinnings of the ability to differentiate various tastes—with sour, bitter, salty, and sweet long known as the primary colors of the taste buds. The most recent scientific success was, apparently, finding the gene (or perhaps *a* gene) that enables humans to identify sweet tastes.

The first major notice of this finding occurred on April 28, 2001, in a press release issued by *Nature Genetics* in advance of the article's publication in that journal. The press release included the following:

> Preference for sweetness over bitterness is not just a matter of taste. *Bitter compounds are often deadly, whereas sweet ones are rich in carbohydrates with high nutritive value* . . . Until now the identity of the "sweet" taste receptor has been a mystery. Robert Margolskee and colleagues . . . have now identified the first candidate receptor for sweetness. (Press release, 2001; italics added)

This was work done with mice; those with a mutation that impaired the function of the *T1R3* receptor gene were unable to identify sweetness.

It should be noted that the press release explicitly states the adaptive value of the ability to perceive sweetness. In addition, the gene that is thought to be associated with this species-typical behavior was isolated by creating an abnormal version of it that impaired its function. Further, I want to stress that this ability is essentially passive—one does not *act* in a way that leads to perceiving sweetness. Yet, when this science got reported in the media, all three of these key points were reversed or ignored.

> Wonder why you prefer a fudge brownie for dinner to spaghetti and meatballs, or can't resist grabbing those last few M&Ms? Maybe you should blame your sweet tooth on your genes (hereditary material in cells). Scientists . . . discover[ed] a gene that's expressed . . . in rodent sugar lovers, but not in others . . . scientists were able to pinpoint the corresponding human gene, called T1R3. The next step: to learn how to switch the gene on or off. [According to] Dr. Y. Gopi Shanker of Mount Sinai, "If we can control the proverbial sweet tooth, it might be of great help to people suffering [diabetes and obesity]." From *Science World* (Morgan 2001)

> Some day, scientists might . . . be able to switch that receptor gene to an "off" position . . . It might also mean that people . . . who tend to eat . . . a bit too much sugar will have a great new excuse around major holidays. Indulgence without guilt. From *Time Magazine* (Reaves 2001)

Thus, the ability to perceive sweetness morphs into a preference for sweet tastes and from there to an action—"grabbing those last few M&Ms." The mice reported on are, in fact, the "normal," wild-type sugar-perceivers, but the story suggests that it is they, not their non-sweetness-perceiving compatriots with the laboratory-induced mutation, who have some special form of the gene. And both stories then move directly to the hope of gene therapy, which will somehow turn off this (normal and adaptive) gene and thus help people seen to be suffering from diseases linked to overconsumption of sweets—itself a medical stretch.

How is one to explain this? It is easy to call it bad reporting, but it seems much more accurately to be an example of the combined influences of social construction, medicalization, and geneticization. One need not belabor the point of the ongoing American obsession with diet and weight, and the recent discovery of an "epidemic" of obesity that promises to soon overshadow the national obsession with tobacco, to see how even the ability to taste, and be pleased by, sweetness can become a danger from which only gene therapy can save us.

None of the above necessarily implies bad science, as long as the hype remains in the media and not with the geneticists interested in the physiology of taste. It is meant rather to demonstrate how the social environment surrounding a trait, and the focus of contemporary medicine in general, might lead behavioral genetics astray.

Another interesting, and more serious, example is that of shyness. While shyness as an aspect of personality has long been known, named, and discussed, it was not until quite recently that shyness became redefined and subsumed under the rubric of social anxiety disorder. This diagnosis was first recognized by the American Psychiatric Association in 1980 and appears with diagnostic criteria in the DSM-IV (American Psychiatric Association, 1994). It is characterized as "a marked and persistent fear in social situations in which the person believes he or she will do something embarrassing or have anxiety symptoms (e.g., blushing or sweating) that will be humiliating."

The critique of social anxiety disorder as an example of both social construction and medicalization has been made explicitly by others (Horwitz, 2002). Nevertheless, the scholarly and self-help literature on social anxiety disorder is very large, and the sense of this as a serious disorder in need of diagnosis and treatment seems increasingly entrenched. The recently claimed usefulness of selective serotonin reuptake inhibitors (e.g., Paxil) for treatment of social anxiety disorder suggests that shyness as a disorder is ripe for behavioral genetic investigation. And, in fact, while behavioral geneticists assume that there are important environmental triggers to shyness, various research also supports a view that this is a trait with a significant degree of heritability (e.g., Eley et al., 2003; Fyer, 1993) and the search for genetic underpinnings has commenced (Arbelle et al., 2003; Roberts et al., 2004; Melke et al., 2003; Osher et al., 2000).

Certainly equally compelling cases could (and have) been made for the social construction and medicalization of other traits falling under the behavioral genetics purview, for example, attention deficit disorder (e.g., Conrad and Potter, 2000), alcoholism (e.g., Appleton, 1995), anorexia (e.g., Way, 1995), and homosexuality (e.g., McIntosh, 1968; Foucault, 1992). Shyness, however, is perhaps a better example of another facet of the argument presented here—that the reification of a fluid, continuous, and essentially normal part of the human behavioral repertoire as a bounded entity is a necessary precondition for a behavioral genetics investigation.

The extent to which shyness was used by novelists of past eras as part of their repertoire of description for characters is striking. A quick perusal of some of these indicates that shyness was often seen as a normal reaction to certain situations but that in both its state and its trait aspects, it could be either lauded or condemned, depending on the appropriateness of the reaction to the social situation, the status, or the gender of the individual; it also seemed to be a characteristic that might say something or reveal something about an individual, rather than being an inherent or fixed aspect of personality worthy of note in itself.

In *The Age of Innocence*, Edith Wharton writes:

> Into this dimly-lit and dim-featured group May Archer floated like a swan with the sunset on her: she seemed larger, fairer, more voluminously rustling than her husband had ever seen her; and he perceived that the rosiness and rustlingness were the tokens of an extreme and infantile shyness. (1986, 198)

For Wharton, May Archer's shyness reveals a character flaw not seen before, but is not one in itself.

In *The Egoist* George Meredith writes:

> "They expect us any day, but it will be more comfortable for papa," was her answer. She looked kindly in her new shyness. She did not seem to think he had treated her contemptuously in flinging her to his cousin, which was odd. (2003, 464)

Here shyness is both something that can be acquired ("her new shyness") and something that can represent an improvement in character.

And in *One Basket* Edna Ferber writes:

> If they could have talked it over together, these two, the girl might have found relief. But the family shyness of their class was too strong upon them. (1947, 85)

Here shyness is an inevitable outcome of a discrepancy in social class position between two parties in an interaction.

All of these uses of shyness suggest a quite different view of personality, one that sees human personality as fluid, contextual, and holistic. Such a view may, in fact, be less accurate than the current one in which personality and behavioral traits and disorders are parsed, categorized, and identified in the *Diagnostic and Statistical Manual*. The point is that it is difficult to imagine a behavioral genetics search for the genetic underpinnings of shyness until this fluid trait was reified, bounded, and medicalized.

Respected behavioral geneticist Robert Plomin contrasts behavioral genetics with other sciences that look at humans from a "species typicality perspective." By this he means that many scientific fields seek to define what is normal or typical for a human being in regard to a particular realm of physiological functioning. Western medical education is built on such a perspective, as training is based on understanding the pathophysiology of those traits that cause disease and disorder by being outside the normal range. In contrast, says Plomin, behavioral genetics, grounded in an "individual differences perspective," *assumes* differences in individual functioning. The field's focus is thus on how to account for this natural and inevitable variation, stressing the fact that almost all human traits exist on a continuum with no bright line that demarcates "normal" from "abnormal." Yet, even the most sincere invocation of this individual differences perspective appears to be swimming upstream against the process of medicalization, as codified in such places as the *Diagnostic and Statistical Manual,* or the enthusiasms described under the rubric of geneticization.

Thus, for example, as medical evidence of the harmful health effects of smoking became irrefutable, cigarette smoking as a behavior became reified, pathologized, and medicalized, and now the genetic underpinnings of addiction to nicotine and to the addictive behavior of smoking are sought. While important research continues on the genetics of developing lung cancer when exposed to cigarette smoke (Ariyoshi et al., 2002), much of the academic action and public interest involves research on the genetic underpinnings of smoking behavior. In fact, many studies of genetics and lung cancer begin with a hypothesis that the gene variant under investigation will exhibit an effect on both smoking behavior and disease (e.g., Tyndale and Sellers, 2002; Raunio et al., 2001; Tan et al., 2001; Oscarson, 2001). Research studies often begin by recruiting a study sample of nonsmokers, former smokers, and current smokers, as though those were actual categories of human beings. Interest is focused on the pathology of smoking behavior and genetic differences are sought among the groups. In one recent study that follows this model (Sabol et al., 1999), a particular allele of a dopamine transporter gene (SLC6A3) was seen to correlate with greater success in quitting smoking and also with low scores on a paper-and-pencil measure of novelty seeking. The authors hypothesize that "individuals carrying the SLC6A3-9 polymorphism have altered dopamine transmission, which reduces their need for novelty and reward by external stimuli, including cigarettes" (Sabol et al., 1999, 7). Thus, in order to conduct molecular genetic research—in which an individual either has, or does not have, a particular allele—the investigators created a study design comprising individuals with three discrete types of relationships to smoking behavior and correlated these with alleles that were biologically, not merely conceptually, discrete.

All of this reinforces the medicalization and geneticization of smoking and works against claims of an "individual differences perspective." But this study actually does something more. In linking smoking behavior with another, highly questionable phenotype—"novelty seeking"—it increases the likelihood of yet another, nonreplicated gene finding.

But perhaps one of the most compelling critiques of behavioral genetics from a social constructionist viewpoint has to do with the profound and unique role of human cognition and self-reflexivity in regard to behavior. Because of this, it seems difficult to overstate the difference between seeking the genetic underpinnings of susceptibility to lung cancer in the face of cigarette smoke, and seeking the genetic underpinnings of the behavior of cigarette smoking. Specifically, a genetic vulnerability to lung cancer is outside the "knowledge of ourselves" but smoking behavior is not. Smoking behavior is, rather, available for self-knowledge, self-reflection, and can be imbued with volatile and profound personal and social meaning.

Perhaps one of the most remarkable things that has happened in the years since the surgeon general suggested a link between tobacco and adverse health consequences is the way that cigarette smoking has become a marker of social class. To acknowledge that fact is to move in the direction of a social constructionist inquiry about smoking that would query the causes and meaning of differential smoking rates among different social class groups. To ignore this social reality while searching for "addiction genes" is probably to guarantee limited, if any, scientific success, while further stigmatizing those who smoke. Since smoking behavior is available for self-reflection, it is even possible that all of this will actually increase rather than decrease the behavior itself.

Why Does Any of This Matter?

If researchers search for the genetic underpinnings of traits that are mistakenly seen as concrete, bounded "things in the world," then we might expect those searches to fail. Some behavioral geneticists have suggested that, even if this occurs, it is unsurprising and not particularly troubling. For example, in a discussion of the belief of early-twentieth-century geneticists in the heredity nature of a desire for a seagoing career (termed *thalassophilia*), one behavioral geneticist conceded that conflating familial and class traditions of seafaring with genetic predisposition probably led to a construct validity problem and made a search for a "seafaring gene" quixotic and likely doomed to fail. But, he continued, is this not simply an example of the routine practice of science, in which some hypotheses don't work out? (Turkheimer, personal communication). However, while thalassophilia sounds quaint to our ears, for all the reasons mentioned above it seems probable that the search for traits that are not bounded and/or do not represent accurate descriptions of reality, is a systemic, rather than occasional, issue for behavioral genetics. It thus suggests that financial and human resources may be repeatedly spent on research that is likely to fail, or at least, fail to be replicated. A greater awareness of the problems of construct validity might slow down the rate of genetic searches with low probabilities of success.

But the most serious consequences are not for the field of behavioral genetics. The most serious consequences are for society as a whole. Ian Hacking (1990) approaches this point through a discussion of the philosophical concept of "dynamic nominalism," which argues "that numerous kinds of human beings and human acts come into being hand in hand with our invention of the categories labeling them [and thus] our spheres of possibility, and hence ourselves, are to some extent made up by our naming and what that entails" (87).

Psychiatrist Leon Eisenberg (1988) has made a similar point, saying that there is a paradox to sciences involving humans, that "what is believed to be true about behavior affects the very behavior which it purports to explain" (1).

It is in just this way that genetics searches are powerful—even when they are not and cannot be successful. The most obvious consequence is that there is a feedback cycle that occurs when a behavior that has been reified and brought under the medical gaze becomes a candidate for a search for its genetic underpinnings. That is, the very process of looking for a "gene for" a behavior reinforces the sense of the reality and medicalized nature of that behavior or disorder. In some cases, it may even help create a social role—a way for a person to *have* or *be* that category. Once available, this role is easier to choose, and an individual, health care providers, a family, society, support groups, all may increasingly sort through feelings and behaviors in a way that reinforces and coalesces the "syndrome." To the extent that behavioral genetics contributes to such medicalization processes, behavioral genetics will contribute to the creation of what I take to be harmful social effects.

In fact, many of the observations made in this chapter are, perhaps surprisingly, quite compatible with the concerns expressed in chapter 4 of this volume by behavioral geneticist Eric Turkheimer. In that chapter, Turkheimer addresses what his colleague, Robert Plomin, calls the "gloomy prospect": the possibility that human behavior will always be too complex, and too prone to the idiosyncratic influences of feedback loops, to yield much to the reductionistic approaches of behavioral genetics. One of the most important points about which Turkheimer and I agree may be as much esthetic as theoretical. While Plomin, as a behavioral scientist, reports on the gloom he would feel if his reductionism failed to illuminate complex human behaviors, someone with a more anthropological or holistic perspective would see an affirmation of the insight regarding human life's messy specificity and complexity. In a way, the scientifically gloomy prospect is, as Turkheimer himself has said, "refreshingly humanistic" (Turkheimer, chapter 4 of this volume). In accord with this, it is possible not to feel gloomy about recognizing the limitations of reductionistic efforts to investigate complex behaviors but instead to take a certain pleasure in realizing that human behaviors may be too complex to be captured fully by reductionistic strategies.

But, unlike Turkheimer, I nevertheless do feel both gloom and concern about the potential power of behavioral genetics searches. This is, perhaps, most clearly illustrated by the following: One day, while driving the LA freeways, I heard an advertisement, part of a series of "spots" intended solely to sell California State Lottery tickets. Each ad in the series asked a winner about the first thing he or she had done after finding out about winning this enormous sum of money. The woman in this particular ad said, "I always thought I'd buy a house or some clothes, or plan a vacation, but what I did was I quit smoking." To me this ad spoke with startling eloquence about the ineffable effect of *feeling* a suddenly open future. It moved me to imagine what the world and various choices felt like from the perspective of life chances very different from mine. This was both a particular and a sociological exercise, and from both those perspectives, the medicalizing and pathologizing of smoking and the concomitant search for the genetic underpinnings of this behavior felt both disrespectful and, politically, conservative.

While not doubting for one second the commitment of behavioral geneticists to relieve the suffering they see around them (nor how much suffering *has* been averted by understanding that conditions such as schizophrenia or autism have genetic bases), I nevertheless feel gloom and concern about the ways that behavioral genetics contributes to the ever-expanding power and purview of the medical gaze; to the institutionalization of Western views of personality and culture as universal norms; to the emphasis on the individual and the genetic over the social and the political. Thus, while I am not gloomy about the limited results I suspect many behavioral genetics investigations will ultimately yield, I am mightily concerned about the mischief that may be caused by the untimely and exaggerated rumors of their successes.

REFERENCES

Ajzenstadt, M., and B. E. Burtch. (1990). "Medicalization and Regulation of Alcohol and Alcoholism: The Professions and Disciplinary Measures." *International Journal of Law and Psychiatry* 13(1–2): 127–47.

American Psychiatric Association. (1994). *Diagnostic and Statistical Manual of Mental Disorders.* 4th ed. Washington, D.C.: American Psychiatric Association.

Appleton, L. M. (1995). "Rethinking Medicalization: Alcoholism and Anomalies." In J. Best, ed. *Images of Issues: Typifying Contemporary Social Problems.* 2nd ed. New York: Aldine de Gruyter: 59–80.

Arbelle S., J. Benjamin, M. Golin, et al. (2003). "Relation of Shyness in Grade School Children to the Genotype for the Long Form of the Serotonin Transporter Promoter Region Polymorphism." *American Journal of Psychiatry* 160(4): 671–76.

Ariyoshi, N., M. Miyamoto Y. Umetsu, et al. (2002). "Genetic Polymorphism of CYP2A6 Gene and Tobacco-induced Lung Cancer Risk in Male Smokers." *Cancer Epidemiology Biomarkers and Prevention* 11(9): 890–94.

Conrad, P. (1992). "Medicalization and Social Control." *Annual Review of Sociology* 18: 209–32.

Conrad, P., and D. Potter. (2000). " From Hyperactive Children to ADHD Adults: Observations on the Expansion of Medical Categories." *Social Problems* 47(4): 559–83.

Costa, P. T., and R. R. McCrae. (1986). "Cross-sectional Studies of Personality in a National Sample: 1. Development and Validation of Survey Measures." *Psychology of Aging* 1(2): 140–43.

Eisenberg, L. (1988). "The Social Construction of Mental Illness." *Psychological Medicine* 18: 1–9.

Eley, T. C., D. Bolton, T. G. O'Connor, S. Perrin, et al. (2003). "A Twin Study of Anxiety-related Behaviours in Pre-school Children." *Journal of Child Psychology and Psychiatry* 4(7): 945–60.

Ferber, E. (1947). "Un Morso doo Pang" [1919]. In *One Basket: Thirty-one Short Stories.* New York: The People's Book Club.

Foucault, M. (1992). "The Perverse Implantation." In E. Stein, ed. *Forms of Desire: Sexual Orientation and the Social Constructionist Controversy.* New York: Routledge: 11–23.

Foucault, M. (1994). *The Birth of the Clinic: An Archaeology of Medical Perception.* New York: Vintage.

Fyer, A. J. (1993). "Heritability of Social Anxiety: A Brief Review." *Clinical Psychiatry* (suppl. 54): S10–S12.

Genetic News. (2001). Press Release, Nature Genetics (hum-molgen: April, 28 2001.

Ginsburg, F., and R. Rapp. (1991). "The Politics of Reproduction." *Annual Review of Anthropology* 20: 311–43.

Hacking, I. (1990). "Making Up People." In E. Stein, ed. *Forms of Desire: Sexual Orientation and the Social Constructionist Controversy.* New York: Routledge: 69–88.

Hacking, I. (2000). *The Social Construction of What?* Cambridge, Mass.: Harvard University Press.

Horwitz, A. V. (2002). *Creating Mental Illness.* Chicago: University of Chicago Press.

Jang, K. L., W. J. Livesley, and P. A. Vernon. (1996). "Heritability of the Big Five Personality Dimensions and Their Facets: A Twin Study." *Journal of Personality* 64(3): 577–91.

Johnson, A. M., P. A. Vernon, J. A. Harris, and K. L. Jang. (2004). "A Behavior Genetic Investigation of the Relationship between Leadership and Personality." *Journal of Personality and Social Psychology* 86(4): 615–28.

Kleinman, A. (1988). *The Illness Narratives: Suffering, Healing and the Human Condition.* New York: Basic.

Labinger, J. A,. and H. Collins, eds. (2001). *The One Culture? A Conversation about Science.* Chicago: University of Chicago Press.

Lippman, A. (1991). "Prenatal Genetic Testing and Screening: Constructing Needs and Reinforcing Inequities," *American Journal of Law and Medicine* 17(1–2): 15–50.

McIntosh, M. (1968). "The Homosexual Role." *Social Problems* 16: 182–92.

Melke J., L. Westberg, S. Nilsson, et al. (2003). "A Polymorphism in the Serotonin Receptor 3A (HTR3A) Gene and Its Association with Harm Avoidance in Women." *Archives of General Psychiatry* 60(10): 1017–23.

Meredith, G. (2003). *The Egoist.* The Pennsylvania State University *Electronic Class Series.* Jim Manis, ed. Hazelton: Pennsylvania State University, www.hn.psu.edu/faculty/jmanis/gmeredith/Egoist.pdf page 464.

Mezzich, J. E., L. J. Kirmayer, A. Kleinman, et al. (1999). "The Place of Culture in DSM-IV." *Journal of Nervous and Mental Diseases* 187(8): 457–64.

Morgan, J. (2001). "Sweet-Tooth Gene—Brief Article." *Science World* (September 17).

Moussa, H. (1992). *The Social Construction of Women Refugees: A Journey of Discontinuities and Continuities.* Ed.D. diss., University of Toronto.

Onishi, N. (2004). "The Struggle for Iraq: The Hostages; Freed from Captivity in Iraq, Japanese Return to More Pain." *New York Times* (April 23): 1.

Oscarson, M. (2001). "Genetic Polymorphisms in the Cytochrome P450 2A6 (CYP2A6) Gene: Implications for Interindividual Differences in Nicotine Metabolism." *Drug Metabolism and Disposition* 29(2): 91–95.

Osher, Y., D. Hamer, and J. Benjamin. (2000). "Association and Linkage of Anxiety-related Traits with a Functional Polymorphism of the Serotonin Transporter Gene Regulatory Region in Israeli Sibling Pairs." *Molecular Psychiatry* 5(2): 216–19.

Plomin, R., et al. (2003). *Behavioral Genetics in the Postgenomic Era.* Washington, D.C.: American Psychological Association.

Press Release. (2001). *Nature Genetics* 28(1).

Raunio, H., A. Rautio, H. Gullsten, et al. (2001). "Polymorphisms of CYP2A6 and Its Practical Consequences." *British Journal of Clinical Pharmacology* 52(4): 357–63.

Reaves, J. (2001). "Is Sweetness in the Genes of the Beholder?" *Time Magazine* (April 23).

Riska, E. (2000). "The Rise and Fall of Type A Man." *Social Science and Medicine* 51: 1665–74.

Roberts, R. L., S. E. Luty, R. T. Mulder, et al. (2004). "Association between Cytochrome P450 2D6 Genotype and Harm Avoidance." *American Journal of Medical Genetics* 127B(1): 90–93.

Sabol, S.Z., M. L. Nelson, C. Fisher, et al. (1999). "A Genetic Association for Cigarette Smoking Behavior." *Health Psychology* 18(1): 7–13.

Sokal, A. (1996a). "Transgressing the Boundaries: Toward a Transformative Hermeneutics of Quantum Gravity." *Social Text* 46–47: 217–52.

Sokal, A. (1996b). "A Physicist Experiments with Cultural Studies." *Lingua Franca* (May–June): 62–64.

Stein, E., ed. (1992). *Forms of Desire: Sexual Orientation and the Social Constructionist Controversy.* New York: Routledge.

Tan, W., G. F. Chen, D. Y. Xing, et al. (2001). "Frequency of CYP2A6 Gene Deletion and Its Relation to Risk of Lung and Esophageal Cancer in the Chinese Population." *International Journal of Cancer* 95(2): 96–101.

Tyndale, R. F., and E. M. Sellers. (2002). "Genetic Variation in CYP2A6-mediated Nicotine Metabolism Alters Smoking Behavior." *Therapeutic Drug Monitoring* 24(1): 163–71.

Verweij, M. (1999). "Medicalization as a Moral Problem for Preventive Medicine." *Bioethics* 13(2): 89–113.

Way, K. (1995). "Never Too Rich . . . Or Too Thin: The Role of Stigma in the Social Construction of Anorexia Nervosa." In D. Maurer and J. Sobol, eds. *Eating Agendas: Food and Nutrition as Social Problems.* New York: Aldine de Gruyter.

Wharton, E. (1986). *The Age of Innocence.* New York: Collier.

Wiebe, W., E. Bijker, T. P. Hughes, and T. Pinch, eds. (1987). *The Social Construction of Technological Systems: New Directions in the Sociology and History of Technology.* Cambridge, Mass.: MIT.

Zola, I. K. (1972). "Medicine as an Institution of Social Control." *Sociological Review* 20(4): 487–504.

CHAPTER SEVEN

Behavioral Genetics and Explanations of the Link between Crime, Violence, and Race

Troy Duster, Ph.D.

Behavioral genetics has always been about differences. Especially in its classical mode, and more recently with the application of molecular techniques, behavioral genetics seeks to understand how genetic differences help to explain phenotypic differences *within* a group. Behavioral geneticists are increasingly attempting to find genetic markers (and sometimes even coding regions) that they can associate with complex behavioral phenotypes, such as criminality, risk taking, violence, intelligence, alcoholism, manic-depression, schizophrenia, and homosexuality. In the past five years, we have seen claims linking DNA regions to cognitive ability in children (Chorney et al., 1998), crime (Jensen et al., 1998), violence (Caspi et al., 2002), and attention deficit hyperactivity disorder (Smalley et al., 2002).

New developments in population genetics now promise to explore the contributions of genetic differences to phenotypic differences *between* groups. The haplotype map, for example, is designed to discern how different populations tend to carry different patterns of small genetic mutations called single nucleotide polymorphisms (SNPs). The stated purpose of that research is to increase the efficiency of efforts at identifying disease-related gene variants. (In this context the dream of "customized drugs"—tailored to treat individuals with particular genetic differences—is often invoked.) But the same research methods can be aimed at identifying gene variants that are thought to be associated with complex behaviors like violence and impulsivity. When researchers start to correlate markers of genetic ancestry by what is now called "continent of origin" with behaviors such as violence and impulsivity, we are poised to usher in a whole new era of scientific justification for theories of racial and ethnic differences and social hierarchies.

Genetic research on humans is always influenced by social and cultural factors, beginning with the foundational question of why certain behaviors are chosen for genetic analysis. During the past decade, the pages of scientific and popular literature have propagated overly simplistic "genetic explanations" for a variety of complex social issues such as sexual preference, risk-seeking behavior, shyness, alcoholism, and even homelessness. Moreover, there is a history of using genetic explanations to account for and justify differences in social stratification and the behavior of those at the bottom of the economic order (Black, 2003; Reilly, 1991; Kevles, 1985). These converging preoccupations and tangled webs interlace crime and violence, race, and genetic explanations. The purpose of this chapter is to anticipate the social issues now arising from our increased ability to conduct research on between-group differences with respect to complex and socially sanctioned behaviors—in a society where race has played a dominant role in sorting and stratifying its members.

The Human Genome Project and the "Turn to Between-Group Differences"

In the first decade of the Human Genome Project (circa 1988–98), the major focus was on how the mapping and sequencing process could be done *on any one human,* precisely because we are all so alike at the level of our DNA. Any two persons, chosen randomly across the globe, share 99.9 percent of the exact same sequence of the nucleotides (cytosine, guanine, adenine, and thymine) that are the building blocks of the DNA throughout the genome. That similarity was so overwhelming that it became the rationale for the conclusion that *anyone's genome would do* for generating the map. At the White House news conference announcing the completion of the first draft of the full human genome on June 26, 2000, Francis Collins (director of the Human

Genome Project) and Craig Venter (who headed the rival private mapping and sequencing venture at Celera) agreed that human similarities at the DNA level were so dramatic that "race is of no significance" at the level of the DNA (Human Genome News, 2000).

By the mid-1970s, it had become abundantly clearly that there is more genetic variation within the most common socially used categories of race than between these categories (Polednak, 1989; Bittles and Roberts, 1992; Chapman, 1993; Shipman, 1994). One important conclusion that some population geneticists drew is that races do not exist (Smith and Sapp, 1997). A consortium of leading scientists across disciplines from biology to physical anthropology issued a "Revised UNESCO Statement on Race" in 1995 that concludes in terms of "scientific" discourse, there is no such thing as a "race" that has any scientific utility (Katz, 1995). In May 1998, the American Anthropological Association issued a statement on race that attempted to address myths and misconceptions. According to the statement, "physical variations in the human species have no meaning except the social ones that humans put on them" (American Anthropological Association, 1998).

However, formulating the matter so that "it is only the social meanings that humans provide" implies that mere lay notions of race provide a rationale for domination, but have no other utility. This is a profound misunderstanding of the implications of a social constructivist notion of social phenomena. How persons identify themselves matters for their subsequent behavior. "Race" as social construction can and does have a substantial effect on how people behave.

Moreover, a series of articles have appeared in the scientific literature over the past seven years looking for genetic markers of population groups that coincide with commonsense, lay renditions of ethnic and racial phenotypes. While there are approximately three billion base pairs of complete overlapping similarity, that recurring figure of 99.9 percent also means that, with only a 0.1 difference, there are still approximately three to five million points of difference in the DNA between any two people. With the use of new supercomputers, it is now possible to take a closer look at these points of difference. Some alleles appear with more frequency in specific population groups reflecting genetic variation inherited in common from ancestral populations (Bahmshad and Olson, 2003; Kittles and Weiss, 2003). These differences, though very slight, may be relevant to understanding susceptibility to certain diseases. When researchers try to make probabilistic identifications about which group a person belongs to, they look at variation in several different locations in the DNA—usually from three to seven loci. For any particular locus, there is an examination of the frequency of that allele at that locus and for that population. In other words, what is being assessed is the frequency of genetic variation at a particular spot in the DNA in each population.

The question as to whether race is a legitimate concept for scientific inquiry is currently quite controversial. Without commenting in detail here, it may be useful to mention my position. I believe that the elimination of racial and ethnic classifications in the routine collection and analysis of data is neither practicable, possible, nor even desirable. Rather, our task should be to recognize, engage, and clarify the complexity of the interaction between any taxonomies of race and biological, genetic, neurophysiological, social, and health outcomes. Whether or not race is a legitimate concept for scientific inquiry depends upon the designation of the unit of analysis of race, and will in turn be related to the analytic purposes for which the concept is deployed (Duster, 2002).

Criminality and Behavioral Genetics

Of the hundreds of thousands, even millions of different kinds of behaviors that humans engage in across time and space, why are some of those behaviors selected as the subject of a genetic explanation? For the layperson, the first answer that usually comes to mind is that some behaviors seem to "run in families." But lots of behaviors that run in families (working for the railroad versus on the police force, styles of humor, political persuasion) are not conceived as explainable by the genotype. Conversely, some behaviors that do not seem to run in families do get subjected to a genetic analysis.

If we leave the laity and move to the scientific literature, the primary, first-order question remains, even if stated in different terms, namely: What is the *theoretical* warrant for designating certain behaviors the subject of behavioral genetics while ignoring or dismissing others as unlikely to be caused by a genetic condition? Indeed, the mere suggestion for designating an occupational choice such as seafaring as best explained by genetics would now be dismissed as ludicrous, a blind alley, a waste of time and effort—a fruitless, unproductive pursuit. However, ninety years ago, it was commonly proposed in both scientific and lay circles that there was a genetic explanation for seafaring (Kevles, 1985). The reason for exploring this idea was simple and straightforward, namely, that of all the men going out to sea as sailors, a very high proportion had fathers and grandfathers who went out to sea. That is hardly a theoretical warrant. Rather, it is an observation of an empirical regularity, followed by the search backward from the behavioral manifestation, or phenotype (seafaring), to the envisioned explanatory gene, the genotype.

Contemporary scientists are not searching for seafaring genes—but some are searching for a genetic explanation of violent, antisocial, and criminal behavior. The reason resides as much in the *Zeitgeist* as in the state of scientific knowledge. Within the boundaries of scientific inquiry, there is a second common answer to the question of why certain substantive arenas are subjected to a genetic prism: there exists a body of literature on the topic, a body of empirical research.[1] But this is an empirical context, not a theoretical warrant. This is about tradition and careers and habits of the mind—not conceptually driven theorems, axioms, and interlinked hypotheses guided by a general theory of why some behaviors are more likely than others to be explicable genetically. Furthermore, this is a second-order frame to the answer because it does not address the prior question of why that body of empirical work on a specific behavior was generated as a first-order question.

While there is no single or simple answer to the question of why certain behaviors are subjected to a genetic explanation and others are not, there is a major avenue that is undertheorized, unexplored, and less appreciated for the rich potential for getting at the answer(s). Again, an impressive array of different kinds of data strongly suggests that the answer lies in what the Germans call the *Zeitgeist,* roughly translated as "the spirit of the times." If this begs the question of why "in these times," then that is precisely the point of entry for an explanation of what it is about "these times" that makes for the selection of particular behaviors as genetically explorable and explainable. Behavioral genetics has long been interested in "the genetics of criminality." At the same time the prospect of discerning a relationship between genes and violent behavior has been very contentious.

Critics have raised a variety of issues. One concern is whether violent behavior is a well-defined classification amenable to scientific analysis (see chapter 6 in this volume, and Wachbroit, 2001). Crime, by definition an act or the commission of activity that is forbidden, is socially constructed; that is, the very categorization of an act as criminal depends on social standards of behavior, the identity of the actor, and the environment in which it takes place. Criminal behavior can be a one-time phenomenon (impulsive homicide after discovery of adultery), or it can be a profession (the cat burglar—the professional thief, or the "hit-man" specialist for organized crime). The theoretical warrant for examining the impulsive homicide as having a completely different etiology than the professional thief is well developed (Wolfgang, 1958; Polk, 1994). In the case of the latter, the empirical literature on both the professions and professional thievery is predictive of the manners and patterns of routinized behavior (Black, 1988; Friedson, 1974). That is in sharp contrast to the literature and conceptual framework with which one approaches an understanding of most homicides (Polk, 1994), where even if impulsivity sometimes gives way to planning, patterns of jealousy, shame, and rage predominate. Crime can be an occasional diversion from one's ordinary life, such as depicted in Cameron's (1964) classic study of shoplifting, or it can be a compulsive-neurotic habituation (sexual abuse of the young by adults); alternatively, crime can be a rational, calculated decision (stealing a loaf of bread to feed one's family), or a routine occupational imperative, as was the case with the price-fixing scandal among the largest electrical companies in the United States (Geis, 1982). Crime can be a bureaucratic response to turf invasion, such as with organized crime during Prohibition (Tyler, 1962), or a violation of existing social stratifying practices, such as the crime of teaching a slave to read— or assisting a slave to run away (Harding, 1983).

In short, what is criminal is as variable, and as variably explained, as any wide range of human behaviors that are legal. To place in the same taxonomic system the theft of bread, exposing oneself in public, cat burglary, and euthanasia, as a single, examinable phenotype is to engage in a breathtaking mystification of the classification of crime. The theoretical warrant in each of these instances is both well articulated and highly differentiated in the best empirical work in criminology. As noted above, Cameron's (1964) research on shoplifting remains the standard and the classic—distinguishing and documenting how and why this form of crime is primarily performed by "amateurs." In so doing, Cameron explained why shoplifting has the lowest rate of recidivism when the perpetrator, almost always (over 90%) the "amateur," is confronted. At the other end of the continuum is the pickpocket, almost always a professional who works with groups of other professionals—where the rate of recidivism is, by contrast, extraordinarily high. The pickpocket regards arrest as an occupational hazard, and has strategies for minimizing its effect on his (usually) behavior. The arbitrary features of the social fabrication of the criminal law comes to us more clearly by looking back to a much earlier time. In late-eighteenth-century England, for example, stealing linens from a linen factory was a crime punishable by death. With the hindsight of two centuries, we now see this more clearly as a narrow, politically and economically motivated specification of a "serious crime." But that is because we have a few centuries' hindsight. Today, we place in the same criminal category someone who leaves lethal nerve gas on a subway station (anonymous killings) and someone who shoots in the back a doctor working in an abortion clinic. Fifty years from now, if some researcher went through the police records to show whether adoptees had a similar "inclination to commit crime" as did those in their biological families, someone might point out the quite reasonable objection that the system of classification was constructed in such a way as to make any claims about a genetic basis for these crimes highly problematic. The search for a genetic explanation for such a demonstrably variegated "phenotype" (criminal) requires a theoretical warrant that has never been delivered. The closest that one can come is in the abstracted notion of an "antisocial personality," but even for this abstracted version, the obstacles to linking phenotypes and genotypes are huge. That is, given this demonstrably high empirical variability (sometimes arbitrary, sometimes systemic reach of the criminal justice system) in what constitutes a crime, and even more demonstrably high empirical variability in what constitutes "antisocial behavior" across social time and space, how is it possible to search for a genotype? The answer, and the conclusion, provide strong reasons for deep concern.

It is therefore not possible to study criminal behavior without taking the circumstances in which the behavior takes place into account. The very classification of criminals or criminal behavior as a biological category may also affect the way people understand a particular kind of behavior. The sheer knowledge of such categories can have a looping effect. That is, it may affect people's attitudes and behavior in a way that feeds back on the classification scheme itself (Hacking, 2001).

Studying Incarcerated Populations

Yet another problem is that so-called genetic studies of criminality have a heavy dependence on incarcerated populations. Thus, for example, one of the more controversial issues in the "genetics" of crime concerned whether males with the extra Y chromosome, or XYY males, are more likely to be found in prisons than are XY males. The first research suggesting a genetic link came from a 1965 study in Edinburgh, Scotland. While all of the 197 males in the account of prison hospital inmates were described as "dangerously violent," seven had the XYY karyotype. The seven males constituted about 3.5 percent of the total. But since estimates are that only about 1.3 percent of all males have the XYY chromosomal makeup, the authors in the study posited that the 3.5 percent rate found in the prison population might be 20 times higher than the frequency in the normal population. They then generalized from that meager data to claim that men with 47 chromosomes were mentally subnormal and had a tendency to hyperaggressivity and violence (Jacobs et al., 1965). The studies of men with the XYY genotype that followed in the 1960s all chose as subjects men who were defined as problematic rather than those who were functioning normally within society and, unsurprisingly, tended to confirm these results. Given this bias in methodology, recent evaluations do not find this body of work credible. XYY individuals have been shown to be no more aggressive than average, but they may be taller and less intelligent, hyperactive, and more impulsive (Rutter et al., 1998). Nevertheless, the claims made managed to stigmatize a generation of XYY males and apparently led to the abortion of a significant number of fetuses with that karyotype.

Although the XYY controversy was not about race, the logic and reasoning behind this kind of study provide fertile ground for a racial theory of violence, crime, or homicide to take root. The method of the XYY study was to compare the characteristics of those incarcerated with those outside prison. If one thinks there's a genetic explanation for why some men are in prison and others are not (i.e., some have an extra Y chromosome and others don't), and if one observes that African Americans are in U.S. prisons at seven times the rate of whites, then one might—erroneously—infer that there's a genetic explanation for the higher incarceration rates of African Americans.

The fallacy of such an inference is shown by the fact that it is only since 1933 that the incarceration rates of African Americans in relationship to whites have gone up in such a striking manner. The gene pool among human beings takes many centuries to change. No genetic change can explain why blacks were incarcerated at only twice the rate of whites in 1933 but seven times the rate of whites in 1995. Moreover, one can only make inferences about high heritability estimates and between-group phenotypic differences by assuming that the environments of blacks and whites are equal (for more on this point, see Parens, 2004). But looking at the factors leading to differential incarceration rates, it is clear that the equal environments premise is ludicrous. Incarceration rates are a function of social, economic, and political factors. In the past decade, the United States has been building more prisons and incarcerating more people than at any other moment in its history. Indeed, in the period from 1981 to 1991, the U.S. prison population went from 330,000 inmates in state and federal prisons to 804,000. That rate constitutes substantially more than a doubling in a single decade, the greatest rise in a prison population in modern history.

Converging on this development is the racial patterning of those arrested and serving time. African Americans are currently incarcerated at a rate approximately seven times greater than that of Americans of European descent, but this is a very recent development. Incarceration rates and the coloring of our prisons are a function of dramatic changes in the past half century. In the past three decades, the War on Drugs has produced a remarkable transformation of the U.S. prison population. If we turn the clock back just about 60 years, whites constituted approximately 77 percent of all prisoners in America, while blacks were only 22 percent (Hacker, 1992). In 1933, blacks were incarcerated at a rate approximately twice that of whites. In 1950, the ratio had increased to approximately four times; in 1970, it was six times; and by the mid-1990s, it was seven times that of whites.

The War on Drugs played the dominant role in this story. It affected the races quite differently with regard to respective prison incarceration rates. According to the government's own best statistics, during the height of the war, blacks constituted only 15 to 20 percent of the nation's drug users (Flanagan and Jamieson, 1990), but in most urban areas, they constituted approximately one-half to two-thirds of those arrested for drug offenses. Indeed, in New York City, African Americans and Latinos constituted 92 percent of all those arrested for drug offenses (Clark Foundation, 1992). In Florida, the annual admissions rate to the state prison system nearly tripled from 1983 and 1989, from 14,301 to nearly 40,000 (Austin and McVey, 1989). This was a direct consequence of the War on Drugs, since well over two-thirds of these felonies were drug-related. The nation gasped at the national statistics reported by the Sentencing Project in 1990, citing the figure that nearly one-fourth of all young black males 20 to 29 years of age were either in prison, in jail, on probation, or paroled on a given day in the summer of 1989.[2] This figure was recited so often and inured so many that only (relatively) a collective yawn greeted an announcement in mid-1992 that a study of Baltimore revealed that *56 percent of that city's young black males were under some form of criminal justice sanction on any given day* in 1991 (Miller, 1992). Indeed, of the nearly 13,000 individuals arrested on drug charges in Baltimore during 1991, more than 11,000 were African Americans.

While racial profiling often seems to be characterized as a local police practice, the phenomenon of young minority males being "just stopped by the police" was actually a national strategy first deployed by the Reagan administration. In 1986, the Drug Enforcement Administration initiated Operation Pipeline, a program designed in Washington, D.C., that ultimately trained 27,000 law enforcement officers in 48 participating states over the ensuing decade. The project was designed to alert police and other law enforcement officials of "likely profiles" of those who should be stopped and searched for possible drug violations. High on the list was young, male, African Americans and Latinos driving in cars that signaled that something might be amiss. For example, a 19-year-old African American driving a new Lexus would be an "obvious" alert, because the assumption would be that the family could not have afforded such a car and the driver must therefore be "into drugs."

The most striking figure showing the shift in the racial composition of prisoners in the state of Virginia. In 1983, approximately 63 percent of the new prison commitments for drugs were white with the rest, 37 percent, minority. Just six years later, in 1989, the situation had reversed, with only 34 percent of the new drug commitments being whites and 65 percent minority. It is not just the higher rate of incarceration, but the way in which the full net of the criminal justice system, all the way through mandatory sentencing, falls selectively on blacks. For example, powder cocaine is most likely to be sold and consumed by whites, while blacks are more likely to sell and consume crack (Flanagan and Jamieson, 1990). Need it be said which activity is more likely to lead to incarceration?

Implications of the Genetics of Between-group Differences

What, then, is the significance of efforts by geneticists to try to understand the relevance of genetic variations for understanding between-group differences? One often-promised outcome is the creation of drugs that will be developed and marketed to meet the needs of specific racial groups. In 1999 leading figures in the field of pharmacogenomics published, in *Science,* the claim that "all pharmacogenetic polymorphisms studied to date differ in frequency among ethnic and racial groups" (Evans and Relling, 1999). According to the authors, "The marked racial and ethnic diversity . . . dictates that race be considered in studies aimed at discovering whether specific genotypes or phenotypes are associated with disease risk or drug toxicity" (488).

In March 2001, a company touted as having produced the "first ethnic drug" received a green letter of approval from the Food and Drug Administration, purposefully aimed at a putative difference of population groups (Winslow, 2001). The drug, BiDil, which is being developed by the pharmaceutical company Nitromed, is currently in clinical trials. The company chief executive officer Michael Loberg explicitly stated that the African American population will be the marketing target for the drug, indicating that "BiDil, a heart failure product, reduced mortality in 66% of African Americans, but proved of very little benefit to whites" (*Financial Times,* March 9, 2001, 16). This is highly contested terrain, and the fields of pharmacogenomics and pharmacotoxicology are engaged in fierce internal battles as to the appropriate role of race in diagnostics and treatment (Xie et al., 2001; Braun, 2002; Frank, 2001; Lee et al., 2001; Risch et al., 2002; Kahn, 2003). This is not the place to address this dispute.

Research on the role of the *MAOA* gene in predicting violent behavior is relevant here. Until recently researchers had identified only one genetic variation ostensibly closely associated with criminal behavior, in one family. In 1993, a team of gene hunters conducted a study of a Dutch extended family in which 14 men, but none of the women members, were characterized by engaging in various forms of antisocial behavior, including acts of aggression, arson, attempted rape, and murder. The fact that all the affected males were related through unaffected females suggested X-linked recessive inheritance, and genetic analysis found that the males had an abnormal gene, the normal form of which codes for monoamine oxidase A, an enzyme that breaks down neurotransmitters in the brain. On that basis, researchers surmised that an accumulation of neurotransmitters might be one possible cause of the violent behavior. Nevertheless, they were cautious about their findings, acknowledging that their study did not conclusively demonstrate a causal relationship between the defective gene and the behavioral disturbances (Brunner et al., 1993).

Then in the last half of 2002, *Science* published a report of research in which different authors made another claim related to functional polymorphisms in the *MAOA* gene, namely, that it moderates the impact of early childhood maltreatment on the development of antisocial behavior in males. According to the article, 85 percent of cohort males having a low-activity MAOA genotype and who were severely maltreated developed some form of antisocial behavior. The authors went on to suggest that these findings could inform the development of future pharmacological treatments (Caspi et al., 2002).

The notion that one can intercept, and then treat with pharmaceuticals, presumes a much higher "correlation" in subsequent replication studies than this study has reported. There is also a remarkable slippage here, between attempts to analyze and interpret markers for an individual's DNA and the attempted operationalization of the concept of *antisocial*. The former rests entirely upon measures that look at the individual, while both the ideas of "antisocial" and "maltreatment" are interactional. Some substantially greater attention to the interactional dynamics needs to be a part of any larger framing of attempts at early identification and, even more significant, breaking down the components of antisocial. Getting in trouble with the criminal justice system is partly about individuals, but it is substantially about individuals with membership in particular social groups, where the criminal justice system has a greater focus of its lens and apparatus. For example, the War on Drugs, which accounts for more than half of all those incarcerated in U.S. jails and prisons, has been remarkably disproportionately aimed at African Americans and Latino (Mauer, 1999; Miller, 1996; Cole, 1999; Reinarman and Levine, 1997).

Race and DNA: Tensions and Current Tendencies Relevant to Behavioral Genetics

Miami, Florida, was the scene of the most notorious and widespread DNA dragnet of the past decade. Between September 1994 and January 1995, six women were killed and their bodies were left just outside the Miami city limits on a street known as the Tamiami Trail. More than 2300 men were stopped by the police as they drove down streets in the area, each asked to provide saliva samples to determine a possible DNA match (Pan, 1998). The so-called Tamiami Strangler was identified through other means, but this dragnet is of particular interest because (1) almost all of the men who were asked for DNA samples were African Americans, and (2) their DNA samples were stored. These stored samples can be used in subsequent criminal investigations, of course, but they can also be used in behavioral genetics research, with its new turn to the molecular level of DNA markers associated with different behavior.

It is important to address the serious implications for behavioral genetics of having race reenter the scientific and medical literature through the DNA, particularly in research linking proclivities to violence, impulsivity, and crime with between-group differences. Some forensic scientists now claim they can make an "ethnic estimation" of the suspect's probable identification with some specific population group from DNA evidence at a crime scene. As we will see, this often means "race" or an effective proxy for race. Others are pursuing work in forensic science with the hope of finding particular allelic frequencies more common in one group than another (Lowe et al., 2001). (Readers interested in pursuing these arguments for the merits of the case should consult the following literature: Braun, 2002; Risch et al., 2002; Rosenberg et al., 2002; Frank, 2001; Lee et al., 2001; Evans and Relling, 1999.)

The use of this technology in these high-profile cases has led to a full set of arguments for widening the net of the DNA database, so that more and more samples can be included, ranging from convicted felons to suspects to arrestees to the whole population. What more objective way could there be of exculpating the innocent and convicting the guilty? However, this conflates three quite distinct strategies and practices of the criminal justice system that need to be separated and analyzed for their disparate impact on different populations. The first is the use of DNA in postconviction cases to determine whether or not there was a wrongful conviction, the kind of situation that would help to free the innocent. The second is the collection of DNA of "suspects" or arrestees in pretrial circumstances to increase the DNA database, which in turn is designed to help law enforcement to determine if there is "match" with tissue samples left at some unsolved crime—the net to catch the guilty. The third is the advocacy of increasing the collection of DNA from a wider and wider band of felons and misdemeanants in the postconviction period, so that there is a record on file in the event of recidivism.

Much like the current situation in which the police can stop a driver and determine whether there are outstanding warrants or traffic ticket violations that have piled up, the new technology would permit authorities to see if the DNA of the person stopped and arrested "matched the DNA" on file for someone at an unsolved crime scene. This is not hypothetical. In early 2000, the New York Police Department began a pilot project experimenting with portable DNA laboratories (Flynn, 2000). The police take a buccal swab—some saliva from inside the cheek of the person stopped—and place it on a chip the size of a credit card. They then put this card through a machine no larger than a hand-held compact disc player, where the DNA is read via a laser in two minutes, isolating about 13 DNA markers to create a profile of the suspect. When this task is completed, the police can then transmit these data to a central database, where it currently requires about 12 minutes to determine if there is a "match" with a sample. Who could possibly be opposed to the use of these technologies for such crime-fighting purposes?

The answer is a bit complex, but it has to do with (1) some hidden social forces that create a patterned bias determining that certain populations will be more likely subjected to DNA profiling, and (2) the resuscitation of some old and dangerously regressive ideas about how to explain criminal behavior. To provide the context for the discussion of the expanding DNA databases, it is important to point out yet again two factors. The first is the systematic bias, by race, of a full range of behaviors displayed across the criminal justice system, from the decisions by police at the point of stop, search, and arrest, through the sentencing guidelines and practices, to incarceration. The second is the forensic science literature that claims to be able to predict "ethnic affiliation" from population-specific allele frequencies. It is the relationship between these two developments that is the source of easily crafted DNA-based research programs with the consequent misattribution of genetic causes of crime.

Background to "Ethnic-Affiliation Markers" at the DNA Level

At the level of the DNA, recall that the mappers and sequencers of the Human Genome Project assure us that humans are 99.9 percent alike. But if humans are 99.9 percent alike and "race" is purportedly a concept with no scientific utility, what are we to make of a series of articles that have appeared in the scientific literature over the past decade, looking for genetic markers of population groups that coincide with commonsense, lay renditions of ethnic and racial phenotypes? It is the forensic applications that have generated much of this interest. Devlin and Risch (1992a) published an article on "Ethnic Differentiation at VNTR Loci, with Specific Reference to Forensic Applications"— a research report that appeared prominently in the *American Journal of Human Genetics*. They wrote:

> The presence of null alleles leads to a large excess of single-band phenotypes for blacks at D17S79 (Devlin and Risch, 1992b), as Budowle et al. (1991b) predicted.

This phenomenon is less important for the Caucasian and Hispanic populations, which have fewer alleles with a small number of repeats. (540)

And:

It appears that the FBI's data base is representative of the Caucasian population. Results for the Hispanic ethnic groups, for the D17S79 locus, again suggest that the data bases are derived from nearly identical populations, when both similarities and expected biases are considered . . . For the allele frequency distributions derived from the black population, there may be small differences in the populations from which the databases are derived, as the expected bias is .05. (546)

The work of Devlin and Risch (1992a, 1992b), Evett et al. (1993, 1996), Lowe et al. (2001), and others suggests that only about 10 percent of sites in the DNA are "useful" for making distinctions. This means that at the other 90 percent of the sites, the allele frequencies do not vary between groups such as "Afro-Caribbean people in England" and "Scottish people in England." But it does not follow that because there is no *single* site where allele frequency matches some phenotype that we are trying to identify (for forensic purposes, we should be reminded), that there is no purpose in trying to locate *multiple* sites (four, six, seven, now 13). It is important to understand that the purpose of this work is to aid the FBI, Scotland Yard, or the criminal justice systems around the globe in highly probabilistic statements about suspects, and the "likely" identification of the ethnic, racial, or cultural populations from which they can be associated—statistically. Determining the boundaries of discrete categories of race and ethnicity is irrelevant for these purposes.

Thus, there is a surface contradiction between molecular biologists asserting that "race has no validity as a scientific concept" and forensic experts (and various others) using allele frequencies in specific populations that correspond to common public uses of racial categories. It is possible to sort out and make sense of this, and even to explain and resolve the apparent contradiction, but only if we keep in mind the difference between using a taxonomic system with sharp, discrete, definitively bounded categories, and those that show patterns (with some overlap), but which may prove to be empirically or practically useful. When representative spokespersons from the biological sciences say that "there is no such thing as race" they mean, correctly, that there are no discrete categories that come to a discrete beginning or end, that there is nothing mutually exclusive about our current (or past) categories of "race," and that there is more genetic variation within categories of "race" than between. While all this is true, it is a discussion more appropriate to abstract theorizing in the logic and philosophy of science, and bears little relevance to the practical matter of helping to solve a crime or the practical application of molecular genetics to health delivery via genetic screening. In both real world sets and settings, there is always the messy overlapping of categories. When Scotland Yard or the Birmingham, England, police force, or the New York police force want to narrow the list of suspects in a crime, they are not concerned with tightly constructed taxonomic systems of classification that have no overlapping categories. Their interest is in probabilities.

In the July 8, 1995, issue of the *New Scientist* entitled, "Genes in Black and White," some extraordinary claims were made about what it was possible to learn about socially defined categories of race from reviewing information gathered using new molecular genetic technology. In 1993, a British forensic scientist published what is perhaps the first DNA test explicitly acknowledged to provide intelligence information along ethnic lines for investigators of unsolved crimes. Ian Evett, of the Home Office's forensic science laboratory in Birmingham, and colleagues in the Metropolitan Police, claimed that their DNA test could distinguish between "Caucasians" and "Afro-Caribbeans" in nearly 85 percent of the cases. Evett's original work (1993) was published in the *Journal of Forensic Science Society* and drew upon apparent genetic differences in three sections of human DNA. Like most stretches of human DNA used for forensic typing, each of these three regions differs widely from person to person, irrespective of race. But by looking at all three, the researchers claimed that under select circumstances it is possible to estimate the probability that someone belongs to a particular racial group. The implications of this for determining, for practical purposes, who is and who is not "officially" a member of some racial or ethnic category are profound.

In more recent years, the technology has moved along, and forensic scientists are now using VNTR loci and investigating 12 to 15 segments of the DNA, not just the earlier 3 to 7. The current computer chip revolution will permit research on specific populations to achieve a single nucleotide polymorphism (SNP) profile of such a group (Hamadeh and Afshari, 2000). There is a dangerous seduction when deploying the technology in this fashion. The computer will inevitably be able to find some patterns for a group of, say, 3000 burglars.

But this is a mere correlation of markers, and it is far from anything but a spurious correlation that will explain nothing, while it will have the seductive imprimatur of molecular genetic precision.

The Dangerous Intersection of "Allele Frequencies in Special Populations" and "Police Profiling via Phenotype"

The conventional wisdom is that DNA fingerprinting is just a better way of getting a fingerprint. That is wrong. The traditional physical imprint of your finger or thumb provides only that specific identifying mark, and it is attached to you and you alone.[3] Quite unlike the actual fingerprint, the DNA contains information about many other aspects than simply a marker for identification. It contains information about potential or existing genetic diseases or genetic susceptibilities one may have, and also contains information about your family. These can involve data of interest to one's employer and, of course, to insurance companies. For these reasons, law enforcement officials claim that they are only interested in that part of the DNA that will permit them to provide identifying markers that are not in coding regions. Coding regions are only 10 percent of the DNA, and it is in these regions that the nucleotides code for proteins that might relate to a full range of matters of concern to researchers, from cancer or heart disease to neurotransmission and thus, for some, to possible "coding" for "impulsivity" or biochemical outcomes that might relate to violence.

While the FBI and local and state law enforcement officials tell us that they are only looking at genetic markers in the noncoding region of the DNA, 29 states now require that tissue samples be retained in their DNA databanks after profiling is complete (Kimmelman, 2000). Only one state, Wisconsin, requires the destruction of tissue samples once profiling is complete. The states are the primary venues for the prosecution of violations of the criminal law, and their autonomy has generated considerable variation in the use of DNA databanks and storage. Even as late as the mid-1980s, most states were only collecting DNA samples on sexual offenders. The times have changed quite rapidly. All fifty states now contribute to the FBI's Combined DNA Index System (CODIS). Moreover, there has been rapid change in the interlinking of state databases. In just two years, the database went from a total of nine states cross-linking "a little over 100,00 offender profiles and 5,000 forensic profiles" to 32 states, the FBI, and the U.S. Army now linking "nearly 400,000 offender profiles, and close to 20,000 forensic profiles" (Gavel, 2000). States are now uploading an average of 3000 offender profiles every month. If this sounds daunting, computer technology is increasingly efficient and extraordinarily fast. It takes only 500 microseconds to search a database of 100,000 profiles. As we increase the numbers of profiles in the databases, there will be researchers proposing to provide SNP profiles of specific offender populations. Twenty states authorize the use of databanks for research on forensic techniques. Based on the statutory language in several of those states, this could easily mean assaying genes or loci that contain predictive information. Tom Callaghan, program manager of the FBI's Federal Convicted Offender Program, refused to rule out such possible uses by behavioral geneticists seeking a possible profile for a particular allele among specific offender populations, including especially violent offenders and sexual offenders (Kimmelman, 2000). It is useful to note here that this is the wedge that inevitably extends to other crimes and even misdemeanors. Indeed, in 1999 Louisiana was the first state to pass a law permitting the taking of a DNA sample for all merely arrested for a felony, but has now been followed by four other states. Seven states now require DNA data banking on *all* felons, including white-collar felons. In the fall of 1998, Governor Pataki proposed that New York State include white-collar convicts in the DNA database, but the state legislative assembly balked and forced him to jettison the idea. Perhaps they were concerned that some saliva might be left on the cigars in those backrooms where price fixing and security exchange fraud occur. Today, nearly half the states include some misdemeanors in the DNA databank. So we can now see that what started as "sex offenders" has now graduated to misdemeanants and arrestees. While 39 states permit expungement of samples if charges are dropped, almost all of those states place the burden on the individual to initiate expungement.

Population-wide DNA Database

It is now relatively common for scholars to acknowledge the considerable and documented racial and ethnic bias in police procedures, prosecutorial discretion, jury selection, and sentencing practices, of which racial profiling is but the tip of an iceberg (Mauer, 1999). Indeed, racial disparities penetrate the whole system and are suffused throughout it, all the way up to and through racial disparities in seeking the death penalty for the same crime. If the DNA database is primarily composed of those who have been touched by the criminal justice system, and that system has provided practices that routinely select more from one group, there will be an obvious skew or bias toward this group.

Some have argued that the way to handle the racial bias in the DNA database is to include everyone, not just those accused of crimes. But this does not address the far more fundamental problem of the bias that generates the configuration and content of the criminal (or suspect) database. If the lens of the criminal justice system is focused almost entirely on one part of the population for a certain kind of activity (drug-related, street crime), and ignores a parallel kind of crime (fraternity cocaine sales a few miles away), then even if the fraternity members' DNA samples are in the databank, they will not be subject to the same level of matching, or of subsequent allele frequency profiling research to "help explain" their behavior. *That behavior will not have been recorded.* That is, if the police are not stopping to arrest the fraternity members, it does not matter whether their DNA is in a national database or not, because they are not *criminalized* by the selective aim of the artillery of the criminal justice system. Thus, it is imperative that we separate arguments about bias in the criminal justice system at the point of contact with select parts of the population from "solutions" like "cold hits." It is certainly true that if a member of that fraternity committed a rape and left tissue samples at the scene, and—because he was in a national DNA database—the police could nab him with a "cold hit," that would be the source of justifiable applause. But my point here is that by ignoring powder cocaine and emphasizing street sales of cocaine in the African American community, the mark of criminality is thereby generated, and this is not altered by having a population-wide DNA database. Moreover, the surface fiction of objectivity will lead to a research agenda on the DNA database about which I would now like to issue a warning. There is a serious threat of how these new technologies are about to be deployed that is masked by the apparent global objectivity of a population-wide DNA database.

I am referring to the prospects for SNP profiling of offenders. As noted, even if everyone were in the national database, this would not deter the impulse to do specific and focused research on the select population that has been convicted. An article appeared in the *American Journal of Human Genetics* in 1997 that claimed:

We have identified a panel of population-specific genetic markers that enable robust ethnic-affiliation estimation for major U.S. resident populations. In this report, we identify these loci and present their levels of allele-frequency differential
between ethnically defined samples, and we demonstrate, using log-likelihood
analysis, that this panel of markers provides significant statistical power for ethnic-
affiliation estimation. (Shriver et al., 1997, 17–18)

As in the earlier work by Devlin and Risch (1992a), one of the expressed
purposes of this research is its "use in forensic ethnic affiliation estimation"
(Shriver et al., 1997). While Devlin and Risch were quite circumspect, even
skeptical, about the ultimate utility of such attempts, Shriver and colleagues
(1997) and Lowe and colleagues (2001) claim the viability of this methodology. This research agenda is likely to produce a significant challenge to the
communitarian claim of a common public safety interest. The right of the individual to remain in a community while she has a contagious disease such as
smallpox or tuberculosis is trumped by the state's right to protect the general
public health of the citizenry. But molecular biology has played a powerful role
in fracturing the public health consensus. While we could all agree that it is in
our common interest to mainly rid society of cholera, yellow fever, tuberculosis, infectious meningitis, and smallpox, this communitarian consensus has
been dramatically undermined as we have learned that some groups are at
higher risk for a genetic disorder than others. Cystic fibrosis is a genetic disorder that can affect the upper respiratory system in a life-threatening manner,
but only those from north European ancestry are at significant risk. Beta-
Thalassemia is a blood disorder primarily associated with persons with ances-
tors from the southern Mediterranean region. Sickle cell anemia is primarily
associated, in the United States, with Americans of West African descent. And
so it goes. In the 1970s, the public health consensus about general health
screening was disrupted by this development, as group interests began to
emerge to demand more funding for research and genetic testing of the gene
disorder most associated with "their group" (Duster, 1990).

If molecular genetics and the emergence of group-based research agendas
fractured the public health consensus, we can expect an even more dramatic
parallel development when it comes to discussions of the public safety. It is almost inevitable that a research agenda will surface to try to find patterns of
allele frequencies, and then SNP profiles of different types of criminals. One

could do a SNP profile of rapists and sex offenders, and find some markers that they putatively share. As I have noted above, "ethnic-affiliation estimations of allele frequencies" is high on the research agenda in forensic science. But like the phrenology of the nineteenth century, these markers will be precisely that, markers and not explanatory of the causes of violent crime. Even if the many causes of criminal violence (or any human behaviors) are embedded in the full panoply of forces that begin with protein coding, there is interaction at every level, from the cellular environment all the way up through embryological development to the ways in which the criminal justice system focuses on one part of the town and not another when making drug busts. We are bemused today about tales of nineteenth-century scientists who sought answers to criminal behavior by measuring the sizes and shapes of the heads of convicted felons. The new IBM computers can make 7.5 trillion calculations per second for biological chip analysis. These are sirens beckoning researchers who wish to do parallel correlational studies of population-based allele frequencies with ethnic estimations and groupings of felons—a recurring seduction to a false precision.

Conclusions

The high variability of rates of crime for any one group, and the high variability for what constitutes antisocial behavior across time and space, will make it easy for geneticists to make erroneous inferences about links between criminal behaviors and members of particular racial and ethnic groups. This has long been a concern, but it is exacerbated by the wedding of new molecular investigations into criminal behaviors with high-speed computers to analyze DNA samples of those caught up in the net of the criminal justice system. Because that system, in the United States, has become increasingly focused on African Americans and Latinos in the past half century, the collection of stored tissue samples will be remarkably skewed toward these segments of the population.

In the last quarter of the nineteenth century, the search for correlations with the behavior of criminals generated highly respected scientific work on the head shapes of criminals. Within a few decades, that work fell into disrepute. Indeed, the sciences of phrenology and craniometry are now routinely ridiculed as pseudo-science. In the first quarter of the twenty-first century, we can expect to see publications in scientific journals that report a *somewhat successful* search for correlations with the behavior of criminals and DNA markers. High-speed computers analyzing 3 million "points of difference" (single nucleotide polymorphisms) will generate correlations with selected markers. As noted, every era is certain of its facts, and its leading proponents often ridicule earlier eras as pseudo-scientific. Sometimes, they are correct. But close scrutiny and skepticism should be the posture toward behavioral research where the "search warrant" involves correlations to unexamined outcome data (trouble with the authorities) and noncoding regions of the DNA. This could easily become the phrenology of the twenty-first century.

NOTES

1. When I raised this question at a conference on behavioral genetics at Cold Spring Harbor in the winter of 1995 (Banbury Conference, March 5–8), the responses ranged from focusing on human suffering to the existence of a body of literature already in place on a topic. While the grounds may be noble, humanistic, or practical, none really addressed the theoretical warrant. As I pointed out, there are many forms of human suffering that are not presumed to have a genetic base, and the existence of a body of literature on a topic is a matter of tradition and career ladder, not a conceptual frame.

2. Reported in the *New York Times,* February 27, 1990.

3. Simon Cole (2001) published a book challenging some of the long-held beliefs about the infallibility of the physical fingerprint, but that is another story.

REFERENCES

American Anthropological Association. (1998). Statement on Race, approved by the Executive Board, May 17, 1998, retrievable at www/ameranthassn.org/racepp.htm.
Austin, J. S., and A. D. McVey. (1989). "The Impact of the War on Drugs." *Focus,* 4. San Francisco, CA: The 1989 National Council of Crime and Delinquency Prison Population Forecast, 39 (December: 1–7).
Bamshad, M. J., and S. E. Olson. (2003). "Does Race Exist?" *Scientific American* 289(6): 78–85.
Bittles, A. H., and D. F. Roberts, eds. (1992). *Minority Populations: Genetics, Demography and Health.* London: Macmillan.
Black, E. (2003). *War Against the Weak: Eugenics and America's Campaign to Create a MasterRace.* New York: Four Walls Eight Windows.
Black, J. (1988). *You Can't Win: The Autobiography of Jack Black, Professional Thief.* New York: Amok. (Originally published by Macmillan, 1926.)

Braun, L. (2002). "Race, Ethnicity, and Health: Can Genetics Explain Disparities?" *Perspectives in Biology and Medicine* 45(2) (Spring): 159–74.

Brunner, H. G., M. Nelen, X. O. Breakfield, et al. (1993). "Abnormal Behavior Associated with a Point Mutation in the Structural Gene for Monoamine Oxidase." *Science* 262: 578–80.

Cameron, M. O. (1964). *The Booster and the Snitch*. New York: The Free Press.

Caspi, A., J. McClay, T. E. Moffitt, et al. (2002). "Role of Genotype in the Cycle of Violence in Maltreated Children." *Science* 297(5582): 851–54.

Chapman, M., ed. (1993). *Social and Biological Aspects of Ethnicity*. New York: Oxford University Press.

Chorney, M. J., K. Chorney, N. Seese, et al. (1998). "A Quantitative Trait Locus Associated with Cognitive Ability in Children." *Psychological Science* 9(3) (May): 159–66.

Clark, E., McConnell Foundation. (1992). *Americans Behind Bars*. New York, May.

Clipper, S. E. (1998). "Huntington's Disease: Hope through Research." Bethesda, Md.: Office of Scientific and Health Reports, National Institute of Neurological Disorders and Stroke, National Institutes of Health.

Cole, D. (1999). *No Equal Justice: Race and Class in the American Criminal Justice System*. New York: New Press; distributed by W. W. Norton.

Cole, S. A. (2001). *Suspect Identities: A History of Fingerprinting and Criminal Identification*. Cambridge, Mass.: Harvard University Press.

Devlin, B., and N. Risch. (1992a). "Ethnic Differentiation at VNTR Loci, with Specific Reference to Forensic Applications." *American Journal of Human Genetics* 51: 534–48.

Devlin, B,. and N. Risch. (1992b). "A Note on the Hardy-Weinberg Equilibrium of VNTR Data by using the Federal Bureau of Investigation's Fixed-bin Method." *American Journal of Human Genetics* 51: 549–53.

Duster, T. (1990). *Backdoor to Eugenics*. New York: Routledge.

Duster, T. (1998). "Persistence and Continuity in Human Genetics and Social Stratification." In Ted Peters, ed. *Genetics: Issues of Social Justice*. Cleveland: Pilgrim Press: 218–38.

Duster, T. (2002). "The Concept of Race in Science." Paper presented at the University of Minnesota on March 14, 2002. (It can be accessed by going to www.lifesci.consorium.umn.edu and then to Conferences/Lectures, and then to March 14, 2002.)

Dwyer, J., P. Neufeld, and B. Scheck. (2000). *Actual Innocence: Five Days to Execution and Other Dispatches from the Wrongly Convicted*. New York: Doubleday.

Evans, W., and M. Relling. (1999). "Pharmacogenomics: Translating Functional Genomics into Rational Therapeutics." *Science* 286: 487–91.

Evett, I. W. (1993). "Criminalistics: The Future of Expertise." *Journal of the Forensic Science Society* 33(3): 173–78.

Evett, I. W., I. S. Buckleton, A. Raymond, et al. (1993). "The Evidential Value of DNA Profiles." *Journal of the Forensic Science Society* 33(4): 243–44.

Evett, I. W., P. D. Gill, J. K. Scranage, et al. (1996). "Establishing the Robustness of Short-Tandem-Repeat Statistics for Forensic Application." *American Journal of Human Genetics* 58: 398–407.

Flanagan, T. J., and Kathleen Maguire, eds. (1990). *Sourcebook of Criminal Justice Statistics 1989*. Washington, D.C.: U.S. Department of Justice Statistics, USGPO.

Flynn, K. (2000). "Police Gadgets Aim to Fight Crime with 007-Style Ingenuity." *New York Times* (March 7): A21.

Frank, R. (2001). "A Reconceptualization of the Role of Biology in Contributing to Race/Ethnic Disparities in Health Outcomes." *Population Research and Policy Review* 20: 441–55.

Friedson, E. (1974). *Profession of Medicine: A Study of the Sociology of Applied Knowledge.* New York: Dodd, Mead.

Gavel, D. (2000). "Fight Crime through Science." *Harvard Gazette* (November 30).

Geis, G. (1982). *On White Collar Crime.* Lexington, Mass.: Lexington Books.

Gibbard, A. (2001). "Genetic Plans, Genetic Differences, and Violence: Some Chief Possibilities." In D. Wasserman and R. Wachbroit, eds. *Genetics and Criminal Behavior.* Cambridge: Cambridge University Press: 169–98.

Hacker, A. (1992). *Two Nations: Black and White, Separate, Hostile, Unequal.* New York: Scribner's: 197.

Hacking, I. (2001). "Degeneracy, Criminal Behavior, and Looping." In D. Wasserman and R. Wachbroit, eds. *Genetics and Criminal Behavior.* Cambridge: Cambridge University Press: 141–68.

Hamadeh, H., and C. A. Afshari. (2000). "Gene Chips and Functional Genomics." *American Scientist* 88: 508–15.

Harding, V. (1983). *There is a River: The Black Struggle for Freedom in America.* New York: Vintage.

Hay, D., P. Linebaugh, J. G. Rule, et al. (1975). *Albion's Fatal Tree: Crime and Society in Eighteenth Century England.* New York: Pantheon.

Human Genome News, Human Genome Program, U.S. Department of Energy. (2000). (v11n1–2).

Jablonski, N., and G. Chaplain. (2002). "The Evolution of Skin Color." *Scientific American* (October): 75–82.

Jacobs P., M. Bruton, M. M. Melville, et al. (1965). "Aggressive Behavior, Subnormality, and the XYY Male." *Nature* 208: 1351–52.

Jensen, P., K. Fenger, T. G. Bolwig, et al. (1998). "Crime in Huntington's Disease: A Study of Registered Offences Among Patients, Relatives, and Controls." *Journal of Neurology and Psychiatry* 65: 467–71.

Kahn, J. (2003). "Getting the Numbers Right: Statistical Mischief and Racial Profiling in Heart Failure Research." *Perspectives in Biology and Medicine* 46(4): 473–83.

Katz, S. H. (1995). "Is Race a Legitimate Concept for Science?" *The AAPA Revised Statement of Analysis and Commentary.* University of Pennsylvania, February.

Kevles, D. (1985). *In the Name of Eugenics: Genetics and the Uses of Human Heredity.* New York: Knopf.

Kittles, R. A., and K. M. Weiss. (2003). "Race, Ancestry, and Genes: Implications for Defining Disease Risk." *Annual Review of Genomics and Human Genetics* 4: 33–67.

Kimmelman, J. (2000). "Risking Ethical Insolvency: A Survey of Trends in Criminal DNA Databanking." *Journal of Law, Medicine and Ethics* 28: 209–21.

Lee, S. S., J. Mountain, and B. A. Koenig. (2001). "The Meanings of 'Race' in the New Genomics: Implications for Health Disparities Research." *Yale Journal of Health Policy, Law, and Ethics* 12(15): 33–75.

Lowe, A. L., A. Urquhart, L. A. Foreman, et al. (2001). "Inferring Ethnic Origin by Means of an STR Profile." *Forensic Science International* 119: 17–22.

Mauer, M. (1999). *Race to Incarcerate.* New York: New Press; distributed by W. W. Norton.

Meierhoefer, B. S. (1992). "The General Effect of Mandatory Minimum Prison Terms: A

Longitudinal Study of Federal Sentences Imposed." *Federal Judicial Center.* Washington, D.C.

Miller, J. G. (1992). *Hobbling a Generation: Young African American Males in the Criminal Justice System of America's Cities.* Alexandria, Va.: National Center on Institutions and Alternative.

Miller, J. G. (1996). *Search and Destroy: African-American Males in the Criminal Justice System.* New York: Cambridge University Press.

Pan, P. P. (1998). "Prince George's Chief Has Used Serial Testing Before." *Washington Post* (January 31): B1.

Parens, E. (2004). "Genetic Differences and Human Identities: On Why Talking about Behavioral Genetics Is Important and Difficult." *Hastings Center Report Special Supplement* 34(1): S1–S36, at S10–S15.

Polednak, A. P. (1989). *Racial and Ethnic Differences in Disease.* New York: Oxford University Press.

Polk, K. (1994). *When Men Kill: Scenarios of Masculine Violence* . New York: Cambridge University Press.

Reilly, P. R. (1991). *The Surgical Solution: A History of Involuntary Sterilization in the United States.* Baltimore: Johns Hopkins University Press.

Reinarman, C., and H. G. Levine. (1997). *Crack in America: Demon Drugs and Social Justice.* Berkeley: University of California Press.

Risch, N., E. Burchard, E. Ziv, et al. (2002). "Categorizations of Humans in Biomedical Research: Genes, Race and Disease." *Genome Biology* 3(7): 2007.1–2007.12 (also available at www.genomebiology.com/2002/3/7/comment/2007.1).

Rosenberg, N. A., J. K. Pritchard., J. L., Weber, et al. (2002). "Genetic Structure of Human Populations." *Science* 298: 2381–85.

Rutter, M., H. Giller, and A. Hagell. (1998). *Antisocial Behavior by Young People.* Cambridge: Cambridge University Press.

Shipman, P. (1994). *The Evolution of Racism: Human Differences and the Use and Abuse of Science.* New York: Simon and Schuster.

Shriver, M. D., M. W. Smith, L. Jin, et al. (1997). "Ethnic-Affiliation Estimation by Use of Population-Specific DNA Markers." *American Journal of Human Genetics* 1(60): 957–64.

Smalley, S. L., V. Kustanovich, S. L. Minassian, et al. (2002). "Genetic Linkage of Attention-Deficit/Hyperactivity Disorder on Chromosome 16p13, in a Region Implicated in Autism." *American Journal of Human Genetics* 4: 959–63.

Smith, E., and W. Sapp, eds. (1997). *Plain Talk about the Human Genome Project.* Tuskegee, Ala.: Tuskegee University.

Taylor, K. A. (2001). "On the Explanatory Limits of Behavioral Genetics." In D. Wasserman and R. Wachbroit, eds. *Genetics and Criminal Behavior.* Cambridge: Cambridge University Press: 117–40.

Tyler, G. (1962). *Organized Crime in America.* Ann Arbor: University of Michigan Press.

Wachbroit R. (2001). "Understanding the Genetics-of-Violence Controversy." In D. Wasserman and R. Wachbroit, eds. *Genetics and Criminal Behavior.* Cambridge: Cambridge University Press: 25–26.

Wasserman, D., and R. Wachbroit. (2001). "Introduction: Methods, Meanings, and Morals." In D. Wasserman and R. Wachbroit, eds. *Genetics and Criminal Behavior.* Cambridge: Cambridge University Press: 23–46.

Wilson, J. F., et al. (2001). "Population Genetic Structure of Variable Drug Response." *Nature Genetics* 29: 265–69.

Winslow, R. (2001). "FDA is Prepared to Approve Heart Drug Intended for Treating African Americans." *Wall Street Journal* (March 21).

Wolfgang, M. (1958). *Patterns of Criminal Homicide.* Philadelphia: University of Pennsylvania Press.

Xie, H. G., R. B. Kim, A.J.J. Wood, et al. (2001). "Molecular Basis of Ethnic Differences in Drug Disposition and Response." *American Review of Pharmacology and Toxicology* 41: 815–50.

CHAPTER EIGHT

Impulsivity, Responsibility, and the Criminal Law

Harold Edgar, LL.B.

In response to the question, What difference may the genetics of impulsivity make for how the legal system views legal responsibility? the only sensible answer is, It all depends. Of course, no one can confidently say on what it depends. Because law is ultimately political, it can change rapidly, through both legislation and judicial interpretation. Legal changes are shaped, however, by broader cultural responses to patterns and specific events that occur in unpredictable fashion.

Who could have guessed in 1954 that legislators 50 years later would take seriously a claimed right to carry handguns in American cities, or that a court would find its state constitution violated by laws limiting marriage to persons of opposite sex? (*Goodridge v. Dept. of Public Health,* 2003).

New scientific understandings can and do impact many aspects of law. Over the past 50 years, the "new biology" has transformed the definition of death and the law of death and dying. Reproductive technology and forensic DNA have had a major effect on family law. Are the core concepts of criminal law at comparable risk over the next half century? I do not think so.

The proposition that most people are responsible most of the time is central to law and will not change easily, no matter what the science shows. Among their other functions, ideas about free will are bound up in the civil liberties protected by criminal law's limits. We too often think of criminal law as a set of prohibitory commands—do not murder, rape, or rob—and fail to appreciate the ways its core requirements protect us from state power. The state cannot take action against a person who is claimed to have dangerous propensities until these propensities manifest themselves in conduct, because conduct involves choice, and until the actor chooses, we cannot know what he will do. Therefore, the state must prove that I—not some hypothetical offender, but I, the author of this chapter—engaged in prohibited conduct before the state convicts me. If I can avoid acting so bizarrely that psychiatrists diagnose me as mentally ill, and not engage in conduct prohibited by laws already on the books, I can arrange my affairs with reasonable confidence that the government will not forcibly remove me from home and family. I think I can do *that* whether or not I have "free will," and I greatly value the security it inspires. Moreover, this freedom is essential to true political liberty. It was hard won as a historical matter, and is absent in many authoritarian societies.

By contrast, the criteria for deciding who are the relatively few people who are *not* responsible for their actions is a peripheral matter whatever its complexities, and nowhere near as important to law's purposes. It can and does change. For example in 1992, a federal jury drawn from the District of Columbia juror pool ruled that John Hinckley was insane, and thus was not guilty of shooting President Ronald Reagan and others. In response, some states abolished entirely their insanity defense, a defense that has a 600-year history in Anglo-American law (Perlin, 1990). More important, Congress and many other states sharply limited the scope of this responsibility doctrine, including abolishing the "irresistible impulse" component of the test for insanity, which as formulated in contemporary language by the American Law Institute's influential Model Penal Code, asked the jury to decide whether a defendant lacked "substantial capacity" to conform his conduct to law (American Law Institute, Model Penal Code §4.01(1), 1962). Had these 12 jurors convicted Hinckley, and perhaps even if Hinckley had been from impoverished rather than privileged background, this *volte face* in legal policy most likely would not have occurred. The change in policy also would not have happened but for widespread belief that crime rates were too high and excuses too easy.

The chance event, however, turns ideas and proposals that might otherwise drift among the intellectual currents of the time into statutes and rules. The upshot is that in most states, one of the three current legal doctrines that might accommodate some genetics defense in criminal law (i.e., the insanity defense) is almost surely foreclosed. It is foreclosed, that is, unless and until public mood changes enough to spark legislative revision or dramatically different judicial interpretations.

What might change the public mood? The genetic science is relevant, and particularly relevant is whether the boundaries the science draws are sharp, and how many people are claimed to be special. But science will never be dispositive, particularly in a country where, for example, many schools give creationism equal billing with evolution. Therefore, it is important to know whether data about the genetic aspects of impulse control come at a time of rising or falling crime rates, and whether crime policy sharply divides our politics. Is there is a realistic medical or behavioral intervention for those identified as genetically disabled? How sympathetic are the cases that focus media attention on the new data?

Finally, although I focus here on the criminal law, the old adage that law is a seamless web is true, and important. Responsibility and neighboring concepts like capacity have wide applicability throughout the legal system, and new findings about impulsivity might affect how these concepts are understood and applied in a variety of contexts. For example, some consumer sales and loans are already subject to rules permitting the consumer to be released from a contract for a limited period of time (e.g., Truth in Lending Act, 15 U.S.C. §1635(a)). This protects consumers from impulsive and ill-considered decisions to purchase. Might we develop doctrines limiting impulsive changes made to longstanding testamentary documents, such as wills? Will new data lead us to say impulsivity is a disability for the purposes of antidiscrimination law? Is impulsivity relevant in deciding who should be the custodial parent of minor children in divorce proceedings? These are all questions about responsibility, and how law resolves them can be shaped not only by whether particular persons are labeled this rather than that, but also by how prevalent we believe the condition to be in the population at large. We would do many things differently if half the population were colorblind. In turn, the way law treats issues like these has a feedback effect on the question of how the criminal law reacts when responsibility is at issue.

Venturing Predictions

Having stressed the long-term uncertainties, let me nonetheless venture some predictions. First, the current work on the genetics of impulsivity is unlikely to have an impact on the criminal law's responsibility doctrine. In the somewhat longer term, it might influence legal development. Numbers count. If a few offenders are identified as having peculiar genetic conditions that make it extraordinarily difficult for them to comply with the law on the occasion that they broke it, they can be excused from criminal responsibility by manipulation of current voluntary act or mens rea doctrine—the other two doctrinal harbors along with insanity that might plausibly shelter such a defense—without doing serious violence to current rules. By no means is it clear that courts would permit the required doctrinal adaptations, the nature of which I will sketch later. It is, however, relatively easy to proffer novel excuses at the trial level, and some trial judges are likely to permit the defense to explore them, and perhaps even charge the jury to consider them. Jury behavior is hard to predict.

Such a development, if it occurs, would not, however, require the criminal law to rethink substantially or abandon its current reliance on popular notions of responsibility and free will (Morse, 1994). If acquitted, these defendants would be judged not to have had free will. Whether the genetics research would have ended up benefiting these defendants is also highly uncertain. If, as seems likely, the genetically based impulsive condition greatly increases the likelihood that the defendant would do a similar act again, then legislatures might respond as they have done with sexual psychopath laws, providing indefinite and potentially lifetime confinement for those judged unable to control their sexual impulses. This probable response is the dilemma of the impulsivity work that I will return to. Society will be torn between its impulse to compassion and its impulse to collective self-protection.

This brings me to my second prediction. If treatment is available; or if the environmental cue that triggered the behavior is highly unusual, by which I mean that the criminal behavior is not likely to be repeated; or even if the behavior is likely to be repeated, it is not particularly dangerous; then individuals afflicted with these impulsivity-related disabilities will likely benefit from favorable exercises of discretion throughout the criminal justice system. This accommodation will happen, I believe, even if the genetic research identifies as special substantially larger numbers of defendants.

One of the weaknesses of the behavioral genetics literature about law that I have read is that it focuses so much on legal doctrine, and speaks little to criminal justice administration (Coffee, 1993; Denno, 1996; Johnson, 1998). The majority of known criminal incidents are not prosecuted. And those that are prosecuted are overwhelmingly settled by agreement between the state and the defendant, and turning on the particular state you are in, an agreement among state, defendant, and judge. Trials are the relatively rare blip on the legal radar screen. To be sure, in these agreements, people act, to some extent, "in the shadow of the law," reaching results that reflect what they believe the litigated outcome will be. But criminal law systems grapple with the fact that they threaten more punishment than they inflict, and choices must be made about relative degrees of seriousness and how to process efficiently the less serious cases.

Behavioral genetics is likely to have its main impact on these largely unreviewable sorting questions, with its impact likely to be a function of the boundaries it can draw. By boundaries, I mean questions like how many people are affected and how easy is it to determine the effect and predict the future from it. To be sure, legal doctrine is influenced by these same boundary questions. The law does not permit voluntary intoxication as a general defense because so many people can claim it, and determining degrees of drunkenness is so difficult.

The individuals who administer the law are, however, particularly sensitive to these boundary questions because they make discretionary decisions every day, and constantly are agreeing to exact less punishment than the law theoretically permits. They ask, "Is this defendant's story true, and how do I know it is true?" Here findings from genetics research could help. Let's assume we know that the defendant has the set of genes that predisposes him to impulsive behavior. Only some small percentage of such persons acts criminally. However, only one in a 100 or 1000 or 10,000 can open the door to a story like this one in the first place. What do I do as a prosecutor if I believe the story? If a person's having a particular set of genes turns out to make it harder for him to obey the law, and, for example, regularly taking a drug would dramatically improve the situation, then I deal with his relatively minor offenses by conditioning nonprosecution or probation on his taking treatment. Prosecutors can make discretionary decisions that the individual was out of control for reasons not within his control; that threatening serious punishment will not influence similar people very much; and that the social harm caused by these individuals is not so extraordinarily grave. It is not that these cases are decided because defendants have climbed doctrinal hurdles, that is, that they had a good chance of acquittal on insanity grounds, but because prosecutors have exercised discretion and acted leniently.

Like prosecutors, judges also frequently exercise discretion in cases involving these issues. Boundary issues affect whether a judge chooses a lighter rather than a heavier sentence. For most crimes, the judge's sentence choice can be more important in terms of time served than whether a defendant can formally mitigate punishment by proving his innocence of the more serious of two degrees of the same crime, say, aggravated versus simple robbery. Despite Congress's abolition of the volition prong of the insanity defense, a federal appellate court has held (*United States v. McBroom,* 1997) and the Federal Sentencing Commission has affirmed (U.S Sentencing Guidelines Manual §5K2-13 com 1, 1998) that a federal trial judge may reduce a defendant's otherwise required sentence in a nonviolent crime if his volitional controls were impaired. In other words, a consideration deemed irrelevant in deciding guilt or innocence can impact sentence.

As the behavior gets more serious, the prospects of treatment or intervention more remote, and the likelihood of repetition more certain, the probability that these very same discretionary decisions will work against volitionally impaired offenders gets higher and higher. No one wants to be the official who treated lightly the person who committed multiple murders at a time when he would have been in prison had an authorized prosecution been undertaken or a sentence imposed. Indeed, the federal sentencing treatment of mentally impaired offenders illustrates the point. From a "fairness" perspective, whether the impaired offender manifests nonviolent or violent behavior should be irrelevant in deciding whether the disability deserves a break. It is not irrelevant from a societal perspective.

The Free Will Debate and the Criminal Law

The question that most excites the literature is, What do we do if all or nearly all behavior is shown to be "compelled" by genetic makeup interacting with the cumulative effect of prior environmental experience? In other words, we are all "path-dependent" creatures: our behavior today is inevitable given the boundaries set by genetic makeup and past experience. For those who posit this view, current research into genes associated with impulsivity provides a window into human behavior generally, just as Freud used his patients' pathologies as the foundation for theories about everyone's behavior.

Surely any demonstration that all behavior is "compelled" (even in the interactionist's sense) is far in the future, and if I understand it right, nothing in the present impulsivity science adds to the plausibility of this account. The strength of the determinist argument is the theoretical claim that everything in the physical world, at least if large enough, has prior causes that fully account for it, and because human behavior is ultimately physical, it, too, must be reducible to such explanations. If the culture as a whole came to believe in such total determination, I believe it might change the rationales we use to justify punishment, but not the practice. Indeed, it's worth remembering that intellectual elites believed in the late nineteenth and early twentieth centuries that much criminality was hereditary, or at least beyond the control of the offender (Rafter, 2001). The belief changed some penal practices—separating young from hardened offenders; more use of parole—but did not shake the elite's belief in punishment. Their perception of why it was just to punish criminals, however, did not stress moral condemnation the way our current literature does. Indeed, it is one of the ironies of contemporary criminal law theory that after World War II, American intellectuals abandoned prior utilitarian precepts because they could not answer questions Nazism posed about the limits on positive law, only to embrace retributive positions emanating from the German philosophic tradition.

I discuss the free will issue first because it facilitates talking about criminal law generally, and then I return to current criminal law responsibility doctrine.

Free Will, Criminal Law, and "Ordinary" Folks

Criminal law is a multipurposed institution. Obviously, it serves the community's interest in maintaining order, and order, taken in the broadest sense, is a necessary condition for human flourishing through cooperative activity in groups. Maintaining order by inflicting sanctions on offenders is, however, only a piece of what the criminal law does. The larger task is to influence the vast majority of people who are never convicted to limit their involvement in crime. To this end, law must punish some offenders just to prove it keeps its promises. The direct threat of punishment and accompanying social humiliation does part of this work, and the hoped for incorporation of criminal law norms into the social fabric of acceptable behavior does the rest. Such an incorporation happens some of the time—think of the evolution in contemporary thought about date rape as a social problem or computer hacking—but by no means inevitably, as Prohibition demonstrated. A contemporary test case is whether young people's attitude toward computer file sharing in violation of copyright laws can be shaped by threats of criminal punishment.

The debate about whether free will is a meaningful concept exaggerates the law's interest in punishing offenders as against shaping broader behavior, and mistakenly assumes that the law's central commitment is to inflict punishment only when it is "just." There are many instances where law compromises on moral justice in pursuit of other ends. For example, the criminal law's continuing use of strict liability, its refusal to allow a defense based upon reasonable mistakes of law, and its refusal to adjust the "reasonable person" to individuals' capacities are all such instances. The central issue is whether most people's behavior can be shaped by threats, and secondarily whether formalized social disapproval adds anything over and above the threatened penalty itself. For these purposes, whether people have free will is irrelevant. Indeed, in a fully determined world, threats are part of the environment that determines behavior. The point is obvious, but too often ignored. Similarly, people's desire to avoid social humiliation does not go away simply because they and everyone else knows that the social humiliation is morally undeserved. You know this is true if you can remember high school. Do dogs have free will in a morally relevant sense? Dog owners routinely take advantage of dogs' genetic propensity to bond to a leader by training them using expressions of disapproval. "Bad dog" adds weight to the rolled-up newspaper.

Law will not abandon threats and disapproval, but the path by which it integrates new understandings about human psychology into its moral universe is unpredictable. We could all become compatabilists and treat practical reasoning as the free will that justifies moral condemnation (see chapter 10). More likely, I believe, the society would return to notions that punishment is appropriate when persons of bad character do bad acts, and that character is the result of countless small decisions along life's way, and that even if each of these is compelled, the cumulative effect warrants condemnation now, perhaps on the restitutionary theory that prior actions that should have been disapproved were not. Surely professors and the society would talk less about moral condemnation in criminal law than we do now, and I believe that would be a good thing. There is something grotesque about society's moralizing in the face of prisons stuffed with poor and minority offenders raised in broken homes in brutal neighborhoods and schooled in armed camps. I do not mean to excuse such offenders, and still less to deny the necessity of their restraint. Nonetheless, that so many people can overcome these handicaps and the political indifference that accompanies them is the miracle.

The significance of free will, however, is not only its relationship to a theory of moral condemnation. Such ideas are an important prop to vital personal freedoms anchored by criminal law's doctrinal core. Through criminal law, society strikes at dangerous people, but criminal law says you can know "ordinary" people are dangerous only if they commit a prohibited act. "Being dangerous" is not an independent crime, and cannot constitutionally be punished. We pay a price in death and damage to hold to this rule. A number of people get killed each year because the police lack authority to intervene until the violence a potential victim fears is put into motion by a person not subject to restraint. Of course, criminal law doctrine is constantly seeking ways to identify dangerous people before they do all the damage they are capable of, hence the criminalization of possession of burglars' tools, attempts to kill and conspiracies, and many other examples. Still, you have to formulate the criminal prohibition by identifying some conduct that an individual on notice of the prohibition might avoid. (And such identification can be very difficult, as drafters of antistalking or gang intimidation laws know—*Chicago v. Morales,* 1999.) Failing a psychological test is not conduct in this sense, because we understand the test-taking behavior as revealing character or disposition, and not as harmful conduct in and of itself (Packer, 1968).

The power of this model is illustrated by the widespread opposition by lawyers, across the political spectrum, to the extended detention of Jose Padilla without filing criminal charges against him. Padilla was believed to have met abroad with high-ranking terrorists, and to have returned home to Chicago with an intent to make and set off a so-called dirty bomb, spreading radioactive material. It is easy to sympathize with administration lawyers who were reluctant to release a person they believed was intent on making and detonating such a bomb. But without some way of showing preparatory conduct, or at least an agreement to do it, the mere desire is not an offense. Hence, the lawyers' necessity to argue the president had a right to detain Padilla as an enemy warrior, not a criminal. Briefs amicus curiae opposing this end run were filed in the U.S. Supreme Court on Padilla's behalf from organizations as ideologically diverse as the ACLU, the Association of the Bar of New York, and the Cato Institute (*Rumsfeld v. Padilla*, 2004).

Free Will, Criminal Law, and Those Who Are "Not Ordinary"

Criminal law cannot be used against "ordinary" people unless they have committed a prohibited act. But if it can be shown that someone is mentally ill and is a danger to herself or others, then society may impose restraints without using the criminal process. If it were easy to seize ordinary citizens, let alone political agitators, and call them mentally ill and dangerous to others, the freedom the criminal law's conduct rule secures would become relatively trivialized. In fact, however, securing such mental health commitments is difficult in the absence of manifested dangerous conduct. In a difficult case permitting lifetime civil commitment of "sexual psychopaths," the U.S. Supreme Court in *Kansas v. Hendricks*, 521 U.S. 346 (1996) suggested that prior conduct might be a constitutional requirement for long-term civil confinement. Although its practical significance lies in connection with sentencing and post-sentence proceedings, I will describe *Hendricks*, and a subsequent decision, *Kansas v. Crane*, 534 U.S. 407 (2002), here.

In *Kansas v. Hendricks*, the Supreme Court upheld the constitutionality of Kansas's sexual psychopath statute. The statute permitted the state to "civilly" incarcerate, potentially for life, individuals like Hendricks who had been determined to have a "mental abnormality" or "personality disorder" that made them likely to engage in "predatory acts of sexual violence." The statute defined a mental abnormality as a "congenital or acquired condition affecting the emotional or volitional capacity which predisposes the person to commit sexually violent offenses" (Kansas Stat Ann §59–29a01 et seq., 1994). The statutory procedures for determining whether Hendricks was such a mentally abnormal person included trial by jury and proof beyond reasonable doubt despite the ostensibly civil nature of the proceedings. Most important for my purposes, however, the statute could only be applied to persons convicted of sexually violent offenses and scheduled for release, or those who had been judged incompetent to stand trial for such crimes, or not guilty of them by reason of insanity. In other words, no one whose propensity to engage in sexual violence had never been acted upon, as against merely diagnosed, could be reached by the law.

The Supreme Court of Kansas had held the statute was unconstitutional on due process grounds, reasoning that the definition of "mental abnormality" was a legislative invention designed to circumvent the fact that Hendricks, a long-time pedophile, was not mentally ill in a conventional sense. He repeatedly molested children, but that alone did not make him ill, any more than a person who regularly commits larceny is ill. The only evidence of "illness" was the behavior itself. Having served his criminal sentence, he was entitled to his freedom. The Kansas court thus ruled that prior bad conduct, even in the presence of predicted dangerousness from a person who conceded he was unlikely to control his behavior, was an unconstitutional basis for locking someone up through a civil commitment, particularly when there was no realistic treatment for him.

The U.S. Supreme Court unanimously reversed the Kansas court on this point. It ruled that a person guilty of past sexual offenses, and abnormal in a way that impaired his behavioral control and made future offenses likely, could be detained indefinitely. The justices differed, however, on the extent to which legislatures could define "mental abnormality" without regard to medical opinions. Justice Thomas, writing for himself and four others in the Court's conservative majority (Rehnquist, Stevens, O'Connor, Kennedy), said the statute was constitutional because the definition of abnormality "narrows the class of persons who are eligible for confinement to those who are unable to control their dangerousness" (521 U.S. at 358). Hendricks's "admitted lack of volitional control, coupled with a prediction of dangerousness, adequately distinguishes Hendricks from other dangerous persons who are perhaps more properly dealt with exclusively through criminal proceedings" (521 U.S. at 360). According to the majority, the legislature could define mental abnormality in ways that did not mirror the beliefs of the medical profession. If the legislature wants to say mental abnormality equals absence of volitional control, it may do so. Justice Thomas, however, included this cautionary language: "The statute thus requires proof of more than a mere predisposition to violence; rather it *requires evidence of past sexually violent behavior* and a present mental condition that creates a likelihood of such conduct in the future if the person is not incapacitated" (521 U.S. at 357; emphasis added).

Justice Breyer and three colleagues concurred in upholding the statute against the due process challenge. They differed with Justice Thomas's granting carte blanche to legislatures by stressing three facts. First, the psychiatric profession itself considers pedophilia a serious personality disorder, and it debates among itself whether pedophilia should be called a mental illness. Thus, Justice Breyer argued that the Kansas legislature had chosen to favor one side of a medical debate over another; it was not inventing new categories. Second, Hendricks admitted to a highly unusual inability to control his actions, an inability similar to what might have grounded an insanity acquittal under the prior "irresistible impulse" prong of the defense. Third, he was unquestionably dangerous. The legislature could therefore decide that conditions like this one fell within the constitutional requirements that limit "mental illness" as a legal category (a limit Justice Breyer did not further explicate).

A more recent case, *Kansas v. Crane,* 534 U.S. 407 (2002), involves the same state sexual psychopath statute. The U.S. Supreme Court for a second time ruled unanimously that the Kansas Supreme Court misapplied federal due process law by setting the bar to indefinite civil commitment too high. In *Crane,* the Kansas court read Justice Thomas's *Hendricks* opinion to require a specific finding that a sexual psychopath is "completely unable to control his behavior." Justice Breyer wrote in *Crane* that requiring total or complete lack of control goes too far. But he simultaneously narrowed *Hendricks* by writing that the constitutional application of the statute requires a "lack of control" determination. It is not enough to find that a person has a mental abnormality, and is likely to commit future offenses. There must also be a determination that the abnormality affects the ability to control behavior. Otherwise states could civilly commit likely recidivists. The Constitution thus requires drawing a line between the "impaired and dangerous" and the simply dangerous.

Legal policy pronouncements toward mentally impaired persons have thus taken another odd twist in the road, illustrating the serendipity I earlier remarked on. The irresistible impulse test was removed from many jurisdictions' insanity doctrine because the counterfactual inquiry it required—whether an impulse that was not resisted could have been resisted—was perceived to be unmanageable. Now, a variant of the same inquiry—the extent to which an "abnormality" interferes with a person's ability to control future behavior—is a constitutionally required determination if these kinds of civil commitment statutes are employed.

I draw two lessons for the behavioral genetics debate from the sexual psychopath litigation. First, the Supreme Court's insistence in *Crane* on the necessity of distinguishing the "abnormal" from the simple recidivist is driven, I believe, by the Court's recognition of the civil liberties implications of the criminal responsibility model. To permit long-term detention of people outside the criminal law based on what they might do must be guarded against, and given very narrow approval, if approval at all.

Second, nothing in these cases, or the Court's recent jurisprudence generally, suggests limits on the criteria for imposing punishment *within* the criminal justice model. In *Hendricks,* for example, no justice doubted that the legislature could have authorized and a judge imposed a life sentence on him for his repeated sex crimes. No justice hinted that Hendricks was so strongly predisposed to criminal behavior that he could not be held criminally responsible for a future crime. More generally, in criminal law, legal doctrine never has and does not now offer much protection against the use of predictions of dangerousness to select sentences for persons who are convicted. Even in its death penalty jurisprudence, the Court has refused to consider whether people have the capacity to predict accurately. It upheld Texas legislation that makes juries' predictions of offenders' future dangerousness, a capricious enterprise at best, a basis for execution (*Jurek v. Texas,* 1976). And the legislature can largely do what it wants, outside the field of capital punishment, in designating maximum sentences for crimes (*Harmelin v. Michigan,* 1991).

I come back to the point, then, that the domains of prosecutorial and judicial discretion are where the social policy implications of behavioral genetics must be appraised. Present legal doctrine presents few hurdles to judges or legislatures using pseudo-science, let alone solid scientific work, to select or require long sentences if individuals are believed to have a particularly high likelihood of recommitting the same serious crime that accounts for their current convictions. This proposition is less true for judges in federal criminal proceedings and states where guideline sentences more sharply limit judicial flexibility, although the rules about guideline sentencing are now, for other reasons, in transition (*Blakely v. Washington,* 2001). The great bulk of violent crime is prosecuted at the state level, however. In any event, legislators are free to credit what science they choose. Once a person is proved to have done some criminal act, he no longer fits the category we most identify with, namely, we and our friends, and the law's concern for false positives—the criminal believed dangerous when he really is not—ebbs.

It is in this context that public conversation about behavioral genetics is most important. Science in the United States gets funded when it promises success at solving problems. The National Institutes of Health (NIH) budget gets doubled, while the National Science Foundation (NSF) crawls along. Some scientists will be cautious about projecting the implications of their findings, but it is foolish to think all will be, because researchers want to be funded and prominent. Would Congress have funded the Human Genome Project if James Watson and others had been more realistic about the likely timelines to major medical benefits flowing from doing the whole thing at once? We see the same process at work today in the trumpeting of stem cell research. At the same time, saying that people should not do science because its findings may be misused is contrary to our deepest cultural traditions, even if we know that social dynamics favor misuse.

Finding language and professional institutions that can frame the implications of the scientific work against the backdrop of similar problems with which people are more familiar, and in contexts that stress the political and cultural values that are bound up in the social practices that are candidates for change, is the difficult task ahead.

Behavioral Genetics Research and Efforts at Exculpation

Nothing in the literature I have read to date about genes and their relationship to impulsive behavior makes me believe the work is close to influencing criminal law responsibility issues at the doctrinal level. Even the most enthusiastic interpretation of the behavioral genetics literature suggests only a probable association between genetic endowment and a propensity to act impulsively, where impulsive behavior itself correlates with the likelihood of arrest or conviction for crime. The biological pathways that underlie the first association are unknown, and the relationship between impulsivity and getting apprehended or convicted as a criminal has many possible explanations.

There are two core problems. The correlations demonstrated are not particularly strong, and the "story" the science tells is completely consistent with other stories we know to be true that have never been treated as excuses in law. The point is a familiar one in the behavioral genetics literature (Baron, 2001). The twin studies themselves show that identical genes and extremely similar environments do not produce identical outcomes. A person is cumulatively formed by the interaction of endowment with the environment's minute-by-minute lessons. The fact that genotype does not control phenotype gives ample room for a theory of choice, including the putative defendant's successive choice of environments that shaped his character. The law often uses a person's past decisions to justify punishment even though she may have little control of her present behavior. Intoxication provides an example, for the theory is you take the risk of losing control when you start drinking. Similarly, there is a very high probability that a person presently addicted to cocaine will at some time in the next few days possess cocaine. The correlation between present condition and future behavior is so strong, one might infer it as a cause. He has no defense to a charge of cocaine possession. Moreover, many environmental factors over which the actor had almost no control are known to increase the likelihood that individuals will be arrested or convicted of crime. Childhood victimization, extreme poverty, and early education failure all correlate to crime. They are not excuses, because the law regards them as influencing the likelihood that people will yield to temptations and not as determinants of conduct.

From the standpoint of criminal law's major purpose, reducing the occurrence of prohibited behavior, the law should be toughest precisely when the impulse to violate it is strong. At one time the military executed wartime deserters because the impulse to avoid battlefield death is so great. To be sure, the law's readiness to be tough is constrained by many other considerations, from the monstrous economic and social expense of incarcerating people to the unwillingness of those who administer the law to impose penalties they regard as wildly excessive. Still, there is nothing about the presence of strong temptation alone that makes law stay its hand or limit criminal responsibility doctrine. And the fact that some people with the same genetic endowment and raised in very similar environments *do not* offend powerfully supports the idea that behavior is chosen rather than compelled.

What new science might it take to overcome the present legal predisposition to find persons responsible for their actions? From the standpoint of abstract justice, I see no difference between the person whose involuntary exposure to an environment predictably influences his behavior toward committing crimes and a person whose genetic disposition does the same. The law, however, is rarely shaped by abstract principle alone. The problem with "I had a tough life" defenses is that many people, including the jurors to whom the appeal is made, have had tough lives too. If I deal with my troubles without doing serious crimes, you can too. So long as the free will model dominates our sense of baseline expectations, this is the likely response. There may be no better way of showing the impact baselines have on us than to recall the XYY controversy, where much was made of the claimed high imprisonment rates of men who carried two Y chromosomes. What was not discussed much was that the first Y chromosome is extraordinarily criminogenic, so great was the disparity in imprisonment of men and women. Second, environments shade into one another in a way that makes them a matter of more-or-less. Your father hit you, but how often, how bad, and for what? Third, you (and your lawyer) have every incentive to overstate the horrible things that happened. But for being caught red-handed, your defense would likely be that there is no evidence linking you to the crime.

As noted, a genetic source of the problem does not alter the moral equation much if at all. The one possible moral difference is that even young children arguably have some choice over their environments, and obviously everyone has more such control as they get older. But the other factors are largely the same. Genetic endowments are also likely to shade into one another, as impulsivity surely involves many genes, with different variations having somewhat different effects. Second, the defendant's ability to lie about how little control he experienced himself having is also the same. Third, there is no a priori reason to believe that therapeutic or other interventions with persons with genetic "dispositions" are more likely successful than with persons habituated by bad environmental influences.

There is a difference, however, in the processes by which we believe that there really is something we should take seriously. To make it plausible, I have to assume that the science gets better and better, and refines the information that identifies particular combinations of genes that correlate with a high likelihood of impulsive behavior. Assume further that people with this condition, when they act, or act in response to particular cues, use different gene pathways than do large numbers of ordinary persons, including persons who engage in similar criminal behavior in roughly similar circumstances. This taxonomic process is the way science operates, showing first that "cancer" is not one disease but many, and then that particular cancers within the same diagnostic category activate different genes, and these differences in turn predict different outcomes.

The difference between this "genetic" story and the environmental story is (1) the capacity to diagnose it independently of the subject's easily manipulable responses and (2) the relative standardization of criteria for determining its presence. (To be sure, it is not impossible to imagine environmental exposures having the same differential impact that can be picked up by increasingly sensitive imaging devices. If so, however, I think we will be more likely to conflate genetics with environment and treat both as irrelevant.) What these preliminary assumptions do, of course, is provide ways of insulating the possible defense from undercutting the ordinary responsibility creating rules as well as freeing those who administer the law from the fear that the defense rests solely on diagnostic criteria that defendants may manipulate or present through expert testimony that cannot be appraised. If these criteria are met, what may happen?

A lawyer looking for exculpatory grounds must first look to the insanity defense. The defense is formulated differently in the federal jurisdiction for crimes against the United States, and in various states. Consider two such patterns. The Insanity Defense Reform Act of 1984 (18 U.S.C. §17) states in part: "It is an affirmative defense to a prosecution under any Federal statute that, at the time of the commission of the acts constituting the offense, the defendant, as a result of a severe mental disease or defect, was unable to appreciate the nature and quality or the wrongness of his acts. Mental disease or defect does not otherwise constitute a defense."

This post-Hinckley enactment substituted in federal prosecutions for the Model Penal Code standard, a standard still employed in a minority of states. The Model Penal Code §4.01(1) declares that a person is not responsible for criminal conduct if "as a result" of "mental disease or deficit" he lacks "substantial capacity" either to appreciate the criminality of his conduct or to "conform his conduct to law."

Under both the pre- and post-Hinckley standards (the Model Penal Code and Insanity Reform Defense Act), the starting point is whether scientific or medical testimony can move the genetic endowment in question into the category of "mental disease or defect." In the federal context, there is an additional burden to show it is "severe." Is it a problem to show either fact? A prosecutor could argue that because the particular genes are present in every cell, the affliction is not peculiarly mental; and the law should be slow to characterize genes as a "disease or defect."

I do not believe these problems are serious ones. To be effective, however, the genetic evidence must link the presence of some genes (or absence of others) to the absence of effective ability to control behavior. This inability to control behavior, and not the genes that produce it, will be called the "mental" disease. We would not stop calling schizophrenia a mental disease just because we found a genetic basis for it. A whole sociology surrounds the labeling of conditions as diseases, and some assert that such labeling is just the increasingly assertive stance of medicine when there is a remedial product to be sold.

Personally, I do not believe such matters are quite so subject to pharmaceutical company control, but they obviously present cultural issues as well as purely scientific ones. If the science proves, for example, that people with particular gene variants provably process information differently, and do not use brain centers used by almost everyone else, I believe a judge would characterize the condition as a mental disease or defect.

There is still little or no chance, however, for exculpation by virtue of insanity under federal law. No exculpation is possible because the "disease" or "defect" does not affect cognition. Impulsive people have the capacity to appreciate what they are doing, and they know right from wrong. I will return to this point later.

Under the Model Penal Code, however, the expert could testify whether the criminal action was the "result" of the disease or defect, and whether its impact on the capacity to control was substantial. The formidable problem here is that even impulsive people commit criminal offenses rarely. What is the basis for saying that a person who is law abiding most of the time (and thus controls his impulses) was moved to action here by a medical cause that does not affect him most of the time, even though the genetic condition that causes it is always present? I get back to the problem that made the "irresistible impulse" formulas so hard to administer. How does a fact-finder distinguish the person who cannot control his impulse from the person who will not resist temptation? Again, I can postulate scientific findings that help, for example, that under stress, as produced in laboratory settings, brain waves go this way rather than that, and then saying that such stress is rare. If you could write the scientific script any way you want, you could fashion a defense without violating any proposition we now know to be true.

Essentially similar problems confront the other two other criminal law doctrines—no conduct and no culpability—that a defendant might employ. The defendant has an additional incentive to try them. Insanity acquittals result in most places in automatic civil commitments for indefinite periods, so the issue for the person judged innocent is the label and place of incarceration. For this reason and others, defendants are often very unwilling to have insanity presented as a defense on their behalf. By contrast, in most places an acquittal because a person did not commit a voluntary act, or acted without mens rea or culpability, results in outright acquittal or conviction of a much less serious crime. And, for this reason, many jurisdictions require that a defendant asserting a defense of mental abnormality do so under the rubric of insanity.

Most states have statutes or a common law tradition that persons who act involuntarily or unconsciously cannot commit a crime while in that state. The classic case is the person who kills another while sleepwalking. As formulated in the Model Penal Code §2.01—and enacted in a fair number of states—a person engages in no voluntary action if his behavior is a "reflex or convulsion"; or done while "unconscious or asleep"; or done during hypnosis or under hypnotic suggestion; or "is otherwise not a product of the effort or determinations of the actor, either conscious or habitual" (Denno, 2002).

Very few defendants successfully invoke this defense, because the behavior it contemplates, action not controlled by the conscious mind, causes criminal results so infrequently. (But imagine if snoring otherwise fit the legal standard for the crime of harassment.) As a medical matter, it is clear that consciousness is a matter of more or less, and the law accepts that fact too. Thus, defendants have been exculpated for want of "voluntary" (in this special sense) behavior even when their actions were goal directed, as in some forms of epilepsy. The struggle to bring impulsive behavior under this rubric would be to refashion descriptions of behavior generally. From what I understand from the literature, when most of us act, we decide our action through unconscious processes (Libet et al., 2000). The role of consciousness is to approve or disapprove these behaviors. When we call an action "produced by our will," we mean that it was processed through brain centers that affirmed it or rejected it. Impulsive people—hopefully on some few limited occasions when under stress—do not exhibit the brain waves the rest of us do when we report ourselves conscious. Their behavior is neither ratified nor censored and is not properly called a product of the will. Nor is it properly called "habitual." All our behaviors are formulated unconsciously, and we would not call them all habitual, or the word would distinguish nothing.

Courts might accept such testimony if it were adequately grounded, although any substantial number of cases would surely result in legislative revision to assure at least that there was diagnostic and preventive confinement if juries ruled not guilty.

The third possible defense is to prove the defendant lacked the so-called mens rea or criminal intent required to commit the particular offense with which he is charged. For these explanatory purposes, it suffices to say that nearly all serious crimes are defined to oblige the state to prove not only that particular behavior was done, but also that the defendant had some mental awareness, or at least should have had, about the key features of his behavior that made it violate the particular offense charged. These mental requirements differ among crimes, and indeed differ in terms of various features of the same crime. In New York, for example, to convict a person of any form of arson, the prosecutor must establish that the defendant purposely started a fire or caused an explosion (N.Y. Penal Law §150.01). If the explosion ignited accidentally because the defendant was tap dancing on a steel floor in front of an open propane tank, it is not arson. If the defendant purposely caused the explosion, however, the prosecution seeking conviction of fourth-degree arson need only show she was reckless—consciously disregarding serious risk—with respect to whether or not the explosion was likely to damage a building or car (N.Y. Penal Law §150.05).

The strategy to convert "impulsivity" to a defense would be essentially the same as with voluntary acts. Intention and recklessness presuppose conscious evaluation of behavior. The argument is that this defendant never applied his intellect to his action, and therefore could not have acted with the mental state the law requires. The arguable advantages of framing the excuse this way, rather than in terms of involuntary action, are two. First, the voluntary act rule requires "will," and the classic cases to which the defendant is trying to assimilate his situation are ones in which there is no mind behind the action. While the law exempts "unconscious" behavior, the image it contemplates is behavior done while asleep. Our impulsive defendant controls his action. He is not asleep or epileptic. His behavior is instinctive rather than reflexive. Because mens rea rules require "conscious" behavior, the defense could say the action was volitionally their client's, but he engaged in it without the necessary conscious decisional processes. Second, the most serious crimes, like murder or aggravated assault, have lesser offenses included within them, such as negligent homicide or simple assault. Inasmuch as negligence requires only that a person *should* have known about risks, it can offer a way of providing some punishment, so that the jury is not put in the position of letting the defendant off scot-free.

In many states, and I believe in a majority, this defense will not work, because the law is settled that a "mental" condition can be a defense only if it amounts to insanity. Evidence of lesser abnormalities is specifically inadmissible if offered to prove culpability. The jury is required to assume it is dealing with a normal person.

That brings us back to whether you can possibly call the impulsive actor insane under the cognition test. If the evidence permits the argument that he did not "consciously" act, does that not also argue that he did not "appreciate" what he was doing for purposes of a cognition-based test? Maybe, but I think not. When courts ask whether a person "knows" something in applying mens rea tests, they usually mean that if he were asked, and answered honestly, he would have said, "Yes, I know that." For example, a person who buys a $1000 watch and does not declare it, but is not thinking about it as he hands over his Customs form, "knowingly" smuggles the watch. In judging whether a person knows right from wrong for insanity purposes, the question is his capacity at the time of the act, not whether he thought to himself, "I do wrong now."

To be sure, the defendant could argue that never having contemplated the act, he cannot be said to have appreciated its nature. The question, however, is whether he had the capacity to. While an expert might testify no, relying on capacity at the moment of action, more likely courts would say this smuggles the "volitional" impairment theory of insanity in through the back door.

I have made clear, I hope, that, while new behavioral genetics findings may affect discretionary decisions, I have seen nothing in the scientific literature that presently grounds any of these genetics-based efforts at doctrinal exculpation. At present, any attempt to present them should be barred by a trial judge pursuant to the rules that make trial judges gatekeepers for scientific evidence (*Daubert v. Merrell Dow Pharmaceuticals*, 1993). If strong scientific evidence developed, however, such defenses are not impossible. If the claim is that every third murderer fits this description, then law is certain to reject them by one technique or another.

Conclusions

Behavioral genetics research provides an occasion to revisit the central responsibility doctrines of the criminal law. The present research results, however, pose no realistic challenge to those doctrines. Indeed, the kinds of linkages found to date, because they show that people with particular genetic endowments are more likely to engage in certain behavior than others, but not everyone so endowed acts in the predicted way, do not strengthen the determinist's view of the world. And punishment as a social practice would, in any event, survive hard determinism.

The problem area lies outside the domain of formal doctrine. One task of criminal law is deciding what behavior should be made criminal, and I include as part of that task formulating rules about when people are responsible for their behavior. The second and less glamorous task is deciding what should be done with persons who do offend. To be sure, a lot of formal legal doctrine is present here too. Law sets out maximum and minimum sentences, and distributes authority to judges and probation authorities, along with many other tasks. In administering that system, however, and indeed, in any system imaginable in a complex society, people have to make some individualized assessments about the particular person before them. And people administering law necessarily bring to that task both their moral intuition about responsibility and their concern for future dangerousness.

We do not have in contemporary American society good gatekeeping mechanisms to filter new information into that necessarily informal system. The result is that decisions are likely to be influenced, toward both mitigating and enhancing penalties, by information that has cultural impact beyond its true scientific significance.

REFERENCES

Cases

Blakely v. Washington, 124 S.Ct. 2531 (2004)
Chicago v. Morales, 527 U.S. 41 (1999)
Daubert v. Merrell Dow Pharmaceuticals, 509 U.S. 79 (1993)
Harmelin v. Michigan, 501 U.S. 957 (1991)
Jurek v. Texas, 428 U.S. 262 (1976)
Kansas v. Hendricks, 521 U.S. 346 (1996)
Kansas v. Crane, 534 U.S. 407 (2002)
Rumsfeld v. Padilla, 124 S. Ct. 2711 (2004)
United States v. McBroom, 124 F.3rd 533 (3d Cir. 1997)
Goodridge v. Dept. of Public Health, 440 Mass, 309; 798, N.E.2d 941 (2003)

Publications

Baron, M. (2001). "Genes and Responsibility in Genetics and Criminal Behavior." In D. Wasserman and R. Wachbroit, eds. *Genetics and Criminal Behavior.* Cambridge Studies in Philosophy and Public Policy. New York: Cambridge University Press.
Coffee, M. (1993). "The Genetic Defense: Excuse or Explanation." *William and Mary Law Review* 35: 353.
Denno, D. W. (1996). "Legal Implications of Genetics and Crime Research." In G. Bock and J. Goode, eds. *Genetics of Criminal and Antisocial Behaviour.* CIBA Foundation Symposium. London: Wiley.

Denno, D. W. (2002). "Crime and Consciousness: Science and Involuntary Acts." *Minnesota Law Review* 87: 269.

Johnson, M. (1998). "Genetic Technology and its Impact on Culpability for Criminal Actions." *Cleveland State Law Review* 46: 443.

Libet, B., A. Freeman, and K. Suterland. (2000). *The Volitional Brain: Towards a Neuroscience of Free Will*. Exeter, U.K.: Imprint Academic.

Morse, S. (1994). "Culpability and Control." *University of Pennsylvania Law Review* 142:158.

Packer, H. (1968). *The Limits of the Criminal Sanction*." Stanford: Stanford University Press.

Perlin, M. (1990). "Unpacking the Myths: The Symbolism Mythology of Insanity Defense Jurisprudence." *Case Western Reserve Law Review* 46: 599.

Rafter, N. (2001). "Seeing and Believing: Images of Heredity in Biological Theories of Crime." *Brooklyn Law Review* 67: 71.

CHAPTER NINE

Behavioral Genetics and Equality

Dan W. Brock, Ph.D.

Extraordinary advances in our knowledge of human genetics have been made in recent decades. The Human Genome Project to sequence the entire human genome has been completed. We have already identified genes causing, or that are risk factors for, many diseases such as Huntington's chorea, cystic fibrosis, breast cancer, and Alzheimer disease. However, our knowledge of the functions of most genes remains at a very early stage and we know little about which genes operate to contribute to particular behavioral traits and capacities. Media announcements of the discovery of the "gene for" are regularly followed by challenges to the claims, with further research often leading to their withdrawal. Nevertheless, there is every reason to expect continued advances in future years in our knowledge of the functions of particular genes and how they interact with other genes and particular environmental conditions to shape phenotype.

There is controversy about the degree to which we will ever fully understand the genetic contribution to important human traits or capacities such as intelligence given the complexity of the traits and the likely extraordinary complexity of the genetic contribution to them, no doubt involving many genes interacting with each other and with the environment in complex ways. There is also controversy about the degree to which, and when, it may become possible to intervene to modify the genetic inheritance of future humans. The use of in vitro fertilization (IVF) together with preimplantation genetic diagnosis (PGD) already gives prospective parents some ability to select the traits of prospective offspring, though now principally only the ability to select embryos that do not have genes for particular diseases. It is likely that this or other technologies will at some point in the future enable further interventions to modify the genetic inheritance of children, not just to prevent disease but also to select for or to enhance some normal traits.

Advances in genetic knowledge are already contributing to the development of pharmaceuticals that are now being used by individuals in the absence of disease to enhance normal function. For example, the group of antidepressants known as selective serotonin reuptake inhibitors (SSRIs)—the most familiar of which is Prozac—is used by persons who are not clinically depressed to increase self-confidence and a general sense of well-being, as well as to reduce shyness. The drug Ritalin, used to treat attention deficit hyperactivity disorder (ADHD), is taken by some adults who have not been diagnosed with ADHD in order to increase their capacity to focus attention for sustained periods of time on tasks and activities. Modafilil, a drug used to treat narcolepsy, is used by some adults, such as long-distance truck drivers, to reduce sleepiness and their need for sleep in order to support their lifestyles. In the near term, pharmaceuticals have a much greater potential for modifying normal human traits and characteristics than does genetic modification, whose potential is more uncertain and lies much farther in the future.

In addition to advances in molecular genetics, work in behavioral genetics, much of it employing twin studies, has increased our knowledge of the genetic contribution to many behavioral traits. For example, some behavioral geneticists have concluded that genetic differences contribute in the area of 40 to 50 percent of the variability in general intelligence, although there is controversy both about the estimate as well as how widely and under what environmental conditions it holds. Bipolar disease (manic depression) and impulsivity and its contribution to violent and criminal behavior have also received the attention of behavioral geneticists. While some people may have wished to believe, though often for unsound reasons, that important human variation in behavior was principally or even entirely due to environmental influences, the results of work in behavioral genetics have made such beliefs increasingly untenable.

We face then, both now and in the future, two broad consequences of genetic advances with potential importance for issues of equality. The first consequence is that many natural differences between persons in traits such as intelligence that affect their opportunities in life and well-being may increasingly come to some degree within our control, if and when we gain the ability to manipulate children's genetic inheritance. To the extent that they do come within human control, the distribution of genes will no longer be determined by chance or a "natural lottery," but will depend in part as well on social interventions that we take or fail to take. The distribution of these traits and differences will become subject to assessment by our concepts of equity and justice; elsewhere, I (and my co-authors) called this the "colonization of the natural by the just" (Buchanan et al., 2000). The second consequence is that if our belief in people's equal moral worth and status depends on a belief in their natural equality in some respects, for example, in their sharing a common human nature, then to the extent that behavioral genetics undermines belief in that natural equality between humans, it may undermine in turn the commitment to their moral, social, or political equality. My aim in this chapter is to explore both these possible consequences of genetics and behavioral genetics for equality.

It may be helpful at the outset to make clear that I am exploring concerns about two quite distinct notions of equality in what follows. The first conception of equality is that which figures prominently in one form or another in many conceptions of distributive justice. This conception concerns when inequalities in advantages and disadvantages between persons are morally justified. As the well-known "equality of what" debate makes clear, even among egalitarians there is disagreement about what the proper focus or "space" for egalitarian principles should be—for example, equality of welfare, resources, primary goods, capabilities, opportunity, opportunity for welfare, and so forth (Sen, 1980; Arneson, 1989; Dworkin, 1981; Cohen, 1993; Roemer, 1989). Moreover, there is disagreement about what factors can justify inequalities in these various spaces—for example, need, effort, contribution, merit, and so forth. The point to be emphasized here is that these debates address the criteria for justifying inequalities between persons. The other conception of equality holds that despite various differences between persons in their abilities, character, accomplishments, contributions, and so forth, they all have equal moral worth or equal standing as members of the moral community; sometimes this point is put in terms of the equal human dignity and human rights possessed by all persons simply as persons, or the equal moral concern and respect they all deserve simply as persons. Just what this second sense of equality comes to or implies, as well as what its ground or basis is, are not my concern now, though they will be briefly later. The point now is that the first consequence about natural inequalities coming within our control to change largely concerns the first sense of equality, whereas the second consequence about our belief that persons' natural equality grounds their moral equality largely concerns the second sense of equality. It is important not to confuse them.

Natural Inequalities and Equality of Opportunity

What will be the consequences for our view of justified inequalities between persons of those persons' natural or genetic endowments coming increasingly within our control? I approach this question by first elaborating several different components of the notion of equality of opportunity. Some conception of equality is arguably a component of all moral theories (Sen, 1980; Arneson, 1989; Dworkin, 1981; Cohen, 1993; Roemer, 1989). Moreover, some conception of equality of opportunity is a component of many otherwise different overall conceptions of distributive justice. Equality of opportunity is important in the distribution of scarce benefits or positions when all who want or would benefit from them cannot have them. Giving all an equal opportunity to gain such benefits or roles is typically understood to be a matter of fairness— it gives all a fair chance to obtain the benefit or position when scarcity prevents all from obtaining it. But what more specifically does equality of opportunity require? In answering this question we will see that it is more complex than it might at first seem.

A minimal conception of equality of opportunity is formal equality of opportunity. It attacks legal or quasi-legal constraints on people's freedom to compete for scarce benefits or roles. Formal equality of opportunity is violated by legal rules, or legally sanctioned rules or practices within institutions, that preclude particular individuals or groups from competing for scarce benefits or roles. For example, formal rules that "no blacks need apply" for desirable positions violate formal equality of opportunity; so, likewise, do informal practices that impose quotas on the numbers of otherwise qualified individuals from a particular group who will be selected for the benefit or position, such as a job or admission to a university or professional school. Ensuring formal equality of opportunity has been extremely important historically in the

United States and elsewhere in securing equality of opportunity for groups subject to prejudice and discrimination, but it falls far short of full equality of opportunity.

Fair equality of opportunity adds two other requirements. The first is that the qualifying conditions for a scarce role or position must be reasonably related to performance in the role or position and not such that they unfairly disadvantage otherwise qualified competitors. For example, the Scholastic Aptitude Tests, which are typically very important in admission to selective colleges and universities, have been attacked on grounds that they require knowledge of facts that is unrelated to performance in college and that is likely to be differentially possessed by different socioeconomic, racial, or ethnic groups. Promotion tests in police and fire departments likewise have been attacked on grounds that they test for knowledge that is not reasonably related to performance in the positions to which applicants seek promotion.

The second component of fair equality of opportunity requires the removal of social and environmental barriers to individuals or groups successfully meeting the qualifying conditions within competition for scarce benefits or positions. It is in meeting this requirement that education is of great importance for equality of opportunity. Education is critical in qualifying for a wide variety of desirable positions within modern societies. That is why free public elementary and secondary education is widely accepted as essential to equality of opportunity. Likewise, since a college education has also become increasingly important for access to many desirable jobs and positions, equality of opportunity requires low-cost public colleges as well as financial aid in private institutions to allow poor as well as wealthier young people to obtain the qualifying condition of a college education needed for those jobs and positions. Programs like Head Start to compensate for deprivations in the home environments of very young children and nutritional programs for pregnant women or for their very young children to avoid the adverse cognitive and other effects on children of inadequate nutrition are both examples of efforts to remove social or environmental barriers so all children will have a fair chance at success in later competing for desirable jobs and positions.

It should go without saying that in the United States, and elsewhere, we are far from fully realizing the requirements of formal and fair equality of opportunity. There remain informal quotas directed against some disadvantaged groups, elementary and secondary education available to different socioeconomic groups is often of widely varying quality, many young people cannot

afford even the charges of low-cost public colleges, and many children still suffer the lifelong effects of inadequate nutrition prenatally or in early childhood.
Yet even if formal and fair equality of opportunity were fully realized, there
would still be large differences between individuals in their opportunities and
well-being. Some of these would be due to a variety of good or bad luck—being in the right place at the right time to obtain a benefit or a job, being the
victim of an accident, and so on. But many such residual inequalities in individuals' opportunities and well-being would be due to differences in their natural or genetic endowments—the result of their good or bad luck in the natural lottery.

How should those committed to achieving equality of opportunity view
these residual inequalities resulting from genetically based natural differences
between persons? In John Rawls's influential account of fair equality of opportunity, he accepts that equality of opportunity is compatible with differences in outcomes between persons in their opportunities and well-being
caused by differences in their natural assets (Rawls, 1971). What fair equality
of opportunity requires is equal opportunities for those similarly endowed and
motivated. Moreover, it is not hard to understand why equality of opportunity
is standardly interpreted in this way. We have at this time almost no ability to
intervene to affect people's biological inheritance or genome, though of course
we do have some ability to undertake medical or environmental interventions
that will affect the phenotypic expression of an individual's genome. And, of
course, it is typically impossible to know the degree to which a particular ca-
pability of an individual such as general intelligence is the result of his genetic
inheritance or of environmental influences to which he has been subject,
though we do know that genetic differences are important contributors to individual variation in such traits.

So if individuals protest that they lack equality of opportunity because they
have inferior genetically based natural endowments, the only practical response now is, "Sorry, but there's nothing we can do about that. We have no
control over your genetic inheritance." The most that we can do now is to try
to arrange their environments to maximize the phenotypic expression of desirable traits and/or to compensate in other ways for their bad luck in the genetic lottery. But in the future, though we do not know how soon and to what
extent, it may not always be possible to make that response. Genetic modification or selection is likely to become possible that will enable us to reduce or
remove some genetically based disadvantages in natural endowments that

would otherwise handicap individuals in competition for scarce benefits and roles. It appears that the same kind of moral complaint based in equality of opportunity would then apply to a failure to use these genetic means to remove a disadvantage in natural endowments as is now accepted for failures to remove socially based disadvantages. If a person is at a disadvantage in competing for many jobs because of cognitive limitations due to poor schools, equality of opportunity is violated by a failure to have improved those schools, and if she is at the same disadvantage because of a failure to use a genetic intervention to remove a comparable cognitive limitation, equality of opportunity looks to be equally violated.

As Bernard Williams pointed out many years ago, this seems to collapse equality of opportunity, which is typically assumed to be compatible with inequalities in outcomes, into equality as identity (Williams, 1972). Any characteristic of a person that puts her at a comparative disadvantage with others in competition for scarce benefits or positions seems to violate equality of opportunity if it is within human control to change it so as to remove that disadvantage. The ideal of equality of opportunity thus appears to be that persons suffer no socially caused or naturally caused disadvantages in such competitions, and that would seem to require that there be no social or natural differences between individuals that create such disadvantages. To the extent that achieving equality of opportunity presses in the direction of equality as identity, valuable human diversity and idiosyncrasy would also be at risk.

This is not to say, of course, that U.S. society will be likely to have the social commitment and political will to actually ensure the availability of any such genetic modification to reduce inequality in opportunity any more than it has had the social commitment or political will to undertake the necessary social interventions to change educational and other social institutions to ensure equality of opportunity; the disgraceful quality of many schools in poor urban areas attests to our failure to take action now possible to improve equality of opportunity. My point is only that the same moral complaint seems potentially applicable in the future to the genetic case as is applicable now to the social case of education.

We will also have good reason in some cases to fail to do all that would be necessary to achieve equality of opportunity. Even before the age of genetic engineering, we know that making all the social changes necessary to achieve equality of opportunity would conflict with other important and legitimate aims and values. Perhaps the most obvious example is the institution of the family. Parents, acting on natural and valuable desires to give their children the best chance in life that they can, confer a variety of advantages on their children—nurturing home environments, high-quality education, special opportunities to develop particular talents, and so forth. To avoid these consequences of parents' natural love and concern for their children would require deep intrusions into the family, indeed probably the end of the family as we know it in modern Western societies. We are justified in failing to achieve full equality of opportunity to the extent that doing so is necessary to preserve fundamental and valuable features of the family. So my point here is not that we will have good moral reason, all things considered, to do all that equality of opportunity could require in the future in the way of genetic modifications, just as we sometimes now do not have good reason, all things considered, to do everything by way of social interventions that equality of opportunity would require because of its conflict with other important values and institutions. The point is rather that the scope or reach of the concern for equality of opportunity will extend from the social into the genetic realm as well.

Using a metaphor from sports, equality of opportunity is often characterized as requiring a "level playing field" for competitors for scarce benefits and roles. In work done together with Allen Buchanan, Norman Daniels, and Daniel Wikler, we distinguished two variants of a level playing field account of equality of opportunity (Buchanan et al., 2000). What we called the social structural account roughly matches Rawls's account of fair equality of opportunity (Rawls, 1971). It focuses on removing the opportunity-limiting effects of social barriers and injustices. On the social structural view natural differences between persons are not irrelevant to justice. For example, Rawls's difference principle holds that inequalities in income and wealth are only justified to the extent that they maximize the expectations of the worst-off representative group in society; this principle applies to inequalities in income and wealth arising from natural as well as social inequalities. But his principle of fair equality of opportunity does not require eliminating or reducing natural differences if and when we could do so. What we called the brute luck account, on the other hand, condemns all unchosen inequalities between persons (Cohen, 1993; Arneson, 1989). It holds that persons should not suffer lesser opportunities or be worse off than others through no fault of their own or from factors beyond their control. At the present time one's genetic endowment is a paradigm example of what is beyond an individual's control. The brute luck view draws a distinction between good or bad brute luck and good or bad option luck. Disadvantages that are the result of bad option luck are disadvantages one suffers because of choices one has freely made, knowing, or when one should have known, that the bad outcome was a risk one was taking in making the choice. Disadvantages that are the result of bad brute luck are disadvantages one suffers for which one bears no responsibility and which did not result from one's choices. In the brute luck view, inequalities that are the result of bad option luck are permissible, whereas inequalities that are the result of bad brute luck are not justified.

An example will illustrate the different implications of the two accounts. Intelligence, for example, as measured by IQ tests, has an important effect on one's opportunities in life, and normal intelligence varies within a wide range and in the absence of disease. Consider the case of Adam and Bert, each of whom has an IQ of 90. Adam's is his "native intelligence," reflecting his genetic inheritance and a normal environment. Bert's IQ had been 110, but was reduced by a childhood exposure to a toxin negligently introduced into the environment where he lived. Suppose, fancifully, that a psychopharmacological intervention is developed that would raise their IQs by about 10 points. Is there any moral difference in the claims on grounds of equality of opportunity of Adam and Bert to obtain this medication? On the fair equality of opportunity/social structural account, Adam would have no claim to the medication. His lower than average IQ is not the result of any social barrier or injustice, or any disease; it is only his native intelligence. Now if an environmental intervention that would have raised his IQ, perhaps access to Head Start or other early interventions, could have been made at reasonable cost but was not, then his IQ deficit is arguably the result of social injustice, not simply a natural deficit. The baseline against which to measure natural as opposed to unjustly socially induced deficits is in part morally determined; here it depends on whether there are early interventions that our conception of justice requires that would have raised Adam's IQ. In my example, however, assume that Adam's IQ of 90 is the result after having made all environmental interventions that our conception of justice and equality of opportunity require. What of Bert? His lower than average IQ is caused by an unjust social condition. Equality of opportunity requires removing the harmful condition, or in Bert's case taking steps necessary to rectify its effects on his intelligence and opportunities. Bert then has a claim to the new medication grounded in equality of opportunity. And note that this will be true on the social structural account even if the environmental toxin caused a mutation of the same genes in Bert that are responsible for Adam's lower native intelligence.

From the perspective of the brute luck view of equality, however, this distinction appears arbitrary. Both Adam and Bert suffer from the same disadvantage—their lower than average IQ—and both could benefit equally from the medication that would raise it. The disadvantage in each case is unchosen and no fault of their own. What, then, is the brute luck account of equality of opportunity committed to regarding genetic modifications to remove inequalities in natural endowments such as genetically caused disadvantages in traits like intelligence, if and when they become possible? Is it committed to equalization of natural assets, that is, to any interventions that would remove disadvantages in natural assets?

Equalization of natural assets is not a plausible goal even for the brute luck theorist, and even if the genetic interventions necessary to realize it were possible, for at least two reasons. First, there are no fixed accounts of natural assets, nor more important of their relative value or importance. What count as natural assets depends to a significant degree on the social and economic organization within which individuals live. For example, within an agrarian society in which most labor is physical, physical strength and stamina may be especially important natural assets, whereas in a modern information-based technological society certain cognitive capacities will be of much greater importance. The value of traits changes over time as a society's social, political, and economic framework changes and evolves.

Second, value pluralism about the nature of a good life will give rise to reasonable differences among persons about the relative value of different natural assets; for example, fine motor skills will be of great importance to a musician such as a violinist, but of much less importance to a philosopher. Within limits, our values regarding what is a valuable life will be shaped in part by the particular natural assets that we have and are able to develop; there is no neutral standpoint that gets behind the particular values and plans of life to which we commit ourselves from which to evaluate the relative importance of different natural assets. Moreover, sometimes surface agreement masks deeper disagreement about the value of traits. For example, although initiative might be agreed to be a valuable trait, a particular individual might be described by some as having initiative and by others as being too pushy; although altruism might be agreed to be a desirable trait, some may praise an individual as altruistically concerned for others, while others see her as unduly self-sacrificing and lacking in a sense of her own worth. These disagreements would be compounded if we had to seek agreement on what overall packages of natural assets are of equal value; people would disagree about the extent to which a deficit in one area, for example, intelligence, was compensated for by a relative strength or advantage in another, for example, a "sunny" disposition.

Moreover, a commitment to equalizing natural assets is subject to the "leveling down" problem (Parfit, 1991). If equality is the goal, it could be achieved by reducing the natural endowments of those with exceptional natural assets and abilities when we could not raise the less talented and able to their level. Derek Parfit imagines a community in which half are sighted and half are blind and puts the leveling down objection to equality as follows:

> it would in one way be better if we removed the eyes of the sighted, not to give them to the blind, but simply to make the sighted blind. That would be in one way better even if it was in *no* way better for the blind. This we may find impossible to believe . . . It is not enough to claim it would be wrong to produce equality by leveling down . . . Our objection must be that, if we achieve equality by leveling down, there is *nothing* good about what we have done.

This suggests that our moral concern is not with equality as such, but with improving the condition of the worse off; Parfit calls this the priority view because it gives higher priority to benefiting people the worse off they are.

For all of these reasons, equalizing people's natural assets, even if the necessary control over people's genetic inheritance was within our power, is not a conceptually coherent, ethically defensible, or politically feasible goal. Elsewhere, we suggested that if the distribution of genetic endowments is thought to come within the domain of justice, then a genetic "decent minimum" may be the appropriate goal (Buchanan et al., 2000). The idea would be that none should have significant enough deficits in genetic endowments and the natural endowments they support to be denied a fair share of the range of opportunities available to persons generally in their society.

Inequality and Equal Moral Worth

I claimed earlier that one important consequence of advances in genetics is that people's genetic endowments may come increasingly within our control. Initially, the main effect will be the ability to use genetic testing, either of prospective parents preconception or of a fetus after conception, to determine the risk for, or presence of, serious genetic disease and to avoid the birth of children with such conditions; this practice is already widespread in developed countries. Serious genetic disease is one significant source of inequalities between people to the extent that it impairs their functioning and in turn opportunities and well-being. In this respect, the effect of advances in genetic testing and prevention of genetic disease will be to reduce inequalities in opportunities and well-being between persons. Of course, to the extent that these means of preventing genetic disease in offspring are not available to the millions in the United States who lack health insurance, or who lack insurance that covers testing and the other services such as abortion necessary to prevent genetic disease, genetic diseases may come to be increasingly concentrated in the poor and uninsured. This effect could be even more pronounced internationally, where genetic testing is largely unavailable in poor countries. So even in the context only of preventing genetic disease, it is difficult to predict the likely net effects on inequality of increasing capacity to use genetic testing to prevent disease.

The principal worry of egalitarians about the longer term, however, is that even if genetic testing to reduce the prevalence of disease has the effect of reducing inequality, other inequality-increasing effects of new control over people's genetic endowments may overwhelm that desirable effect. The worry specifically concerns the potential effects of genetic enhancements of normal functions and traits, should they become possible. Suppose, for example, that genetic enhancement becomes possible of people's memory, intelligence, immune system, self-esteem, or need for sleep. These enhancements would all be significant advantages in a variety of work and other contexts. There would undoubtedly be great demand for them. Right now, many persons with no disease or illness already seek out some pharmaceuticals for purposes of enhancement. As noted above, persons who have not been diagnosed as depressed use the new SSRI antidepressants like Prozac to increase their self-confidence in social and other settings and some adults use Ritalin to increase their capacity to focus attention on tasks for sustained periods of time. If germ line genetic enhancements become possible, the effects of the enhancements may potentially accumulate over time and across generations.

Who would be able to obtain these enhancements for their children or themselves? First, it is likely that they would be expensive procedures. Second, they would be unlikely to be covered by health insurance. Health insurance generally uses a "medical necessity" standard for coverage; crudely put, interventions are medically necessary when they are needed to treat disease or injury. Enhancements are by definition not intended to treat disease or injury, but rather are intended to enhance the function of normal, healthy persons. Given their likely expense, there is little reason to believe that health insurers would extend coverage to them. Moreover, they would be difficult to cover with insurance in any case. Insurance is typically used for uncontrollable and unpredictable events and is designed to spread the uneven costs of individuals over a broader pool of persons many of whom, while members of the pool of insured persons, do not suffer the event insured for. Enhancements do not fit this condition of insurability. Nearly everyone would have reason to want such enhancements were they to become possible. Insurance premiums for them would have to be priced at or near the full costs of the procedures, even disregarding insurance administrative costs.

So the result would be that wealthier individuals would be able to purchase genetic enhancements for themselves and their children, while the poor and middle class would find them unaffordable. In poorer developing countries virtually no one would be able to afford them. Privileged members of society already are able to confer various social advantages on their children—high-quality private schools and universities, special lessons and camps, social connections and privileges. They would now be able to confer genetic advantages on their children as well, compounding the inequalities between classes. Frances Fukuyama suggested that new capacities for genetic modification could decrease rather than increase inequality: "it seems highly unlikely that people in modern democratic societies will sit around complacently if they see elites embedding their advantages genetically in their children." Indeed, he sees this as an issue that people will be roused to fight over, not just politically, "but actually picking up guns and bombs and using them on other people" (Fukuyama, 2002, 158). One alternative to avoid this conflict would be to employ regulation to forbid the use of biotechnology for enhancement, but he recognizes that this may be difficult to pass and enforce, or that it might be struck down by the courts. Alternatively, state-sponsored eugenics might resurface not in the old form of discouraging or preventing those thought to have inferior genes from breeding, but in the form of using genetic modification to raise the bottom by breeding children who are "more intelligent, more healthy, more 'normal'" (158). Fukuyama notes that this would require the Left, which has been generally hostile to biotechnology, both to acknowledge the importance of heredity more than it generally has and to be willing to use biotechnology in the service of reducing hereditary inequalities.

At this point in time, of course, one can only speculate about whether the pessimistic or optimistic scenario is more likely. If Fukuyama is correct, then democratic forces in effect will succeed in pressing the brute luck interpretation of the requirements of equality of opportunity into the domain of people's genetic inheritance. This would result in raising the absolute position of the genetically disadvantaged and reducing their relative disadvantage, at least if the genetic gains to the disadvantaged are not outweighed by the gains from genetic enhancements to the better-off. On the other hand, recent experience lends some support to the more pessimistic scenario, at least for the United States. Economic inequality has been increasing in recent decades, not decreasing, in part from the rising role of education and cognitive skills in work. U.S. society exhibits great tolerance of socially and environmentally caused inequalities in education, income distribution, and other conditions that affect people's opportunities and well-being, and it is hard to be confident that it would be intolerant of genetic inequalities.

Moreover, there is an important complexity that will make it difficult, both ethically and politically, to limit the use of genetic enhancements. Consider some examples of traits that it might be possible to enhance through genetic modification in the future—memory, capacity to focus attention more intensely and for more sustained periods, longevity, and general intelligence. Each of these (with the possible exception of longevity) is a trait whose enhancement would have obvious competitive advantages in education, the workplace, and other competitive contexts. In that respect, to be better off than average in any of these traits constitutes a positional or competitive advantage over others who are not better than average in the trait. Being less well off than others in any of these traits is therefore grounds for a complaint based on fairness and equality of opportunity, and we might, as Fukuyama suggests, regulate the use of these enhancements on such grounds. But an enhancement of any of these traits would also constitute a nonpositional or noncompetitive, intrinsic benefit to its recipient. By an intrinsic benefit I mean a benefit that makes its recipient better off without making anyone else worse off. Take the capacity to focus one's attention more intensely and for more sustained periods of time—this could enrich one's life in many ways, such as increasing and deepening one's enjoyment of music, which would not make anyone else worse off. While regulation of this enhancement could be supported on grounds of fairness and equality of opportunity because of its competitive advantage, its regulation could be opposed on grounds of its intrinsic benefit. "Why should you prevent me from using my own resources to make my life better—no one else is made worse off by my greater pleasure from listening to music?" those who seek the enhancement would argue. The complexity for public policy is that most real examples of traits and capacities that we may gain the capacity to enhance and that people will want to enhance will provide complex combinations of positional and intrinsic benefits. This will make the ethical case for limiting their use by regulation more complex and the political task of doing so more difficult.

Suppose, therefore, that the future onset of capacities for genetic enhancement in fact leads to increasing inequalities in many important human traits and capacities, as well as to greater socioeconomic inequalities. How might this affect beliefs about people's equal moral worth and general acceptance of their equal moral worth? How might it affect our belief in human rights, which are rights that all people have simply by virtue of being human and which are an important aspect of their equal moral worth? The question seems to turn on whether the claim of equal moral worth rests on there being at least some limit in the degree of inequalities in the characteristics that would be enhanced. If so, then it might be that if that limit was significantly exceeded by a widespread use of genetic enhancement, the basis for the claim of equal moral worth would be undermined. So what is the basis or ground of people's equal moral worth?

It is unquestionable that the equal moral status of human beings rests on some nonmoral or empirical properties they share, or, as it is sometimes put, on a common human nature. No one argues that it is seriously morally wrong to destroy living bacteria or viruses and that is presumably because they lack the properties that make it wrong to kill or destroy humans. Of course, exactly what those properties are and whether every member of the human species has them, including extremely damaged and impaired members, is notoriously controversial; so also is whether members of any other species share those properties. And even among those who believe it is seriously wrong to kill some nonhuman animals, no one ascribes rights of free speech and expression to animals; virtually no one holds that members of any other species share the full moral rights, claims, and interests of humans. So if all persons deserve equal concern and respect, or have equal moral worth, that must be based on empirical properties in which humans differ from members of other species.

Frances Fukuyama argued that it is the way human language, human reason, human moral choice, and human emotions combine in human beings that give them human dignity. His concept of human dignity, which all humans share, is roughly equivalent to what I mean by equal moral worth. Human dignity rests on human nature, what he calls Factor X, which is a whole that is greater than the sum of its parts.

> If what gives us dignity and a moral status higher than that of other living creatures is related to the fact that we are complex wholes rather than the sum of simple parts, then it is clear that there is no simple answer to the question, What is Factor X? That is, Factor X cannot be reduced to the possession of moral choice, or reason, or language, or sociability, or sentience, or emotions, or consciousness, or any other quality that has been put forth as a ground for human dignity. It is all of these qualities coming together in a human whole that make up Factor X. Every member of the human species possesses a genetic endowment that allows him or her to become a whole human being, an endowment that distinguishes a human in essence from other types of creatures. (Fukuyama, 2002, 171)

Now the claim of this last sentence is false. Some humans have been left so impaired by their genetic endowment that they lack capacities for language or reason or emotion necessary to become a "whole human being" in this sense. And on this line of thinking about human dignity, that raises serious problems about whether human dignity should be attributed to them. However, the moral status of very seriously impaired humans is a difficult problem for any secular moral view and that is not my concern here.

What are the implications of this view for the source of human dignity and in turn of human rights for genetic modification and enhancement that may become possible in the future? Here is Fukuyama's answer to this question:

> What is it that we want to protect from any future advances in biotechnology? The answer is, we want to protect the full range of our complex evolved natures against attempts at self-modification. We do not want to disrupt either the unity or the continuity of human nature, and thereby the human rights that are based on it. (Fukuyama, 2002, 172)

But is this the right answer to the question? I believe it is not. Our species, like other species, is continually evolving and it is not necessary to freeze it in place at where it happens to be at present in order to protect the human nature that grounds human dignity. It is correct that we do not want to modify humans in ways that would destroy or seriously impair important human capacities. But that only means that we must approach any possible genetic modifications with appropriate caution and prior research to understand the full consequences of the modification, and with an appreciation of the limits of our understanding of genetic complexity. This is not dissimilar to the caution needed generally regarding medical interventions in light of the complexity of the human body, or environmental changes in light of the complexity of the environment. Whether it is new pharmaceuticals or new medical procedures and interventions, they should be tested for safety and efficacy before being introduced into use, and the same holds for genetic modifications.

Enhancements, just as treatments, will have risks and uncertainties that need to be appropriately understood and minimized before they are employed, and their risk/benefit ratios will often be less favorable than treatments directed at serious human disease. Successful treatment of serious disease produces substantial benefits that can justify significant risks. Normally functioning individuals do not suffer serious functional impairments that would justify comparable risks. But suppose a trait such as memory, or a particular form of memory, is widely enhanced so that most people have the memory that only a few humans now have who are said to have a "photographic memory." What reason would there be to think this would interfere with human nature in a way that threatens human dignity? And suppose other traits such as general intelligence or human reasoning capacities could be similarly enhanced so that all could be brought up to where those now at the high end of the normal range of these traits are. Again, what reason would there be to think this would interfere with human nature in a way that threatens human dignity? If anything, wouldn't it increase human dignity?

The broader lesson here is that the "natural," or better, what is now the natural, lacks any moral significance or weight just in virtue of being what is natural. And human nature likewise lacks moral significance or weight just in virtue of being what is now natural for humans. This is not to say that typical human capacities such as those to which Fukuyama appeals, like language, reason, and emotion, are not morally significant, but only that retaining them in their present form is not necessary for human dignity or equal moral worth. And in particular, improving any of these capacities would not in itself undermine human dignity or moral worth.

So I believe that modifying what Fukuyama calls the "unity and continuity" of human nature need not threaten human nature if those modifications are truly enhancements of desirable human traits whose safety has been adequately established. Instead, any threat to human dignity must be from these enhancements being only selectively available to some individuals, groups, or social classes and not others, and that is what I suggested above is likely to be the case. So the worry for moral equality must be an increasing inequality between individuals, groups, or classes in important human traits such as intelligence. And these inequalities could compound over time from germ line genetic modifications that are passed down across generations. Now it is important to emphasize that the various capacities that Fukuyama and others believe constitute our common human nature—reason, intelligence, language, emotions, and the like—and ground human rights are now possessed by individuals and groups across a fairly broad range; intelligence is perhaps the most obvious example. This means that the common human nature we now share, and that is thought to ground human dignity and people's equal moral worth, must be compatible with a significant range of variation. Being even near the lower end of that range is enough to possess the human nature that grounds human dignity and human rights. But enhancing some individuals or groups in the future to the higher ends of this range, or even enhancing some above what is now the higher end of this range, will still leave those who are at the lower end of the range where they are now; those at that lower end will still be at a level now considered sufficient for a human nature grounding human dignity, moral equality, and human rights. It might be argued that we are mistaken now in believing that the combinations of the various capacities typical in persons at the lower end of the normal ranges of such capacities are sufficient to ground their human dignity and human rights. But the possibility or reality of genetic enhancements would not support that argument. If we are not so mistaken, then future individuals with the same level of capacities as those who are now at the lower end of the range will still have capacities sufficient to ground their human dignity and rights, even if in that future world some will have substantially enhanced capacities. The degree of inequality should not undermine what is morally owed to those at the lower end of the range of the relevant human capacities, so long as that level remains the same, either now or in the future when the higher end of the range may be substantially raised.

We do know from history that those who have been denied full moral status, whose equal moral worth and human rights have been denied, have often been viewed as subhuman. This was a typical justification for the institution of slavery in the United States in the eighteenth and nineteenth centuries, and it was a central part of the justification offered by the Nazis for their treatment of Jews and disabled persons. But this still was not just a belief that whites were superior to blacks, or Germans superior to Jews or disabled persons, but more specifically that the latter were not fully human, that they did not fall within the range of capacities of normal humans; they were believed not to share a common human nature because they were believed to fall below the range of normal humans. For the reasons discussed earlier, a widening inequality in people's well-being and opportunities from genetic or other enhancements would be unfair and a violation of equality of opportunity, but it will not provide any justification for treating those still at the low end of the normal range any worse than we are justified treating those now at the low end of that range, whom we do in fact accept as sharing in a human nature that grounds human dignity and human rights. So the point is that the human nature that is necessary to ground human rights will still be possessed by the unenhanced even if new enhancement technology raises the capacity of many others above their level.

Nevertheless, it is a truism that people seem to find it easier to mistreat others whom they deem different, and in particular inferior to themselves, and if some groups have significantly enhanced capacities, thereby widening inequalities between themselves and those who have not had access to such enhancements, the degree to which the enhanced will feel and be superior to the unenhanced would increase. It is even possible that if widespread and extremely powerful enhancement technologies are developed, their selective use over time by some classes could widen greatly the normal range of human capacities; some individuals or groups might even come to have capabilities that we cannot now imagine humans having. It is important to underline that enhancement capabilities of this power and scope probably exist only in the realm of science fiction, and if they ever become a reality it will only be in the very distant future. But a wide enough degree of inequality in capacities and capabilities between different groups could undermine humans' important capacity to identify with the needs, suffering, and concerns of other people. This capacity for moral identification with others, our ability to put ourselves in others' shoes and see things from their perspectives, is important to our recognition of others as sharing a common humanity and as deserving of equal moral concern and respect. The unenhanced might come to seem so different, and in particular so inferior in important respects, as to also undermine belief in democratic equality in favor of a natural aristocracy. Those with vastly superior capabilities could come to associate only with others like themselves and to see the unenhanced as inferior and alien beings with whom they had little in common. In the face of such widespread, deep, and pervasive "natural" inequalities, it would be difficult to sustain a true shared moral community or democratic political institutions that respected the human rights of all. Besides the unfairness and denial of equality of opportunity to those without access to the enhancements, this would be a further compelling reason to avoid such greatly increased inequalities that powerful enhancement technologies could make possible.

As I have argued above, it would be a mistake to believe that the unenhanced were undeserving of human dignity and human rights in the face of greatly widened inequalities in capabilities, just as it would be a mistake to deny human rights to those now at the lower end of a much narrower range of human capabilities; those with lesser capabilities in each case have the necessary human capabilities to lead self-governing, worthwhile lives and are deserving of equal moral concern and respect. However, if the mistake would likely be commonly made, then we have strong reasons to avoid the conditions that would lead to it. But I end by emphasizing that the moral objection is not to enhancement technologies in themselves, but only to the selective access to them in ways that would greatly exacerbate social, economic, and moral inequalities.

REFERENCES

Arnes, R. (1989). "Equality and Equality of Opportunity for Welfare." *Philosophical Studies* 56(1):77–73.
Cohen, G. A. (1993). "Equality of What?: On Welfare Goods and Capabilities." In M. Nussbaum and A. Sen, eds. *The Quality of Life*. Oxford: Clarendon.
Dworkin, R. (1981). "What is Equality?" *Philosophy and Public Affairs* 10(3): 185–246 (Part I); 10(4): 285–345 (Part II).
Buchanan, A., D. W. Brock, N. Daniels, and D. Wikler. (2000). *From Chance to Choice: Genetics and Justice*. Cambridge: Cambridge University Press.
Fukuyama, F. (2002). *Our Posthuman Future: Consequences of the Biotechnology Revolution*. New York: Farrar, Straus and Giroux.
Parfit, D. (1991). "Equality or Priority?" The Lindley Lecture. Department of Philosophy, University of Kansas.
Rawls, J. (1971). *A Theory of Justice*. Cambridge, Mass.: Harvard University Press.

Roemer, J. (1989). "Equality and Responsibility." *Boston Review* 20(2): 3–7.

Sen, A. (1980). "Equality of What?" In S. McMurrin, ed. *Tanner Lectures on Human Values*. Cambridge: Cambridge University Press.

Williams, B. (1972). "The Idea of Equality." In P. Laslett and W. G. Runciman, eds. *Philosophy, Politics and Society*. Oxford: Blackwell.

CHAPTER TEN

Behavioral Genetics and Moral Responsibility

Gregory E. Kaebnick, Ph.D.

One unnerving ramification of behavioral genetics is that it might upend some of our usual ways of talking about human agency. In particular, it might seem to make talk about moral responsibility and freedom of the will nonsensical. When we hold people responsible for what they do—assigning either blame or credit—we make an assumption that they have some self-control: they could have done otherwise, and what they did is what they *chose* to do. But discoveries in behavioral genetics sometimes seem to suggest that people were *driven* to do what they did. Given their genetic makeup, they were not able, or were scarcely able, to control their behavior. Their genes made them do it. Tourette's syndrome provides the model. Once the offensive utterances of people with Tourette's might have seemed opprobrious; now, it seems clear, they are not. People with Tourette's say offensive things, and may offend some people, but they do not commit offenses. If all behavior can be explained in the way Tourette's can, what will happen to the very idea of moral responsibility? So goes one line of concern.

Strictly speaking, free will regards our control over what we do. It is about actions—about what agents do. The problem behavioral genetics poses for free will is usually expressed in terms of actions, but it presents itself first as a question about our control over what kind of people we *are*—whether we will be anxious, happy, shy, easily aroused to anger, and so on. These are questions of character or temperament. The challenge that behavioral genetics poses to our control over *who we are* seems, on its face, more serious, but also less revolutionary. It has long been accepted that character and temperament owe a lot to physical makeup—witness the Greek theories about bodily humors. Plainly, genes do not code directly for specific actions. But equally plainly, actions and character are interrelated. One's character inclines one to do certain things. Thus the question about freedom of the will and moral responsibility has this somewhat complicated form: do our genes give us characters, inclinations, that make it all but inevitable that we will on occasion behave in certain ways? Do they make us the sort of people who cannot help but do as we do?

This question is broad in scope. Although the courtroom is often the first thing we think of, there are many occasions in which we speak of responsibility and blame. When children don't pay attention in school, when employees don't work very hard, when friends make promises they don't keep, when opponents don't recognize others' viewpoints, when family members don't think about anybody except themselves, we will often hold them responsible and blame them. In all of these realms, behavioral genetics might affect the kinds of judgments we make. If we concluded that some people are fated by their genes to be narcissistic, the question would arise whether those people can be blamed for being narcissistic, to what extent they can reasonably be expected to overcome the narcissism, and whether special allowances should be granted them in, say, relationships or classrooms.

The problem might also prove hard to contain. The number of conditions that people might be "diagnosed" as having might multiply, and distinctions between diagnosable conditions and normal health might be hard to hold onto. If some people are identified as violent because of a diagnosable condition, and receive special allowances because of it, then others who are violent might wonder what really distinguishes them from the "genetically violent." The science is obviously incomplete; if some violent behavior can be put down to physical causes, then other violent behavior seems likely to have the same sort of explanation. Why should some people get special allowances just because science has made a little more headway in understanding their behavior at the biochemical level? If it begins to appear as if all behavior has biochemical and eventually genetic substrata, why should *anyone ever* be held morally responsible?

All the same, there is an emerging consensus in the philosophical literature that behavioral genetics need not swamp all views about freedom of the will and moral responsibility—that this millennia-old philosophical debate is not about to be solved scientifically. None of the major philosophical positions on freedom of the will must be recast in light of discoveries in behavioral genetics. Those positions rest on metaphysical suppositions, and behavioral genetics offers empirical data that cannot destroy suppositions of that sort; only more philosophical argument could do that (and the interminability of the debate may make one wonder whether even more philosophical argument would do any good). Thus behavioral genetics does not introduce new arguments for supposing that we are not free; rather, it changes the terms in which the old arguments are phrased. The impact of genetics on human agency, and on the philosophical debate about human agency, seems to be analogous to that of environment: in most cases, both environment and genetic makeup predispose a person to act in certain ways; neither determines her actions.

Such is the drift of argument in the philosophical literature on behavioral genetics, and in this chapter. Yet the conclusion requires two significant caveats. First, behavioral genetics may allow us to describe deterministic positions more richly than before, and therefore more persuasively—more attractively. The scientific details offered by behavioral genetics give us a more complete and satisfying way of fleshing out determinism. Second, even if behavioral genetics does not prevent us from talking about freedom of the will and has no uniform and universal effect on the way we ascribe freedom and responsibility, it may have many, diverse consequences about many kinds of cases or contexts: it may change the way we think about many specific psychological states or conditions.

The structure of this chapter is that of a stroll across a landscape. Three primary kinds of philosophical positions have been staked out on the problem of freedom of the will, and the chapter proceeds by touring them. These positions are strong defenses of freedom of the will, which reject determinism; hard determinism, which rejects freedom of the will; and compatibilism, which accepts both freedom of the will and determinism. The chapter concludes by broaching a possible fourth position, attributed mainly to Kant but updated here with Wittgenstein's (probably unwilling) help, according to which freedom of the will and determinism are logically incompatible but can nonetheless be retained because they belong to different modes of thinking and talking about human behavior.

Hard Determinism versus Strong Freedom

The argument for determinism is that every event has a cause, that human actions are events, and therefore that all human actions are caused. A strong thesis about determinism—hard determinism—holds that if human actions are merely nodes in a universal causal network, then the language of "freedom" and "moral responsibility" is mistaken and must be abandoned—at least by the cognoscenti. We might continue to speak of freedom and responsibility in the public square, on grounds that such talk, even if mistaken, is useful for altering the behavior of the uninformed hoi polloi. If we continue to punish people, we will do so because punishing people is a useful way of changing their behavior, not because they *deserve* punishment.

Behavioral genetics may offer insight into the genetic component of complex behaviors. If one is already a determinist, it could certainly give evidence that would change one's view about the contribution that genes make to behavior. B. F. Skinner, one of the best-known hard determinists, held that there was an innate tendency to respond to rewards and punishments in certain ways, but that the pattern of rewards and punishments was the immediate and primary cause of behavioral outcomes. A contemporary popular view of the science of human nature runs the other way, toward holding that behavior is rooted primarily in the genes. Behavioral genetics can affect the balance between these two ways of developing a determinist position.

In short, behavioral genetics *contributes* to the debate over determinism. But it does not introduce new arguments for determinism; it simply means that when we characterize human actions as events with causes, we might be led to characterize those events and causes differently. But detailed claims about genetically acquired predispositions are not necessary for determinism. The hard determinist position requires only very rudimentary claims about human nature—in the behaviorist account, for example, that we respond to stimuli in set ways.

Nonetheless, even if behavioral genetics does not change the basic structure of the argument for universal determinism, it may allow us to set it out in greater detail, and in such a way that the resulting picture squares with our intuitions about human behavior. The Skinnerian behaviorist had only a simplistic and distorted account of human actions. Eventually, behavioral genetics might allow us to describe human actions in considerable detail and richness, to make them part of a long and elaborate story about why people do the things they do, and to set that story alongside many other stories that science gives us about the world. It is this sort of story that Daniel Dennett attempts in *Elbow Room,* his widely read book about human freedom (although Dennett is not a hard determinist). Dennett offers us "Just So Stories" about how humans came to be rational beings, possessed of the capacity to engage in meta-level self-reflection and speak of agents' decisions and responsibility for the effects of their decisions (Dennett, 1984). Painting in the details of the causal pathways by which behavior is controlled would give the determinist thesis more substance, and therefore make for a more attractive and more persuasive story. The argument remains structurally the same, but richer and more satisfying.

Behavioral genetics also does not substantially change the conceptual task involved in a strong defense of freedom of the will. The defense typically starts with the claim that a person is responsible for her actions only if she could have done otherwise. If an action is necessitated by other events, and those events by other events, reaching back to events that precede the person's existence, so that the action is the outcome of events over which the person has no control, then the person cannot really be said to be free. This simply establishes what "freedom" is: freedom is the antithesis of the claim that all human actions are "events" in the determinist's sense. Sometimes, for human actions, the causal chains come to an end.

One strategy of the strong defender of freedom is merely to challenge the general account of causality that the determinist seems to endorse. The determinist seems to suppose that a cause requires its effect, but what do we really know about this "requires"? All we really know is that the effect has always followed the cause. But must it always? William James declares, "The principle of causality [is] but a postulate, an empty name covering simply a demand that the sequence of events shall some day manifest a deeper kind of belonging of one thing with another than the mere arbitrary juxtaposition which now phenomenally appears? . . . All our scientific and philosophic ideals are altars to unknown gods. Uniformity is as much so as is free-will" (James, 1993, 177).

A more daring strategy is to develop a new account of causality, one that distinguishes human causality from natural, fully determined causality. All events have causes, but some human actions are self-caused. In Aristotle's image, "the stick moves the stone and is moved by the hand, which again is moved by the man; in the man, however, we have reached a mover that is not so in virtue of being moved by something else" (1941, 367). There are various ways of trying to distinguish human causation from normal causation. At one end lies dualism: one might try to locate human causation within another ontological realm, as proposed by St. Augustine. More modestly, one might stipulate merely that there are two kinds of causation: "event-causation," such as when billiard balls strike other billiard balls and make them move, and "agent-causation," where we place human choice. And one need not even say that all human behavior is to be understood as *choice:* freedom of the will is still possible even if people do not always act freely. (Someone who was free even in the strongest possible sense could not be blamed for sleeping poorly.) This is the usual modern approach, since it seems to stand a better chance of avoiding dualism's metaphysical excesses.

As with the strong determinist position, nothing about behavioral genetics requires that these lines of argument be retooled. Another way of putting this point is noted by Dan Brock and Allen Buchanan. The different philosophical positions on free will and determinism, they argue, rest on metaphysical claims that no empirical investigation can overturn (Brock and Buchanan, 1999). However one defends free will—whether by positing a distinction between different realms of being, or simply by drawing a distinction between different kinds of causation—one is offering claims that lie beyond the reach of science.

But behavioral genetics may make that defense look thin—or, as Dennett puts it, "desperate" or "forlorn"—just as it makes the determinist position look rich and detailed. In this spirit, Patricia Greenspan points out that revelations about genetic factors in behavior "look" worse than discoveries about environmental factors because they are so blatantly contrary to the explanation of action adopted by agent-causation views (Greenspan, 2001). They make humans look like machines; agent-causation views can tolerate the appearance of machinery, but they must maintain that humans are in fact capable of something else.

Genetic factors look worse than environmental factors because they seem internal to the agent's own capacities of deliberation. Environmental factors can constrain an agent's capacity for deliberation, but because they act on the agent from outside, they seem contingent and remediable. Genetic factors appear to affect an agent's thoughts or deliberations *from within,* and so appear to be innate and unavoidable. They might affect one's desires, for example, or perhaps the ability to fight those desires. But this introduces nothing that reframes the debate about freedom of the will. Defenders of free will are already aware that people have powerful desires of various sorts, against which they must sometimes fight to do what they think is right or best, and that their ability to fight those desires can be attenuated by various circumstances.

Genes versus Environment

In effect, the emerging picture of how genes contribute to behavior presents genes as constraining human action in a way that is conceptually similar to the constraints posed by the environment. This is another reason for supposing that behavioral genetics will not suddenly settle the question about freedom of the will. In the picture developed by contemporary behavioral geneticists, genes can impart *dispositions* to act in certain ways. Having a disposition means that one is *predisposed* to act in a certain way, but not that one is flatly caused to act in that way. But the environment can also impart dispositions, and the philosophical literature on behavioral genetics is replete with comparisons making this point. Marcia Baron offers this illustration:

> Suppose there were a genetic factor in crime and a test that disclosed whether the individual had the marker. The individual who tested positive would simply be genetically *predisposed* toward such behavior . . . The person's position would be exactly the same as that of people whose environment—including, especially, their past environment and, in particular, their childhoods—significantly increased the chance that they would become violent offenders. (Baron, 2001, 202)

Arguing for a similar conclusion, Peter Van Inwagen asks us to compare two societies. In one, there is a "legal, ubiquitous, and very well produced pornography that is essentially a glorification of rape. Even parents with the best wills in the world find it extremely difficult to prevent adolescent boys from being continually exposed to this pornography." In the other, "a certain gene-sequence is very common; it has the following phenotypic effect on those men whose genotype contains it: they experience an inordinately strong urge for immediate sexual release" (Van Inwagen, 2001, 236).

Both genes and environment can influence our desires and deliberative processes. In that sense, both can have an internal influence on choice. Neither genes nor environment leads directly to actions. In that sense, neither is internal to the choice itself. Someone predisposed to act in a certain way might only very rarely act that way. And on any given occasion, she can choose to act differently. In fact, the language of disposition is such that she need not *ever* act that way. A disposition is not to be understood as just a statistical generalization about outcomes. Someone predisposed toward violence is not guaranteed to act violently on any given occasion, and is not even guaranteed to *sometimes* act violently. The predisposition (detectable perhaps with brain scans, or by seeing which circumstances make the person's face flush, or through some other investigation) might never issue in actual violence.

Compatibilism: Freedom and Determinism

Most contemporary philosophers reject the strong defense of freedom. Instead, they favor a compatibilist account, which admits that human behavior might be fully determined by natural laws, but holds that talk of freedom can be upheld nonetheless. We retain the free will thesis by redefining it—or, as the compatibilist would have it, by defining it more accurately, in an ordinary, down-to-earth way, one that relies on everyday observations about the human capacity to think and talk self-consciously about ends and means, rather than on metaphysical speculations about causality and mind. The compatibilist derides the strong defender of freedom of the will as wanting something more grandiose than is either necessary or supported by what we observe about human agency. Typically, the compatibilist defines free actions simply as those which are taken by agents with the capacity for self-reflection about their actions, and which are not forced by circumstances or by other people. This approach is well represented by Dennett:

> What we want when we want free will is the power to decide our courses of action, and to decide them wisely, in the light of our expectations and desires. We want to be in control of ourselves, and not under the control of others. We want to be agents, capable of initiating, and taking responsibility for, projects and deeds. All this is ours, I have tried to show, as a natural product of our biological endowment, extended and enhanced by our initiation into society. (Dennett, 1984, 169)

The form of determinism understood as compatible with this kind of freedom of the will is soft determinism, although the label is something of a misnomer, since it is only the account of freedom that is changed. What was true of behavioral genetics' effect on hard determinism is also true of its effect on soft determinism and compatibilism: behavioral genetics neither dictates a general overhaul of them nor proves them correct, but it may well make them more attractive by making possible a rich and detailed account of human agency.

Because compatibilism accepts a limited free will thesis, however, behavioral genetics can have one effect within it that it cannot have within hard determinism: this is that discoveries in behavioral genetics may well lead a compatibilist to assess many *specific* human actions differently. For the compatibilist, free will has to do with self-reflection and constraint, and the constraints can be either external to the agent—a gun held to the head—or internal—an uncontrollable psychological tic. Thus, part of the compatibilist view is that free actions result from normal human psychological mechanisms: an action is freely done when a person deliberates about it normally, decides to do it, and then successfully turns that decision into action. Understood this way, freedom of the will is tied by definition to normal human functioning, and hence to psychological health. Given this fundamentally naturalistic account of freedom, a compatibilist might well decide, after investigation, that some people who had once seemed free and morally responsible are not, due to genetic predispositions that affect their behavior. In principle, at least, the compatibilist might also sometimes decide the exact opposite: that individuals who once seemed constrained by circumstances should be deemed free and morally responsible. Finally, given the complexity of the human brain, it might even be that an individual would be able to deliberate and act on some matters normally, but not on others. In theory, a person might be declared unable to control his overeating but still be held morally responsible for stealing money from his company. In the compatibilist frame, a free will might not be a single ball of wax; it might instead be behavior-specific.

One of the attractions of the compatibilist account of freedom is precisely that it very nicely accommodates a plausibly complex account of human agency, and the discoveries of behavioral genetics fit comfortably into this frame. Similarly, compatibilism nicely accommodates a plausibly complex account of interpersonal moral attitudes and assessments, as P. F. Strawson famously noticed in a highly influential essay titled "Freedom and Resentment." Strawson called attention to the range of emotional reactions we have toward other people whom we take to be fully participating members of the moral community. These include such things as resentment, gratitude, forgiveness, and hurt feelings (Strawson, 2003, 77–79). Strawson also noted that there are a variety of ways in which we sometimes say that these reactions—which he called "participant reactive attitudes"—should be suspended. Sometimes, even when one is injured, one cannot reasonably be aggrieved. Sometimes, as Strawson explained, the other person is a typical moral agent but the circumstances of the action are abnormal, and we say things like, "He didn't mean to," or "He didn't understand." And sometimes the other person is not a typical moral agent, perhaps because of special circumstances bearing on the person—"He's been under a lot of strain lately"—or perhaps because of standing features of the person's agency—"He's just a child," or "He's a hopeless schizophrenic." If we accept these assessments, we will adopt an "objective attitude" toward the person: we see the person "as an object of social policy" rather than as a full participating member of the moral community (79), and we will concentrate on understanding "'how he works'" (82).

The discoveries promised by advances in behavioral genetics are all grist for the mill here. They could lead to and justify various special assessments of others' moral agency, and they could then help us understand how others work. But they would not lead to anything new in the moral life: these sorts of assessments were familiar to us already. Further, the assessments are of various sorts and are highly context-specific, and if Strawson is to be believed, they do not seem likely to boil down to any one simple underlying thesis of determinism.

One way that genes might contribute to behavior is by influencing desires. If genes contribute toward impulsivity, for example, they might do so simply by imparting especially strong impulses. Of course, strong impulses are a common problem for all deliberators, so unless they are exceedingly strong—capable of overwhelming the agent's deliberative abilities—they do not require us to abandon freedom of the will. The agent can be responsible for the actions, in the compatibilist sense; there are undoubtedly genetic contributions to all impulses, but they are not automatically exculpatory (Van Inwagen, 2001). Depending on the circumstances, though—the strength of the impulse, what the agent has done to resist it, what we know about the statistical correlation between the genes and the behavior, perhaps an understanding at the biochemical level of how the genes actually help *cause* the behavior—we may well feel sympathy for the person, and we might think that the genetic contribution to the behavior is a mitigating, if not exculpatory, consideration. (In all of this, however, as Baron and others have stressed, there is nothing special about the fact that these impulses, this disposition, can be traced to genetic causes [Baron, 2001]. Environmental circumstances might have been mitigating in a similar way.)

Generating impulses is only one way that genes might contribute toward behavior. Research may suggest that in people diagnosed as having impulsivity disorders, for example, genes may contribute toward behavior not by generating especially strong impulses but by giving people weakened mechanisms for self-control (Greenspan, 2001). Impulsive people, such as kleptomaniacs, may have the same impulses as others, but an attenuated ability to resist them. In such cases, the genetic contribution to behavior might be said to consist in an impairment of the deliberative mechanisms themselves. Impulsive people have, as it were, a "localized learning disability"—they are unable to learn how to control themselves. As Patricia Greenspan observes, the genetic contribution "denies the agent the very stuff of self-directed agency" (Greenspan, 2001, 249). Thus, she concludes, genetic science might lead us to hold that an agent lacks freedom of the will *even if* that individual's behavior is *not* flatly determined.

This might be an example of how behavioral genetics could change specific assessments of freedom of the will. Of course, much hangs on how strong the learning disability is. Greenspan's picture seems to be of someone who will reliably fail to resist her impulses. A disposition, however, is only a tendency, and it is only a psychological tendency, not a statistical one—it has to do with what eggs us on, not with rates of different behavioral outcomes. Some people who struggle to learn new material are still able to do it much of the time, by gaining insight into their unique ways of learning and discovering what exacerbates or ameliorates their difficulties, and they may not really be said to have a "learning disability"—not a sufficiently severe disability that it warrants being publicly labeled as such.

The Kantian View

There is perhaps one other way of thinking about freedom of the will. We might argue that claims about moral agents' freedom and the physical universe's natural laws belong to different conceptual frames. Something like this was proposed by Kant, who held that we must, as a practical matter, assume ourselves to be free, even if it does not accord with our scientific understanding of the world. Kant also tried to explain how this practical assumption makes metaphysical sense: roughly, his thought is that the conflict between our science and our working assumption of freedom is a result of the *limits* of metaphysics. We can, in principle (thought Kant), distinguish between things as we perceive them and things as they are in themselves. Things as we perceive them (phenomena) comprise our ordinary physical realm, can be studied scientifically, and adhere to whatever laws we discover through science. People, too, belong to the realm of perception, of course, and when they are understood as belonging to the realm of perception, their behavior can reasonably be understood as determined. Philosophers have always wanted to get past the realm of perception, to understand things not as we perceive them, but as they are in themselves (noumena). Kant assures us that this is impossible. Even when we study ourselves, we must regard ourselves as belonging to the realm of science. Nonetheless, as a logical matter, we must assume that "behind the appearances there is something else which is not appearance, namely, things in themselves" (Kant, 1993, 52). An agent "must necessarily assume that beyond his own subject's constitution as composed of nothing but appearances there must be something else as basis, namely, his ego as constituted in itself" (53). If we sift out everything that we know about ourselves through the world of sense, we are left with a conception of ourselves as pure consciousness, thought in action, as it were: self-acting, autonomous beings, who are necessarily free.

It is possible to see the Kantian position either as an elaborate defense of a strong thesis about freedom of the will, or as an elaborate shrug of the shoulders over the effort to resolve the metaphysics of freedom. Suppose it's the latter. What seems most promising about it is the recognition, first, that we cannot get outside our own perspective on the world—our own way of thinking about talking about the world—and, second, that the limits of our perspective force us to give up trying to integrate into a systematic whole all our different ways of thinking and talking about the world and ourselves. We simply have, it allows, contrary standpoints from which we can regard ourselves, rendered compatible (in a sense) only because we adopt those standpoints at, in effect, different times—in different conversations.

The Kantian resignation about the reach of the human perspective has a modern and metaphysically more palatable analog in the later Wittgenstein's musings about our inability to separate out things as they are in themselves from our ways of thinking about them, and our ways of thinking about them from our ways of talking about them. We are stuck, in philosophy, with studying our words and the ways we use them. And it might be that we engage in different realms of discourse, and that these different realms are not fully compatible with each other. Wittgenstein suggests that our language is like a huge, old city, which is an accretion of innumerable smaller "language games." The whole city is not laid out neatly. Ancient, cramped sections have narrow streets and alleys running in this and that direction, other neighborhoods are laid out in other directions, broader avenues cross here and there, and larger, newer boroughs encircle the whole. And possibly, the overall layout might not be consistent except for the fact that a traveler is always only in one or another portion of the city and must struggle only with the rules that apply in that portion. Similarly, perhaps, we participate in different language games at different times, or for different purposes. I might write a scientific paper that implies a deterministic outlook on human behavior but still believe that it is genuinely an open question whether I'll work through the afternoon—not because I have a single conception of "human choice" that is uniform in my scientific paper and in my decision whether to have a snack and enjoy the sun, but because I am doing different things.

The effect of this line of thought is to turn the question about freedom of the will into a question about reductionism. We make claims in mathematics, biology, physics, sociology, aesthetics, morality, and so on. There is no reason at the outset to suppose that all these different realms can be adequately understood by employing solely the terms of any one of them. If we participate in a range of different language games, it might be the case that what we take as objective fact in the context of one game disappears, or is differently construed, in another game. (Colors might provide one such example: that something has the property of being red might be an objective fact in everyday conversations about the physical world; if we recede into the specialized conversation of physics, colors are but human projections onto the world. Nor is there yet any convincing account of what color is.) That there are real moral constraints on action is taken for granted in everyday conversations about human affairs, but from an evolutionary biological perspective—so it is often claimed—moral constraints are but evolving tools for pursuing self-interest. Similarly, perhaps strong freedom of the will can be spoken of as a fact in some conversations, yet seem a mere fabrication in others. It is tempting to suppose that in each of these pairs, one of the two ways of speaking must be fundamental, must offer a truer reflection of the world as it really is, and the other way of speaking must be reducible to it. But if we cannot get outside our way of speaking and thinking to check the alignment with the world as it is, independent of speaking and thinking about it, then this supposition is but an article of faith.

Conceivably, behavioral genetics could drive a slow evolution in our language about free will, so that we gradually found ourselves abandoning some of our older ways of talking about human agency in favor of newer, more scientific ways of talking about it (Elliott, 1999). But that need not happen, if these different ways of speaking about agency belong to different language games—different realms of the city—so that they do not really come into contact with each other, and if we cannot easily give up those old ways anyway. Probably, here as with the other three views about freedom of the will, behavioral genetics has no sweeping effect. In fact, if the two modes of speaking do not really contact each other, then the comparatively rich picture of causality that behavioral genetics helps us develop need not incline us to regard talk of free will as comparatively forlorn—it might not be a comparison that we make.

In fact, even within our talk of freedom and moral responsibility there seem to be competing strains. David Wasserman has argued that there are contrary ways in which we speak of responsibility, and contrary ways in which discoveries in behavioral genetics could affect our language. If an individual were shown to have an innate flaw that weakens self-control, it seems, on the one hand, to lessen responsibility. Yet it also seems to show a true defect of character, and therefore to merit moral disapprobation. "We punish recidivists more severely not only because they appear to be more dangerous, but because their recalcitrance appears to provide stronger evidence of an antisocial character than any single offense, however serious. We judge the offender not only for his acts, but for the character they reflect" (Wasserman, 2001, 304). The social stereotype of the natural-born killer, after all, is of someone who kills as a result of strong, innate dispositions, and therefore kills without having engaged in normal deliberative mechanisms, yet is nonetheless morally abhorrent (Slote, 2001). Yet behavioral genetics can have diverse local effects, just as it might within the compatibilist approach. There are a variety of ways in which we all see ourselves as constrained by circumstances or limited by nature, dependent on others or on technology, our possibilities variously circumscribed. Among these constraints are genetically influenced conditions. In severe cases, we may decide that the language games that involve free will sometimes cannot be applied to a person. At other times they may be mitigating circumstances. At still other times they may simply be part of the background—not remarkable enough to warrant a change in our talk of free will.

In this way, the question about free will and behavioral genetics comes down to earth. Initially, the question seemed to be about metaphysics—about the nature of rational agency and causality. Reframed in the compatibilist or neo-Kantian mode, the metaphysical issues are put aside, and the pertinent question concerns the particular circumstances under which we would say that someone who has a mental disorder has a lesser degree of moral responsibility, or is simply absolved of moral responsibility. This question is best approached by, on the one hand, pursuing the science, and on the other hand, describing with the help of a range of examples the ways we actually use the language of freedom and responsibility and the kinds of constraints that are taken to condition responsibility and blame.

REFERENCES

Aristotle, *Physics*. R. P. Hardie and R. K. Gaye, trans.. In R. McKeon, ed. *The Basic Works of Aristotle*. New York: Random House, 1941.

Baron, M. (2001). "Crime, Genes, and Responsibility." In E. Wasserman and R. Wachbroit, eds. *Genetics and Criminal Behavior*. New York and Cambridge: Cambridge University Press: 199–224.

Brock, D., and A. Buchanan. (1999). "The Genetics of Behavior and Concepts of Free Will and Determinism." In J. R. Botkin, W. M. McMahon, and L. P. Francis, eds. *Genetics and Criminality: The Potential Misuse of Scientific Information in Court*. Washington, D.C. : American Psychological Association: 67–75.

Dennett, D. C. (1984). *Elbow Room: The Varieties of Free Will Worth Wanting*. Cambridge, Mass.: MIT.

Elliott, C. (1999). *A Philosophical Disease: Bioethics, Culture, and Identity*. New York: Routledge.

Greenspan, P. (2001). "Genes, Electrotransmitters, and Free Will." In D. Wasserman and R. Wachbroit, eds. *Genetics and Criminal Behavior*. New York and Cambridge.: Cambridge University Press: 243–58.

James, W. (1993). "The Dilemma of Determinism." In Dd. Kolak and R. Martin, eds. *The Experience of Philosophy*. Belmont, Calif.: Wadsworth.

Kant, I. (1993). *Grounding for the Metaphysics of Morals*. James W. Ellington, trans. Indianapolis, Ind.: Hackett.

Slote, M. (2001). "Moral Responsibility without Free Will." In D. Wasserman and R. Wachbroit, eds. *Genetics and Criminal Behavior*. New York and Cambridge: Cambridge University Press: 259–72.

Strawson, P. F. (2003). "Freedom and Resentment." In G. Watson, ed. *Free Will*. Oxford: Oxford University Press: 72–93; reprinted from *Proceedings of the British Academy* 48(1962): 1–25.

Van Inwagen, P. V. (2001). "Genes, Statistics, and Desert." In D. Wasserman and R. Wachbroit, eds. *Genetics and Criminal Behavior*. New York and Cambridge: Cambridge University Press: 225–42.

Wasserman, D. (2001). "Genetic Predispositions to Violent and Antisocial Behavior: Responsibility, Character, and Identity." In E. Wasserman and R. Wachbroit, eds. *Genetics and Criminal Behavior*. New York and Cambridge: Cambridge University Press: 303–27.

CHAPTER ELEVEN

Normality and the Significance of Difference

Robert Wachbroit, Ph.D.

The profoundest effects of genetic discoveries are those that affect our self-conception. Concerns about what such discoveries will enable us to do—at what cost and with what risk—are of course important, but their implications for how we should understand ourselves can sometimes matter more. An intense interest in questions regarding free will, for example, often arises whenever scientists identify or even suggest a genetic factor or influence on behavior. We are worried that the existence of such factors or influences might be incompatible with our acting or choosing freely. The belief that we have such freedom is central to our common self-understanding of our behavior. Its centrality is widely recognized (and it is discussed in chapters 8 and 10).

Our understanding of normality—who or what is normal and why—is also central to our self-conception. Its centrality has many sources, but one source surely is a concern over the significance of difference. Classification schemes—whether of genes, behaviors, attributes, or even people—can record a variety of differences. But when some differences are then labeled as normal or abnormal, we touch upon a special interest about how differences should be interpreted. To put it colloquially, we regard normal differences as OK, abnormal differences as not OK (Hacking, 1990). A concern with normality is tied to the anxiety—or comfort—we derive from the thought that normality might be objective, reflecting the way the world is and not just convention or human (social) construction. It is easy to believe, or fear, that discoveries in genetics—those fundamental markers of biological differences—should have important implications for our understanding of normality. The matter, as we will see, is much more complicated.

Claims regarding human normality are also thought to have implications regarding what is human nature. Both human normality and human nature concern differences, but whereas the former is usually about the differences between people, the latter is usually about the differences between people and other things (e.g., other animals). Thus, our understanding of human normality touches on our self-conception as individuals; our understanding of human nature touches on our self-conception as human beings. How these two are connected will occupy us later in this discussion.

The Multiple Meanings of *Normal*

One of the first points to acknowledge in any discussion of normality is that the word *normal* is used in several different senses. Consider, for example, the following quote from a book by distinguished biologists Harold Varmus and Robert Weinberg (1993):

> *Normal* life processes are often directly illuminated by study of the *abnormal*. This book is another testament to the accuracy of that research adage; for the understanding it will record begins not with the beauties of living form, but with cancer, one of nature's aberrations. The fingers of a newborn child or the pattern of a butterfly's wing represent what we *normally* admire in biological systems: form; control; a unity of design and function that favors the survival of the organism. In cancer, all of these virtues are lost. Cancer cells divide without restraint, cross boundaries they were meant to respect, and fail to display the characteristics of the cell lineage from which they were derived. Yet it is from such cells, with their feared consequences for the organism, that biologists have learned many key mechanisms in the drama of *normal* growth and development. To show why and how such mechanisms may fail—and may thereby initiate cancer—requires an initial review of our understanding of *normal* biological function, above all, of the general strategies that organisms use to govern their growth and differentiation. (1; emphasis added)

It is doubtful that *normal,* and associated terms, are all being used in the same sense in this paragraph; that, for example, the sense of normal in "normal admiration" and in "normal biological function" is the same. And, indeed, most people who have written about normality have acknowledged the multiple meanings of normal, though they haven't agreed on the number. Some have claimed that there are seven (Murphy, 1972); others suggest even more (Davis and Bradley, 1996).

The exact number of meanings of normal is not important for our purposes. What is important is that, regardless of the number of different meanings that have been suggested, they can be grouped into three broad categories—statistical conceptions, social conceptions, and biological conceptions.

Statistical Conceptions. Examples of meanings or definitions of normal that fall into this category are easy to identify. They include definitions of the normal as the average (or the mean), as the most common (or the mode), or as falling within two standard deviations of the mean. These definitions characterize normality as a property of a group or population, so that changing the population—even by adding or subtracting just one individual—can immediately alter what constitutes normal. For example, the term *normal height* could be used to refer to the average height of people in a population, the most common height, or a range of heights that characterize 95 percent of the population. Altering the population by just one individual would likely change the average height, though it would require a more extensive alteration to change the common height or the height that characterizes 95 percent of the population.

Statistical conceptions of normality are the clearest and most straightforward. They are not only clear in their applications—determining the average is a straightforward, mechanical procedure—but also in their limitations. Because they are nothing more than mathematical properties of populations, one cannot take what is normal in one population and generalize or extrapolate that to another population. Knowing the average height in one population doesn't tell us, relying solely on the mathematics, the average height in a different or larger population.

Social Conceptions. This category contains a wide variety of conceptions of normality, ranging from ordinary judgments of what is acceptable behavior to sophisticated and nuanced accounts of the constitution of social expectations and deviance, such as that found in Goffman's classic study, *Stigma* (1963). They include explicit pronouncements about what is "weird," as well as implicit though still systematic assessments of social acceptability. Some social conceptions of normality refer to everyday behaviors or conditions; others refer to states that are ideal but unrealizable.

Social conceptions of normality are not as precise as statistical conceptions. And it would be futile to try to characterize in only a few paragraphs a major topic of the social sciences. Nevertheless, the general idea should be clear because it is, in a sense, so familiar. As familiar as the judgment that someone is—or is acting—weird.

Despite differences in precision, it is worth contrasting statistical and social conceptions of normality. First of all, these conceptions are logically independent of each other. What is statistically normal, however that is defined within the category, need not be socially or culturally normal in that population. That is to say, it is logically possible for the socially normal not to be the most common or the average. Consider, for example, sexual behavior. Because of a widespread hypocrisy or ignorance, certain sexual activities might be common but nevertheless be regarded by society as (socially) abnormal. Social norms of beauty or attractiveness might not reflect how most people look.

Statistical conceptions of normality and social conceptions of normality are simply about different things. Nevertheless, although they are logically independent, they may be related by scientific theories or empirical hypotheses, claiming an empirical relationship between the statistically normal and the socially normal. For example, one might hypothesize that, under certain conditions, what is common (e.g., regarding sexual behavior) will be what is socially normal or acceptable. But this is an empirical hypothesis, not a logical or conceptual truth. Specifying the conditions for such interconnections between statistical and social conceptions of normality is, of course, one of the tasks of empirical social science research. Indeed, discoveries that something socially abnormal is nevertheless statistically normal are surprises that can attract popular interest (e.g., an interest in unmasking widespread hypocrisy).

Biological Conceptions. Since biological conceptions of normality are the least familiar, we need to describe them with some care. According to the standard understanding of biology, one of the primary tasks of biological research is to identify the biological function of various items and processes. It is not enough to know how the organ, tissue, cell, or gene behaves or reacts under various conditions. We also want to know its function. What is the purpose of this organ? To circulate the blood. What is the purpose of this gene? To produce a protein essential to protect the lungs against airborne irritants. In identifying the biological function of an object, we have specified what it is for that object to be normal or in a normal state: it is normal insofar as it is performing its function. A normal heart is one that performs its function of circulating the blood. And so forth.

The concept of biological normality is completely intertwined with the concepts of biological function and dysfunction. When you have specified one, you have specified the other. To be performing its function is to be normal or to be in its normal state; to be dysfunctional or malfunctioning is to be abnormal or in its abnormal state. This point is well illustrated by the last sentence of the quote at beginning of this section, where normal biological function is simply biological function. Thus, this idea of normality is as much a part of biological science as the idea of function and dysfunction.

Insofar as a subfield of biology does not engage in the search, identification, or characterization of biological functions, then biological normality has no role or place in that subfield, though statistical or social conceptions of normality may still be appropriately and usefully invoked. Similarly, insofar as one has doubts about the standard understanding of biology and the importance of biological functions, these doubts will translate immediately to doubts about biological normality. Many logical positivists, for example, dismissed biology's appeal to functions as merely a convenient heuristic; apparent appeals to functions in biological explanation were to be analyzed away (Nagel, 1961). Such positivists would have been similarly skeptical of appeals to biological normality.

It is not my purpose here to defend the use of the concept of function in biology; I assume that the concept is as legitimate as any of the other well-entrenched concepts used in biology. Nor do I wish to engage directly in any of the disputes over the meaning or analysis of the concept of biological function. There are some longstanding controversies over the meaning of biological function—such as whether functions are to be understood in terms of the organism's overall ability to survive and reproduce (Boorse, 1976) or whether functions are to be understood in terms of an explanation for why the different parts of the organism evolved the way they did (Wright, 1976). The analysis of biological function adopted will affect one's specific conception of biological normality.

In sum, the concept of biological normality has all the clarity, controversy, ambiguity, and confusion that attaches to the concept of biological function.

Insofar as we are unsure or disagree about the biological function of some entity, we are unsure or disagree about what being biologically normal means for that entity. There are many questions about the nature of functions: How do biological entities (organs, tissues, etc.) with a clear function evolve to perform an entirely different function and how should we characterize the function of the item during the transition? Can biological items have only one function, so that any other beneficial effects of the item are just that—side effects? Or can items have multiple functions? If so, do these functions form a hierarchy of primary and secondary functions? Or are all these multiple functions on a par, so that the claim that the item is dysfunctional must always be understood to be relativized to the failure of a specific activity of the item? And so forth. Each of these questions about biological function raises a corresponding question about biological normality. While the answers to these questions are important for a fuller understanding of biological normality, as we will see, they do not have a significant bearing on the ethical and policy matters to be addressed later. (For more on the relationship between function and normality, see Wachbroit [1994].)

Recall the earlier contrasts noted between statistical and social normality. The same contrasts obtain between biological normality and these other two conceptions. Biological normality is logically independent of either statistical normality or social normality; nevertheless, important empirical connections between these various conceptions of normality may well exist. Let me explain.

Biological differences that do not affect functioning are differences that do not matter to the classification of biological normality. For example, differences in blood type have no effect on the biological function of blood—A-positive blood functions as well as O-negative blood—and so they all fall under the classification of biologically normal. (These differences are sometimes called "variants.") In particular, even though type O-negative blood is rare (i.e., statistically abnormal), it is biologically normal. The opposite—statistically normal but biologically abnormal—is also found, as in the case of a widespread epidemic or dental caries. Even though the disease is statistically normal, it reflects nevertheless some biological dysfunction (i.e., some biological abnormality) because it is a disease.

Nevertheless, we should expect some connection between statistical normality and biological normality. Presumably, the biologically normal is more likely to flourish than the biologically abnormal, and so more likely to be the statistical norm. Even though such things as epidemics can undermine that presumption at a particular time, it does seem reasonable to assume that over the evolutionary history of a species, the biological norm is also the statistical norm. The connection nevertheless is empirical and not logical or semantic.[1]

The logical distinctness of biological normality and social normality is probably sufficiently clear to need no further elaboration. Biologically normal organs, conditions, or features may or may not be socially normal; indeed, depending upon the society, the question of what condition of a particular biological entity is socially normal may not arise or may not even make sense. The distinction between biological and social conceptions of normality is perhaps most evident in discussions over the definition of disease. Although disease can be defined as an abnormality, there is often debate about what sort of abnormality it is. To a large extent, the controversy over the definition of "disease" turns on the question of whether disease should be understood as a biological abnormality, a social abnormality, or some combination of the two. The issue would not make sense unless biological and social conceptions of normality were distinct (Wachbroit, 1998).

The possible empirical connections between biological normality and social normality may involve a more complicated story. Depending on the society, a biological abnormality, especially if it's highly visible and statistically abnormal, may also be deemed socially abnormal—for example, it may be regarded as a stigma, and the person with the biological abnormality may be stigmatized. This association of biological abnormality with social abnormality can be a matter of some concern. It will be a focus of our attention later.

Before concluding this section, I want to repeat a point made at the beginning. This classification—statistical, social, and biological—does not denote three different meanings of normal; the classification refers to three different kinds or families of meanings of normal. Under each term there are several candidate meanings, and so we should not talk about *the* meaning or definition of statistical, social, or biological normality.

Behavior and Normality

Our characterization of the multiple meanings of normality has so far been quite general. But how are they to be understood in the case of behavior?

As we would expect, the idea of statistically normal behavior is straightforward. Once we have a classification of behaviors in place, we can count them and so determine which behaviors are more common. (If, in addition to the classification scheme, we have a system of measuring behavior, then we can also talk of averages.) Conceptually, determining statistically normal behavior rests on little more than an identifying description of behaviors and the frequency of their occurrences.

Determining whether some behavior is biologically normal is a more complicated matter. The same physical movements can reflect a biological abnormality or not. The hand-shaking of someone with Parkinson disease reflects a biological abnormality. The outwardly identical behavior of a violinist executing a wide vibrato does not indicate a biological abnormality. In general, a behavior is biologically abnormal if it is the result of a biologically abnormal condition. The classification reflects the etiology of the behavior. In order to determine the biological normality of some behavior, we need to know its cause; we do not, in general, need to know anything about its causes in order to determine whether the behavior is statistically normal.

Determining the social normality of behavior turns on yet a different type of information—the context in which the behavior takes place. Like biologically normal behavior, socially normal behavior cannot be determined simply from its description. Knowing that the behavior can be described as jumping (or dancing) does not yet determine whether the behavior is socially normal; we need to know the context or circumstances in which this behavior is taking place. But in contrast to biologically normal behavior, we do not necessarily need to know the (biological) causes of the behavior in order to determine whether it is socially normal behavior. If the behavior is unacceptable, inappropriate, or just plain weird, the behavior is likely to be regarded as socially abnormal, even if the behavior is biologically normal. Similarly, behavior can be regarded as socially normal even though it is biologically abnormal. For example, in some cases it seems that lisping is biologically abnormal behavior because it is the result of a biological abnormality. Nevertheless, in some linguistic communities—upper-class English speakers in England or Castilian Spanish speakers in Spain—lisping is socially normal.

Some examples will illustrate the diverse ways normal behavior can be understood. Let's begin with bipolar disorder. It seems that the behaviors associated with that disorder—manic as well as depressive behavior—are abnormal on all counts. Since only a minority of people suffer this disorder, the behaviors are statistically abnormal. The wild and abrupt swings from manic to depressive behavior are not regarded as socially normal, as least not in our society. Finally, because the abnormality of this behavior has a biological basis, because bipolar disorder reflects some biological abnormality, the associated behavior is biologically abnormal.

Unfortunately, this nice convergence of abnormalities in the case of bipolar disorder masks the complexities that can arise in other cases. One of the most important complexities arises from the interaction between the classification of normality and the classification of behavior. There are obviously many ways of classifying or grouping behavior—on the basis of its causes, on the basis of external features (whether it requires any equipment or a particular social structure for its performance), on the basis of manner of execution, and on the basis of type of actor. Some of these ways of classifying behavior will mark significant distinctions for some conceptions of normality but not others. Classifying behaviors on the basis of their use of certain equipment— for example, driving behavior—might fit nicely with a classification of social normality but it might be irrelevant to (bear no systematic relationship to) a determination of biological normality. In other words: there is no one standard or canonical way of classifying or describing behavior. A division of behaviors into social types might not coincide with a division of behaviors into biological types. Consequently, when comparing the social normality of a type of behavior with its biological normality, we should be aware that we may well be altering or redefining the type of behavior under examination, as we move between social and biological considerations.

This point becomes important as we turn to our next example—impulsive behavior. This type of behavior seems to be more or less a matter for social characterization—as well as for its various subtypes: antisocial behavior, aggressive behavior, violent behavior, and so on. Determining the social abnormality of such behaviors—their deviance—seems to be a straightforward matter. The problem with determining their biological abnormality lies in the lack of fit between these social types and biological considerations. If impulsive behavior, understood as a social type, is not also a biological type, then *any* biological characterization of that behavior—its cause, its genetics, it biological normality, and so on—will only be approximate. At best, a biological type is identified or constructed that significantly overlaps with the social type, so that what is said of the biological type of behavior will apply to much, though not all, of the social type of behavior. We should also acknowledge that social classifications of behavior are not static, so that certain social classifications can evolve to coincide more with biological classifications. This appears to be the case with the social classifications of illness: more and more, our social types of an ill person, especially in the case of mental disorders, are giving way or being redefined so as to coincide more with biological types. For example, it seems that over the past few decades the social classification of senility has given way to the more biological classification of Alzheimer disease.

Noting this complexity, let us now put it aside: let us assume that the social types and the biological types coincide, that impulsive behavior, understood socially, is the same as impulsive behavior, understood biologically. What can we say about the normality of such behavior? Although impulsivity does cover a range of behaviors, the kind that has been the most frequent topic of discussion has been behavior that is violent, aggressive, antisocial behavior (i.e., behavior that is both socially and statistically abnormal). Because we do not know the biological basis for such behavior (e.g., whether impulsive behavior arises in part from a distinctive biological process or set of genes), we cannot say whether this behavior reflects a biological dysfunction. Are impulsive behavior and nonimpulsive behavior just variants, much like different blood types, or should some impulsive behaviors be understood as biologically abnormal? That is a matter for biological investigation. Insofar as researchers can identify the biological function of the various biological components of impulsive behavior, an assessment regarding the normality of such behavior is possible. But until that is done, we can only speculate.

Finally, let us consider the example of intelligence. Since intelligence is more a trait than a type of behavior, it might be helpful to divide the example into three cases, corresponding to average, above average, and below average intelligence. The social assessment of these cases seems straightforward: average intelligence is socially normal; low intelligence is socially abnormal. There might be some dispute over the assessment of high intelligence, but it seems to me that in many contexts high intelligence is not regarded as socially abnormal. Turning to the biological assessment of intelligence, we should note that many of the points made about impulsivity can also be made about intelligence. We do not know how much overlap exists between social and biological characterizations of intelligence; we do not know enough about the biological basis of intelligence to make assessments regarding the biological normality of statistically high or statistically low intelligence, or even whether there is something distinctively biological that is common to low intelligence or common to high intelligence. It does seem reasonable to assume that statistically normal intelligence is also biologically normal and that at least some cases of low intelligence—those resulting from a disease—are also biologically abnormal. High intelligence is especially puzzling. If there is a distinct biological basis for high intelligence, it is difficult to believe that it would reflect a biological abnormality or dysfunction. How could something so apparently advantageous as high intelligence be the result of a biological malfunction? While this may seem unlikely if not impossible, we should note that at least in other areas of biology dysfunctions can in certain environments have beneficial effects. Having a physical deformity such as flat feet can enhance one's survivability and longevity by making one ineligible for military service. Having the genetic mutation associated with sickle cell anemia, but only in the heterozygous state, does not result in anemia but does confer the beneficial effect of some resistance to malaria. It may well be that the advantages of high intelligence, which are more pronounced in man-made environments, nevertheless reflect a biological dysfunction. The biological normality of high intelligence is an open question.

Genetic Discoveries and Judgments of Normality

As I have tried to show, there are many areas where, given the current state of biological research, we are not yet able to determine biological normality, particularly with respect to certain behaviors. With the intense focus of genetics research, we can expect this to change: we could well discover that certain behaviors are in fact biologically abnormal. Because the different conceptions of normality are logically independent, we could discover that some socially normal behaviors are biologically abnormal. It might be easier to see that such discoveries are possible if we consider first the situation with non-behavioral traits, such as height. Even though someone might have a height that falls within the normal range, scientists could discover that her height is nevertheless biologically abnormal because it has been affected by a disease (a biological abnormality). If she hadn't suffered the disease, she would have been even taller. Similarly, someone's behavior—for example, regarding its level of aggression or shyness or fastidiousness—might well fall within the normal range of social behavior even though the behavior reflects a biological abnormality. Our earlier allusion to lisping might be an example of this.

The possibility of such discoveries in behavioral genetics can have important ethical and social implications. The idea of three distinct conceptions of normality is not widely recognized, much less explicitly acknowledged. Consequently, we can expect there to be a tendency to conflate assessments of normality: if something is abnormal in one sense, it is abnormal in the other senses as well. In particular, if scientists discover that some behavior is biologically abnormal, there is the danger that it will thereby be considered or relabeled as socially abnormal. In other words, biological discoveries can lead to or extend social stigmatization.

Imagine a person who is somewhat messy—his clothes are a bit disheveled, his workplace looks disorganized, his home is full of clothes and dishes lying about—but all within the socially normal range. Suppose it were discovered that in some cases such behaviors reflect a biological or genetic abnormality—specifically, a mental abnormality. (This may seem farfetched at first until we recall the scientific reports not long ago of an alleged "grooming gene." See Greer and Capecchi [2002].) Because mental abnormalities (i.e., mental illnesses) are often stigmatized, the worry is that this behavior is then relabeled as socially abnormal or is even stigmatized (i.e., the biological discovery could well transform that behavior from socially normal and accepted to socially abnormal and stigmatized).

Just as worrisome are cases where the social acceptability of the behaviors is controversial. A discovery that the behavior is biologically abnormal might well persuade some (and give encouragement to those already convinced) that the behavior is indeed socially abnormal. What would be the social impact of a discovery that homosexual behavior was a manifestation of a biological abnormality (i.e., a disease)?

This phenomenon bears some similarity to the process known as "medicalization," where a social classification (e.g., the elderly, the alcoholic, the drug addict) is transformed into a medical classification and treated accordingly: the problems of the alcoholic are medical problems, solutions are to be found in medical treatment, and the responsibility of an alcoholic for being what is he is somewhat diminished because of his "medical condition." I am certainly not claiming that the medicalization of a social classification is always wrong. Indeed, in some cases, medicalization can arguably be seen as representing moral progress. Medicalizing alcoholism is widely, though not universally, regarded as a good thing. The appropriateness of medicalizing old age is more controversial.

Thus, reassessing a social classification based on discoveries in biology is not always wrong or unjustified; it depends on the specifics of the case. However, reassessing a social classification based on a confusion between kinds of normality is always wrong and unjustified. And that is just what is happening in the first case described above in which a behavior previously considered socially normal is now deemed abnormal simply because of a discovery that it is biologically abnormal. Such relabeling rests on a conflation of distinctly different kinds of abnormalities—social and biological. It is simply a mistake to conclude that a behavior is socially discreditable because of its biological origins.

The risk of such confusions and their adverse social consequences is part of a much larger phenomenon regarding the public reception of scientific discoveries. To what extent can scientific discoveries undermine commonsense beliefs or ordinary social institutions or practices? That is to say, to what extent do our commonsense beliefs and ordinary practices rest on assumptions of a primitive biology or, as Bertrand Russell would put it, a "stone-age metaphysics"? We could ask this question about the threat posed by progress in genetics to our central beliefs and practices: Can genetic discoveries undermine our belief in free will and ordinary practices regarding moral responsibility? Can genetic discoveries challenge our ordinary beliefs regarding what is a fair and just distribution of resources? Can genetic discoveries undermine our ordinary beliefs about who is sick and who is healthy? The general issue is the relationship between science and common sense, between scientific discoveries and ordinary practices, between experts and the public. It deserves much more attention than it has so far received.

The response to conflating kinds of normality is clear, at least theoretically, though challenging in practice to effect. We need to educate the public and, where appropriate, scientists, about these distinctions regarding normality and how to avoid confusing one type of normality with another.

Nevertheless, as suggested above, not all reassessments of social normality based on biological discoveries are unsophisticated conflations of different types of normality. When the response is based on an argument rather than on a simple conflation, the matter is, of course, less straightforward and more controversial. Because of their diverse character, I cannot hope to discuss all such responses. But there is one type of sophisticated response that warrants special attention, which I do want to examine. The logic or argumentation of this kind of response does not so much turn on the idea of normality as on the idea of human nature. It involves claims that discoveries about what constitutes (biological) normality have implications about what constitutes human nature. With a proper understanding of human nature, important conclusions can then be drawn about human dignity and public policy.

The Normal and the Natural

A good illustration of this type of sophisticated response can be found in Francis Fukuyama's book, *Our Posthuman Future* (2002). Fukuyama holds that the relationship between the normal and the natural—specifically, between human normality and human nature—is roughly that of identity: "The definition of the term *human nature* I will use here is the following: human nature is the sum of the behavior and characteristics that are typical [i.e., statistically normal] of the human species, arising from genetic rather than environmental factors" (130). With this definition Fukuyama argues against biotechnological modifications that go against human normality and so against human nature. Such modifications would violate the border that separates humans from other animals. This would be morally objectionable, according to Fukuyama, because our dignity as human beings is based on our human nature. Our sense that we owe a greater moral obligation to human beings than to other animals is based on our shared human nature. The bond we share, our moral community, would be broken if we allowed genetic interventions on human beings that resulted in creatures that no longer had a human nature. Since human nature is our "genetic endowment" (171), scientific discoveries detailing this endowment, specifying human normality, should help identify what genetic interventions are morally permissible.

With this much allegedly at stake, we should look more carefully at Fukuyama's definition. First of all, we should note that he intends this definition to be statistical: "typicality is a statistical artifact—it refers to something close to the median of a distribution of behavior or characteristics" (130). Hence my gloss on the word *typical* as meaning statistically normal. The reason why Fukuyama believes he needs to invoke a statistical concept in his definition of human nature is that he wants the definition to tolerate exceptions or mutations. The existence of mutant female kangaroos born without pouches should not undermine the claim that having a pouch is part of (female) kangaroo nature (135). (I am assuming, as Fukuyama appears to be as well, that being pouch-less in a female kangaroo is an abnormality and not a mere variant of the species.)

Insofar as Fukuyama wants with his definition of human nature to identify what is distinctive of the species *Homo sapiens,* his appeal to statistics is misplaced. If the concept of human nature refers to the identifying features of the species, then there is no need to make any mention of what is typical or statistically normal in the population. As I pointed out earlier, species can undergo hard times, where most of the surviving members of the species suffer disease or trauma, so that, in a sense I have tried to explain earlier, the average member of the species might not be representative of the species.

Thus, not only should the mere existence of a pouch-less kangaroo not undermine what constitutes kangaroo nature, neither should the widespread existence of pouch-less kangaroos undermine what constitutes kangaroo nature: if most current kangaroos were wiped out by a disease, leaving mainly the pouch-less kangaroos standing, we would not conclude that pouches on females were no longer distinctive of the kangaroo species; that pouches were not part of kangaroo nature. That would be to conflate statistical normality with biological normality. Instead, we would say that kangaroos were on the verge of extinction, with primarily abnormals or mutants surviving at the moment, or we might say that a new species, similar to *Macropus rufus* (i.e., kangaroo) was emerging. All this suggests that Fukuyama would do better to employ the concept of biological normality rather than statistical normality in his definition of human nature.

Perhaps a more troubling feature of Fukuyama's definition is the final phrase, "arising from genetic rather than environmental factors." On the literal reading of that phrase, we are to consider those behaviors or characteristics that are caused by genes only, in which environmental factors play no causal role. The difficulty with this reading is that it renders his definition empty. It is a basic principle of genetics that the characteristics of an organism—its phenotype—are the result of a causal interaction between the genes of the organism—its genotype—and its environment. There is no characteristic or behavior that is a product only of genes. Nor is the environment some unimportant or constant background condition. For any characteristic or behavior, it is always possible to identify an environment where, despite the organism's genes, that characteristic or behavior would not emerge or would be significantly altered.

Presumably, this literal reading is not the intended meaning. Perhaps what Fukuyama really meant to write in that last phrase was "arising *more* from genetic than environmental factors." But now two difficulties arise. First of all, it is not at all clear what "more" means in this context. In physics we can easily determine whether one cause is more significant than others and by how much, using such standard techniques as vector decomposition of forces. But no such technique is available in genetics, in part because the impact of genes is not independent of the environment: genes are one factor, the environment is another factor, and, in an important sense, the interaction between genes and environment is yet another factor.

As Kenneth Schaffner explained in chapter 1 of this volume, there are indeed statistical measures of the significance of genetic variation in a population—so-called measures of heritability—where the genetic variation in a population is correlated with the phenotypic variation in that population. Using these techniques we can say such things as: "Seventy percent of the variation in characteristic X in a particular population is correlated to the genetic variation in that population." But, as many scientists have pointed out, these correlations are not claims of causation, and the degree of correlation reveals little or nothing about any causal contribution.

The second difficulty lies in the apparent arbitrariness of "more." Are we to believe that a characteristic that is 51 percent genetic is part of human nature but a characteristic that is only 49 percent genetic is not?

Let's leave Fukuyama's troubled definition and consider a much different understanding of the relationship between human nature and human normality. According to Ian Hacking, in his *The Taming of Chance* (1990),

> "normal" bears the stamp of the nineteenth century and its conception of progress, just as "human nature" is engraved with the hallmark of the Enlightenment. We no longer ask, in all seriousness, what is human nature? Instead we talk about normal people. We ask, is this behaviour normal? Is it normal for an eight-year old girl to . . . ? Research foundations are awash with funds for finding out what is normal. Rare is the patron who wants someone to investigate human nature. (161)

In contrast to Fukuyama, Hacking suggests that the relationship between human normality and human nature is not that of identity, but more like that between oxygen and phlogiston. The scientific concept, human nature, has been shown to be wanting and has been replaced by the scientific concept, human normality.

While it is certainly true that the term *human nature* is rarely used in the current scientific literature, the term has not gone the way of other discarded scientific concepts such as phlogiston or the ether. Every year there seems to be at least a couple of new books and quite a few articles published on human nature. To be sure, these books and articles are either studies in the humanities or efforts at popularizing or interpreting science. Nevertheless, this suggests that the relationship between human normality and human nature is more complex than Hacking suggests.

Part of this complexity is due to there being two interconnected issues that an appeal to the concept of human nature is meant to address. An effort to characterize or articulate human nature is often understood to mean an effort to formulate the scientific laws and principles governing human behavior, emotions, cognition, and the like. Invoking the concept of human nature is thus meant to address such issues as: Are there any interesting scientific laws governing human behavior? What are these laws and how rigid and universal are they? (For some, particularly those in the grip of the so-called nature versus nurture debate, the crucial issue is whether these laws can be specified independently of the environment.) The concept of human normality seems well suited to investigate many of these issues, transforming these questions into ones presumably more amenable to scientific investigation (e.g., what constitutes [biologically] normal human behavior?).

Sometimes, however, the concept of human nature is invoked not so much to refer to the laws governing human beings but more to refer to what is distinctive about human beings. What makes something a human being—rather than a chimpanzee, a tree, or a rock—is that it possesses a human nature. Human nature in this use is intended to refer to what is essential rather than contingent or accidental. Simply identifying the laws governing human beings does not address this issue of distinctiveness unless these laws are shown to be *necessarily unique* to human beings. Insofar as we share a particular property with other animals—for example, aspects of our mating behavior or our reactions to certain kinds of perceived threats—that property cannot be part of the human nature that distinguishes us from other animals. It is no more part of our human nature than is being subject to gravity, a property we share with rocks.

The concept of human normality is not well suited to address these issues. If human nature refers to the essential property of being human, then a human being who didn't possess human nature would be equivalent to a human being who wasn't a member of the human species—that is, a contradiction. Biological normality, however, does not constitute a criterion of identity. An abnormal or malfunctioning heart is still a heart; it is not thereby a different organ. To be sure, we could imagine altering the heart so that it became a different thing altogether, but then we wouldn't call the result an abnormal heart.

A heart that was burned to ashes would no longer be a heart; it would not be an abnormal heart. To put the point more generally, a human being who was not normal would simply be an abnormal human being—but a human being nonetheless.

This is why investigations regarding human normality are aimed at explaining differences between human beings. Findings about the differences between humans do not entail any conclusions regarding the differences between humans and other beings. The intraspecies finding cannot be simply generalized into an interspecies discovery.

Investigations in human genetics can help us better understand human (biological) normality. They can help us determine whether a particular difference between humans is a mere variant or an abnormality. But an investigation in human genetics—such as the Human Genome Project—cannot determine what is essential to being human. For that we would seem to need at least the findings of various ape and chimpanzee genome projects. (We should note that, for some commentators, even the findings of these other projects wouldn't be enough for identifying what is essential to being human because the structure of evolutionary theory complicates the question of what the essential properties of being human are. For more on this, see Sober [1980].)

All this is bad news for those like Fukuyama who want to draw large claims about human distinctiveness from genetic discoveries. Current investigations in human genetics, including those regarding normality, do not seem capable of identifying the essential properties of being human. But even if such properties were discovered, their discovery would not entail social or moral conclusions. We cannot go from a view of what is essential, distinctive, special about humans to a view of what makes humans special. That would be like saying having an atomic number of 79 is what's essential to gold, and so that is what makes gold (financially and esthetically) special. Such a conflation is comparable to the conflation of biological and social normality.

NOTE

1. This point is in contrast to one of Boorse's claims in his oft-cited discussion of health as a biological concept (1977). His main point is to argue that the concepts of health and disease are biological concepts, linked to the concept of normal functioning (what we have called "biological normality"). He also asserts that normal functioning

should be understood in terms of statistical concepts—that is, species typicality. But this second claim, which rests at least on a particular philosophical analysis of biological function, can be rejected without rejecting the idea of biological normality. Unfortunately, Boorse's critics have often not separated these two claims, believing that health, disease, and normality—if they are understood as biological concepts—must be statistical concepts. The point of the text above is that problems with a *statistical* conception of health, disease, or normal functioning do not entail problems for a *biological* conception of health, disease, or normal functioning.

REFERENCES

Boorse, C. (1976). "Wright on Functions." *Philosophical Review* 85: 70–86.
Boorse, C. (1977). "Health as a Theoretical Concept." *Philosophy of Science* 44: 542–73.
Davis, P., and J. Bradley. (1996). "The Meaning of Normal." *Perspectives in Biology and Medicine* 40: 68–77.
Fukuyama, F. (2002). *Our Posthuman Future.* New York: Farrar, Strauss and Giroux.
Goffman, E. (1963). *Stigma.* Englewood Cliffs, N.J.: Prentice-Hall.
Greer, J., and M. Capecchi. (2002). "*Hoxb8* is Required for Normal Grooming Behavior in Mice." *Neuron* 33: 23–34.
Hacking, I. (1990). *The Taming of Chance.* Cambridge: Cambridge University Press: 160
Murphy, E. (1972). "The Normal and the Perils of the Sylleptic Argument." *Perspectives in Biology and Medicine* 15: 566–82.
Nagel, E. (1961). *The Structure of Science.* New York: Harcourt, Brace and World.
Sober, E. (1980). "Evolution, Population, and Essentialism." *Philosophy of Science* 47: 350–83.
Varmus, H., and R. Weinberg. (1993). *Genes and the Biology of Cancer.* New York: Scientific American Library.
Wachbroit, R. (1994). "Normality as a Biological Concept." *Philosophy of Science* 61: 579–91.
Wachbroit, R. (1998). "Concepts of Health and Disease." In R. Chadwick, ed. *The Encyclopedia of Applied Ethics.* New York: Academic.
Wright, L. (1976). *Teleological Explanations.* Berkeley: University of California Press.

III / Promoting Public Conversation about Behavioral Genetics

CHAPTER TWELVE

Creating Public Conversation about Behavioral Genetics

Leonard Fleck, Ph.D.

Why do we need a "public conversation" about behavioral genetics at all? This sounds like the sort of subject matter that is best left to some range of experts, that is, geneticists and neuroscientists and behavioral psychologists, not your average citizen. I agree with this view, at least as far as the formal science is concerned. Further, if the scientific disagreements and debates about behavioral genetics were confined to research labs, then again there would be no need for some broader public to intrude into these debates. But the fact is that the scientists themselves have suggested that their work in behavioral genetics may well have consequences of an ethical and political sort (Beckwith and Alper, 2002; Nuffield Council on Bioethics, 2002). Particular behavioral geneticists may or may not be correct about the social consequences they project as the practical implications of their work. But if there are such possible consequences, *then there ought to be a public conversation about how those social consequences ought to be assessed and regulated and responded to.* This is the central thesis that I will argue for in the first two sections of this chapter.

For at least a decade, scientific articles have periodically reported a connection between some gene locus and some behavioral disorder. *Time* magazine's headline, "The Search for a Murder Gene" (Lemonick, 2003), is representative of how those reports often get translated in the media. Such headlines clearly create public impressions; they are not in obscure scientific journals. But why should such headlines matter?

One short answer is that such headlines create serious distortions in public understanding. But there are numerous distortions of public understanding. Tens of millions of Americans have a distorted understanding of the evolution of the universe. Why should genetic misunderstandings evoke special concern? Again, the short answer is that these misunderstandings could provoke misguided public policy, which is to say that the coercive powers of the state could be used to violate the rights or liberties of individuals whose socially unapproved behavior was "genetically linked," if the public believed that meant such behavior was an irrevocable feature of them as individuals. (See chapter 13 of this volume, which explores the extent to which the lay public is—and is not—likely to make such mistakes.)

One of the distinctive features about behavioral genetics is that it is about essential features of our identity *as agents*. I may have a genotype that predisposes me to early-onset heart disease. But that is something quite accidental and distinct from who I am as a person. However, if there were such a thing as specific genes that were causally related to sexual orientation, that would seem to be importantly related to an essential feature of my identity (Hamer et al., 1993). I would not have the option of simply choosing a heterosexual identity (CNN.com, 2003). Some have found this possibility liberating. If my sexual orientation is not something I have chosen, then I cannot be held responsible or blameworthy for simply being who I am. But something crucial needs to be noted about this conclusion. This conclusion does not represent a scientific "fact." Rather, it is no more than a possible social response. Just as possible would be a repressive or intolerant response.

Lest anyone think that these concerns are merely the product of a fevered academic imagination, the reader should recall the many excesses associated with the eugenics movement from the early twentieth century (Kevles, 1985; Abate, 2003; Nuffield Council on Bioethics, 2002, 13–22). In particular, the eugenics movement was not about removing cancer or heart disease or cystic fibrosis from the human gene pool. Rather, the focus was on what we would recognize today as behavioral genetics, removing from the human gene pool the lazy, the criminal, the feeble-minded, the alcoholic, and the mentally deranged. Sterilization laws and other policy interventions would be the means to accomplish this. (In North Carolina that story gets carried all the way up to 1975 [Schoen, 2003].) As Troy Duster mentioned in chapter 7, more recently, we have witnessed the discrimination visited upon African Americans who were identified as being carriers of the sickle cell trait (mistakenly believed to be afflicted with the disease itself). And there was also the XYY controversy, which started to move in the direction of seeking public policies to require genetic testing to identify those who were "born to be crooks." These are not benign intellectual errors. Nor, I would add, are these errors that could be readily corrected by improving only the quality of the public understanding of the underlying science.

If people really believed that individuals were genetically destined to become crooks, then it is easy to imagine a public clamor for developing a genetic test to identify such individuals, followed by a public policy that would mandate such testing. Universalized use of this test might be resisted, but this would be small comfort. We could imagine instead that only individuals accused of a crime would have to undergo the test. Then, if the test were positive, the obvious question would arise as to whether this was admissible evidence at trial. Some might even wonder whether a trial was necessary. After all, juries are flawed. Individual jurors are vulnerable to clever psychological manipulation by defense attorneys. If we have an objective scientific test that tells us this individual is a crook (immutably), then we are beyond a reasonable doubt. Why give such an individual three strikes when one strike and a genetic test settles the matter?

I want to pass over in silence that very badly distorted way of linking genes and behavior that is reflected in those headlines and in the scenarios above. The more likely relationship of genes and behavior was explored at length in chapters 1–5 of this volume and expressed nicely by Wasserman when he wrote: "What behavioral geneticists generally mean when they claim that a person is genetically predisposed to a given kind of behavior is, in part, that he has genetic features that make him more likely to engage in that behavior in certain environments" (2001, 306). In other words, human behaviors are most often the result of complex interactions among multiple genes, each of which has only a small effect on the behavior of interest.[1] Further, specific environmental factors are necessary as well to elicit specific behaviors. And all of this may be related to a rapidly emerging appreciation of the fact that many effects are "epigenetic"; that is, they occur at the level of the DNA molecule, but they are not simply the result of differences in the sequence of base pairs (Caspi et al., 2003; Dennis, 2003; Blakeslee, 2003).

In the first part of this chapter I will offer a number of scenarios that would suggest some possible public policy changes as a result of what we might come to know about the relationship between genes and behavior. My goal will *not* be to make any policy recommendations. Rather, this discussion will provide a concrete focus for the remaining parts of the chapter. What I want to offer is a rich and diverse array of possible policy problems that would seem to warrant social attention. In the next part of the chapter I will argue that normal "interest group competitive politics," including reliance on expert judgment and public opinion polling, would be the wrong political methods for articulating and legitimating public policy solutions to the problems raised in the first part of the chapter. I will argue instead that we ought to devise methods and practices of rational democratic deliberation[2] for addressing these sorts of issues and legitimating certain policy solutions. In the third part of the chapter I will seek to characterize in sufficient detail what those methods and practices ought to look like in terms of 15 normative criteria that can be used to judge the integrity of these democratic deliberations.

Genes and Behavior: Ethical and Policy Issues

We are going to consider three behavioral genetic disorders that have received considerable scientific attention as well as significant media attention of late. Our "case descriptions" will be excessively succinct, since I have only the modest goal of generating a list of possible ethical and policy issues.

As Jonathan Beckwith mentioned in chapter 3, one recent longitudinal study (Caspi et al., 2003) found that individuals with the short version of the *5-HTT* gene were much more likely to experience depression (and have serious thoughts of suicide) in response to stressful life events than were those who had the long version of this gene. To be more precise, 43 percent of those with two copies of the short version of the *5-HTT* gene experienced depression in response to stressful life events compared to 17 percent of those with two copies of the long version of this gene who experienced the same sort of stressful life event. Serious thoughts of suicide were twice as great among the "short gene" group as opposed to the "long gene" group. There are a number of obvious questions to be raised, such as why the other 57 percent of the "short gene" group did not experience depression in response to stressful life events. But we need to pass over those. Instead, I note a reaction from a psychologist at Vanderbilt University, Steven Hollon, who suggested that people with the vulnerable form of the gene could be identified for purposes of preventive interventions (Vedantam, 2003). I also note a piece of related research (Herman et al., 2003), which reports that this same gene, in its short form, is linked to binge drinking by college students who drank for the purpose of becoming inebriated.

Another study (Barrett et al., 2003) identified a specific gene, *GRK3,* thought to be causally associated with 10 percent of cases of bipolar disorder. The study involved 400 families with a history of bipolar disorder. The specific defect identified in this research is in the promoter region of the *GRK3* gene. Six mutations were identified in that region, but the P-5 mutation seems to be the strongest candidate. That mutation occurred three times more frequently in patients with bipolar disorder than in nonafflicted individuals. The researchers believe that this gene regulates the brain's response to dopamine and other neurotransmitters, modulating that response in a downward direction. Failure in the promoter region results in a more intense response to those neurotransmitters, as if the brain was responding to cocaine. The researchers hope their work will yield new targets for drug therapy. About 2.3 million adult Americans are believed to be afflicted with bipolar disorder.

Our third case study is schizophrenia. One novel approach to thinking about schizophrenia is represented by David Braff, a professor of psychiatry at the University of California in San Diego. Braff is the director of the new Consortium on the Genetics of Schizophrenia. His team is looking at a number of genes that are responsible for six or more brain functions that make one more vulnerable to developing schizophrenia. Their belief is that a cluster of genetic alterations is necessary to evoke schizophrenia in an individual. But those genetic alterations by themselves are not sufficient. Braff notes, for example, that identical twins have only a 65 percent chance of sharing schizophrenia, which suggests that other factors, such as epigenetic ones, might be necessary to achieve that effect (Clark, 2003). If both parents have been diagnosed with schizophrenia, there is a 46 percent chance that any one of their children will have schizophrenia as well. That figure is about 13 percent if one parent is schizophrenic. Roughly two million individuals in the United States are schizophrenic, and the cost of the disease in the United States is estimated at $40 billion annually.

I will just list some possible public policy issues that might be raised in the light of scientific reports linking genes and disorders as complex as the ones I've just mentioned. My goal is to put these issues out for critical assessment to be accomplished later. Depression (unipolar and bipolar), schizophrenia, alcohol and drug abuse are all significant and costly social problems in our society. Premature death and substantial loss in quality of life are consequences for both those afflicted with these disorders and significant others socially attached to these individuals. If these disorders could be prevented, or just substantially ameliorated through, for example, ingenious pharmaceutical interventions, this would be regarded as a major social good. However, these are not outcomes that can be achieved by individuals as such, for the most part. Policy options must be considered. What might they be?

First, should we provide public funding for the rapid development of genetic tests that would identify individuals at risk for any of our case disorders? As already noted, there are extremely high social costs associated with all of these disorders. That would seem to be one consideration that would justify such a social investment. Second, once such tests had been developed, what should our public policies be with respect to the use of those tests? Should all infants be tested at birth? That is, these would be mandatory tests. The goal of such testing would be entirely therapeutic, perhaps in the preventive mode. We might have in mind PKU as an analogy. But is that an accurate analogy, given that for all these behavioral disorders we are talking about susceptibilities and probabilities of actual expression? What would we imagine in the way of very early childhood interventions? Would we imagine either behavioral or pharmacologic interventions in the case of depression? And would we imagine that these would be continuous interventions throughout grammar school and high school?

Obviously, merely testing infants would do nothing about persons born prior to the development of these tests. So there would be the additional policy question of whether children and adults ought to undergo mandatory genetic testing as well for the genes or gene clusters associated with any of our case disorders. Again, many considerations would support such a policy. Societal welfare would be increased through reduced levels of crime and violence linked to any of our behavioral case disorders. The best interests of individuals would be protected by providing therapeutic resources to individuals who were positive for the problematic genotype, thereby reducing their risk of being arrested or fired from a job or suffering the results of ruptured social relationships. But other consequences need to be considered as well, some related to privacy, some related to individual liberty, some related to justice and protecting fair equality of opportunity.

Imagine that this mandatory testing policy were put in place. Who would have a legal right to know the results of these tests? In the case of children, would teachers have a right to know this information? The plausible claim could be made that teachers could be more attentive to such children, meaning that they would not allow the problematic behavior to get beyond the beginning stage before they provided a corrective response. Such preemptive preparation carries with it the clear risk of stigmatization. Further, if these children were regularly directed into some form of behavioral therapy throughout their formal schooling, then their classmates would certainly notice this intervention, as would the parents of those classmates. Such knowledge could have potentially adverse developmental consequences for these children (Florencio, 2000).

These same sorts of issues would arise for adults. Would potential employers have any legal right to know this information, especially if the work required considerable public contact in circumstances where there was frequent opportunity for social friction (e.g., police officer or loan officer at a bank)? Should professional schools (medicine, nursing, social work) have a legal right to know such information about applicants? The overall population risk of any individual having schizophrenia is slightly less than one percent; Wong (2001) reported that Hong Kong put in place a policy that would deny employment in the police force or fire department or emergency services to an individual who had a first-degree relative diagnosed with schizophrenia. Obviously, such social policies would compromise privacy rights. And there would also be the risk of unjust discrimination and loss of economic and professional opportunities. Should a society that cares about justice and respect for individual rights have in place policies that would protect individuals by denying employers the right to access such information? If so, should there be exceptions to that policy, such as situations in which clients or patients must place enormous trust in professionals serving them?

All of our behavioral case disorders have significant risk of having a corrosive effect on a marriage. Does this imply that we ought to make legally obligatory divulging the results of these hypothetical genetic tests to potential marriage partners, perhaps in the hopes of reducing divorce and the adverse effects divorce has on children? Or would such a loss of privacy not be warranted by what we hope for in the way of social gain? Apart from divorce, there are issues related to the welfare of future possible children of "unfortunate" matings. What sorts of social policies ought a genetically responsible society to have in these matters? If two individuals with bipolar disorder marry, is the risk to future possible children such that a responsible society (ultimately respectful of individual liberty) ought at least to fund a strong public education campaign (akin to antismoking campaigns) aimed at creating a social climate that would discourage individuals from having children if there were a greater than 10 percent risk of those children having a serious behavioral disorder? Or should even that indirect an effort to alter behavior in these very intimate life dimensions be regarded as a violation of our liberal political traditions?

Our political traditions assign substantial weight to respect for individual liberties and individual privacy. It might be impossible politically to believe that we would ever mandate genetic testing of such breadth. We can imagine a different scenario, one in which adolescent individuals display behavioral signs of a more serious depression or alcohol/drug abuse or schizophrenia. Should we then have a public policy that would mandate genetic testing of these individuals so that appropriate therapeutic interventions could be offered to them? Perhaps this would still represent too much of a threat to individual rights and liberties to be justified, even with hoped for substantial gains in social welfare. Should our policy then be one in which there is a mandated "offering" of these genetic tests that would then ultimately respect what would be an informed refusal? If there were an informed refusal, would there be a record kept of this? And could that informed refusal have future consequences for individuals should they engage in illegal behavior linked to the behavioral risks for which they could have been tested? Should individuals be able to claim that they have a moral and legal right to remain genetically ignorant about their own genetic endowment, especially if they fear they would be unable to cope with such knowledge? Or should a society judge that such deliberate ignorance in these circumstances is irresponsible, and should be legally culpable as well?

Many will find the policy options in the prior paragraph too threatening to some of our most important political values. But the problem would still remain that it would seem uncaring, maybe socially irresponsible, to do nothing to prevent the adverse consequences associated with these behavioral disorders for both the at-risk individuals and the larger society. Some may think that these individuals did not choose to be born with this genotype and these genetic vulnerabilities. What this suggests is an alternate policy strategy, an "incentives" strategy that is generally regarded as being more congruent with respect for individual rights. We could choose as a society to underwrite the costs associated with offering these tests to individuals whose behavior has suggested the possibility of a genetic vulnerability. We could also choose to underwrite the costs of either drug therapy or behavioral therapy aimed at helping individuals manage these vulnerabilities in ways that were congruent with both their best interests and the larger welfare of society. There would be no social or legal penalties associated with failing to take advantage of these incentives. We might imagine that a program such as this might be modeled on the End Renal Stage Disease (ERSD) program that underwrites the cost of dialysis for all who have the relevant medical need, that is, failed kidneys. Given the very high economic and social costs associated with depression, alcoholism, drug abuse, and schizophrenia, this would seem to be a reasonable and decent and responsible policy response. But then issues of health care justice would need to be raised.

The ESRD program has had its share of critics from the perspective of health care justice, that is, fair treatment or equal treatment. The program, for example, will pay for kidney transplants. But there is no social program that underwrites the cost of heart or liver or lung or other major organ transplants, though there seems to be no morally or politically relevant difference among these needs. This seems intuitively unfair. Likewise, if we underwrite at public expense the cost of genetic testing and therapy for these behavioral disorders, the argument can be made that it seems unfair that we would not do the same for various forms of heart disease or cancer or other such costly major medical disorders that might have just as much in the way of genetic roots as any of the behavioral disorders we have been considering. Rakowski (2002) addresses in broader terms the problems of justice raised by our increasing capacity to shape the genetic endowment of future possible children (see also Parens, 1998).

Public Reason, Public Policy, and Behavioral Genetics

How should we, citizens of a liberal pluralistic democratic society, address the possible policy issues raised above? The short answer, I suggest, is that we invoke the methods of public reason, as those have been articulated by John Rawls in *Political Liberalism* (1993). My goal in this section is to explain what public reason might mean with reference to the policy issues raised by behavioral genetics, and then to justify employing this method for addressing these issues as opposed to any of its rivals.

Rawls introduces the notion of public reason for purposes of addressing the problem of justice in liberal pluralistic democratic societies. I believe the notion of public reason can be usefully invoked for addressing most of the normative policy issues that emerge from the field of health care ethics today. For example, should we have public policies that would ban human cloning? Or that would ban public funding for embryonic stem cell research? Or that would permit physician-assisted suicide? Or that would require genetic testing of all babies for a range of disorders linked to behavioral genetics? The global political problem that Rawls feels our sort of society must address is this. On the one hand, we want to grant as broad a measure of liberty to individuals in our society to choose a life for themselves that they find satisfying and valuable, often in the light of a deep philosophic or religious perspective, what Rawls refers to as a "comprehensive vision of the good." This is what makes our society a "liberal" society, a society that is deeply respectful of individual rights, including the right to determine what counts as a sufficiently satisfying life as judged from the perspective of some comprehensive vision embraced by that individual. But, on the other hand, we do wish to be able to live with one another in peaceful and complexly cooperative relationships. What might prevent that from coming about is if groups of individuals who have one deep philosophic perspective that licenses some social practice (permits their members to choose physician-assisted suicide in the face of terminal illness) is seen by another social group with a very different philosophic perspective as harming their welfare through that practice (many disability advocates would claim that their lives are publicly devalued if physician-assisted suicide is permitted) (Smith, 1997; Bickenbach, 1998; Silvers, 1998). Obviously, individuals should not be allowed to use their rights to engage in behavior that is harmful to others. Does this mean that disability advocates may justifiably use the policy-making process and the coercive powers of the state to outlaw physician-assisted suicide? The answer to this question will turn, in large part, on how we (liberal citizens) characterize what will count as the sort of harm justifiably limited by the state.

Integral to our understanding of what it means to be a liberal society is that we are a pluralistic society. That is, we recognize and respect that there are these deep competing religious and philosophic perspectives that our citizens embrace. However, the state itself may not embrace any one of these religious or philosophic perspectives as a basis for creating public policies under which all of us will live. In political science literature this is what is usually referred to as the "neutrality" commitment of a liberal society. This is the essence of the problem for which Rawls invokes the notion of public reason.

We (liberal citizens) recognize that we are rational and reasonable beings who wish to live peacefully and cooperatively with one another. We recognize that we must be mutually respectful to accomplish that goal. We also recognize the desirability of stable, clear understandings of what we may mutually expect; and consequently, we recognize the need for social practices and social rules that will sustain that expectation. Such social rules, given the pluralistic nature of our society, will frequently result in constraints on the liberty of individuals. Given our rational natures, it is reasonable to expect that we will give one another reasons for such constraints that all who are bound by such constraints will find reasonable. But it would be difficult to meet this condition if the reasons we wished to give for such constraints were very deeply embedded in a particular religious or philosophic perspective. We would in effect be privileging one religious or philosophic perspective over others, which would clearly undermine any rational motivation for those committed to the disfavored perspectives to remain as cooperative members of that society. Social and economic circumstances might force these individuals to remain in (grudgingly) cooperative relationships, but this is hardly a desirable (or stable) state of affairs. The alternative, as advocated by Rawls, is to find or construct public reasons to justify value-laden public policies that are independent of any particular religious or philosophic worldview (Rawls, 1993, chapter VI). Thus, if Hindus were to become a majority of the population of the United States, they would not be justified in using their majoritarian political power to put in place public policies that would ban the sale of all beef on the grounds that cows were sacred. This would not be a public reason, the sort of reason that liberal citizens could not reasonably reject.

There are, of course, all manner of public health policies that shape our lives together. Such health-related reasons would have presumptive political legitimacy from the perspective of public reason. However, we can imagine that vegetarians might achieve majority status in our society. Further, they might wish to ban the sale of beef products because of the deleterious health effects associated with our consumption of beef. Would this be a legitimate public policy? The short answer is that it would not. Granted, we are assuming that no vegetarian philosophy is driving this policy. Still, the problem is that there is no *public interest* that would warrant such a policy in a liberal pluralistic society. A public interest is an interest that each and every citizen in our society has and that we, as individuals or as privately organized groups of individuals, cannot adequately maintain or protect without the coordinated efforts and coercive powers of government. Clean air and clean water that would otherwise be threatened by powerful economic interests represent clear cases of public interests because there is virtually nothing that we as individuals can do to protect our interests in this regard. The risks posed by beef fail this test because we are individually capable of determining whether or not we are willing to accept those risks for ourselves. There are no powerful economic interests forcing us to eat beef. Nor is eating beef analogous in morally or politically relevant respects to our need to breathe clean air or consume clean water.

But there is another critical point that needs to be noted. *How clean* must clean air and water be in order to protect adequately the public interest that is at stake? This question takes us directly to the function of rational democratic deliberation and the reasons why it should be thought of as an essential feature of our political life. In theory we could have air and water that were as pure as the day Native Americans began to populate the continent. However, such a standard would be unreasonable. It would be excessively costly both economically and in terms of the sacrifices we would all have to make in terms of the quality of our lives. This implies that some degree of impure air and water is morally and politically tolerable, even though that might have bad consequences (health-wise) for some members of our society.

What degree of impurity is morally and politically defensible? I would argue that no one best answer can be given to this question. An indefinitely large number of "just enough," "reasonable enough" trade-offs might be made, no one of which is unequivocally superior in all morally and politically relevant respects to all the others. Further, no amount of additional scientific information will alter this conclusion because what is at stake is not just a matter of facts. There are multiple value considerations that somehow need to be weighed and balanced and critically assessed. Further, following the general arguments of moral pluralists (Rawls, 1993; Walzer, 1983), I would contend that there is no one moral or political theory that would identify any uniquely superior moral or political option in this matter. The values at stake are too diverse; the relevant facts are too uncertain or too complicated. We are simply faced with what Rawls refers to as "the burdens of judgment" (Rawls, 1993, 54–58).

Who then should judge? And how should that judgment be justified and legitimated? All of us in this society are potentially affected by the environmental policies (and associated risks and costs) we adopt regarding air and water; and consequently, all of us ought to have the opportunity to make that judgment for ourselves. Of necessity this will be a collective judgment because we have already judged that it is a public interest that is at stake, as opposed to the welfare interests of discrete individuals who had the capacity to protect those interests themselves to the degree they desired. Processes of rational democratic deliberation provide a mechanism for making real a *public* decision regarding that public interest. Public reason, as Rawls uses that term, provides a normative standard for shaping the content and process of that public deliberation so that the results would be morally justified and politically legitimated.

Let me briefly outline what I take to be the core features of this deliberative process. We start by noting that this is a *public* process. Backroom bargaining and secret deals among some group of elite insiders are intrinsically subversive of legitimate democratic deliberation. Next, we note that there is a kind of *political space* within which this deliberative process has its primary application. The defining features of that space have been suggested above. (1) We have a political problem at the core of which is a substantial public interest. That a public interest is at stake means collective democratic deliberation is necessary. (2) There are multiple ways in which that problem could be addressed reasonably, no one of which is clearly and unequivocally superior from the perspective of political morality. This is because there are multiple public values that can be potentially balanced in multiple complex ways depending on how one interprets complex and uncertain social and scientific facts as well as social preferences. This was illustrated above in the first section, where I teased out a range of policy options related to genetic testing for our case behavioral disorders.

But (3) this space is bounded by what I refer to metaphorically as "constitutional principles of political morality" (Fleck, 2002). Policy options that violate any of these metaphorical constitutional boundaries are necessarily not objects of legitimate democratic deliberation.[3] If, for example, a community was considering a site for a new plant that represented 800 jobs (but the plant would produce pollutants that increased cancer, lung disease, and heart disease for those within a range of five miles downwind), and if community leaders chose a site for the plant where the poorest members of the community lived in that downwind range (and were very unlikely to get any of the jobs brought in by the plant), then this option would be "constitutionally flawed" because it would violate the "equal concern and respect" principle of political morality. By way of contrast, if the pollutants from the plant were widely distributed in all directions so that both the risks and the benefits were widely and randomly distributed, then the issue of whether to accept this trade-off would be a legitimate object of democratic deliberation.

(4) The deliberative process is *rational* because it is committed to "reason giving" as the primary deliberative mechanism, as opposed to political bargaining rooted in the capacity to organize political power for the sake of advancing self-interested goals. In its ideal form (which is realizable) it is a matter of mutual civic education and shared social problem solving, very much in contrast to reliance on public opinion polls, which do no more than aggregate the often uncritical, momentary, marginally thoughtful judgments that a particular polling question might trigger from some number of isolated individuals. The focus of the deliberative process will be some number of public interests, which will have the effect of restricting the kinds of reasons and reasoning that can be a credible part of the process. A plant owner who seeks a relaxation of air and water quality standards in order to maximize profits for shareholders (as well as his annual bonus) cannot reasonably expect that those who would suffer the adverse health consequences would see this as a credible or persuasive reason for endorsing his request. What he is seeking is a compromise of public interests to advance private interests. There is no fair sharing of risks and benefits associated with this request.

Finally (5), after there has been a full enough and fair enough and inclusive enough deliberative process, some sort of reasonable and fair aggregating mechanism (some form of voting) needs to be used to achieve decisional closure. In large political bodies it would be utopian to expect consensus. But consensus is not necessary to achieve moral and political legitimacy for a decision. Again, the range of options that are the focus of the deliberative process is reasonable enough and inclusive enough and just enough, which implies that any that might be chosen would have presumptive moral and political legitimacy. This might suggest the thought that the deliberative process is unnecessary, that some random selection device could achieve a legitimate result without the effort and "inefficiency" of the deliberative process. However, that is a false implication because of the value of the educational and transformative and stabilizing effects of the deliberative process itself. The deliberative process itself builds mutual understanding, which in turn may provoke social imaginative processes that will transform the initial available options into novel social responses that will elicit broader and more stable agreement from those potentially affected by that choice.

I now want to turn to the task of exploring the relevance of this model to the potential issues raised earlier in connection with some specific social problems related to work in behavioral genetics. The very first question we need to raise is whether there are any public interests at stake in any or all of our three issue areas. If there were no public interests at stake (potentially adversely affected), then there would be no need for public policy or the deliberative conversations that would shape and legitimate those policies. We would see social problems, but those social problems would be addressed through professional groups or churches or businesses or other relevant private social institutions. However, it does seem obvious both that there are public interests at stake and that they tug in different directions.

We asked earlier whether there ought to be mandatory genetic testing in various social contexts for any of the behavioral disorders I identified. There are at least six relevant public interests that can be identified in that issue area. They are privacy, liberty, justice/protecting fair equality of opportunity, social harm, invidious discrimination, and personal responsibility. Again, each of these items represents a public interest because each and every one of us has these interests but is unable to protect them adequately alone or with other private individuals *in our present social context*. Protecting the privacy of my personal genetic information was not a problem a couple decades ago because there was no capacity to do genetic testing, nor was there the capacity to disseminate that information rapidly in ways unknown to an individual through vast computer networks capable of readily sharing information. But that is no longer true today when we have the capacity to capture thousands of genetic facts about me with a single genetic test that can be done surreptitiously. Hence, mandated genetic tests have the presumptive capacity to affect adversely the privacy rights, liberty rights, and rights to fair treatment of individuals covered by the suggested mandate.

We might say that the easiest way to avoid those threats to those public interests would be to avoid all mandated genetic tests. However, there is the risk of preventable and irreversible serious social harm on the other side of the moral and political equation. If mandated genetic testing could effectively prevent such harm in some range of circumstances (prevent suicide and deaths from impaired drivers), then we might not be able to dismiss mandated testing that quickly. In addition, behavioral genetics seems to raise questions about our social understanding of personal responsibility. The broad question would seem to be: Should we, with regard to our moral and legal understanding of what individuals should be held accountable for, modify our norms and criteria of responsibility when specific behaviors have been influenced by a specific genetic endowment, such as that associated with bipolar disorder or a tendency toward alcoholism? Again, there would be a considerable number of possible policy options for consideration that would represent different complex mixes of trade-offs among relevant social interests (Nuffield Council on Bioethics, 2002, 121–88; Buchanan et al., 2000, 308–45). Some might eventually be recognized as violating one or another constitutional principle of political morality, but it is likely that the deliberative process will be needed to make that clear and acceptable to a broad engaged public. Other options are very likely to be appropriately situated in that political space where rational democratic deliberation is feasible and necessary.

Normative Criteria for Assessing Rational Democratic Deliberations

I have provided so far a partial answer to the question used to title this chapter. I now want to expand that original question to read: How do you create a public conversation about behavioral genetics that is civil and that has moral and political integrity? I have served as co-principal investigator for two National Institutes for Health, Ethical, Legal and Social Implications of the Human Genome Project (NIH ELSI) projects (Fleck, 1996, 1997; Citrin and Fleck, 2001) that have tested slightly different models of deliberative democracy with respect to genetics and public policy. In reflecting on the work of that project I have been able to identify 15 different questions that need to be asked that will serve as useful normative criteria for assessing specific deliberative efforts. I describe and illustrate them below.

First, do individual participants in the deliberative process say that they find themselves *internally conflicted* regarding the particular range of issues under discussion regarding genetics, ethics, and policy? To my mind this is the single most important touchstone for a fair and effective democratic deliberative process. In recruiting participants for these community dialogue sessions we told them what we most wanted to avoid was the bitter ideological divisiveness and intransigence and mindless inflammatory rhetoric that has characterized much of the public debate about abortion. There is certainly the potential for that happening a hundred times over with each moral and political issue that emerges that is linked to our developing genetic knowledge and related technologies. The socially important difference is that the abortion issue is relatively isolated. It touches directly the lives of only relatively small numbers of people, which means that the vast majority of our population can choose to be indifferent or disengaged from the verbal battles. The genetics issues, however, will increasingly affect directly a very large portion of our population in many different ways, which means there is the potential for a manifold increase in the level of corrosive social and political friction.

What we have found in our community dialogue projects is that the single most important goal that must be accomplished is creating in the minds of deliberators this sense of internal conflict. If this can be accomplished effectively in the earliest stages of deliberation, then political or ideological straitjackets will typically be greatly loosened. Individuals will find themselves in a puzzled frame of mind that will more readily dispose them to engage in cooperative social problem solving rather than heated debates where there must necessarily be winners and losers. The tone and nature of the deliberative process is markedly different when many options are being cooperatively assessed for their strengths and weaknesses in addressing a social problem as opposed to having groups of individuals "defend a point of view" to which they are rigidly attached. Mutual education is possible and effective in the former process whereas in the latter process the object is to "score points" against the opposition.

One example we actually used in those community dialogues was that of a 26-year-old male whose father had died of Huntington disease at age 52. He knows that there is a 50 percent chance that he himself has the gene variant for Huntington disease, but after much reflection he concludes that he is better off not knowing his fate rather than taking the test for Huntington disease and knowing his fate. The first question we pose to the group is whether they believe he has a strong right to privacy and a strong right to autonomy, and that these rights ought to be politically protected. In other words, he ought not be coerced into taking a genetic test that he fears might be more personally destructive than constructive; and further, he ought not be forced to reveal this genetic information to others. Typically, 80 to 90 percent of a group will endorse this conclusion when it is just taken in isolation. Then we add that this young man wishes to marry and have children of his own. We ask whether he should be morally and legally obligated to reveal to a future possible spouse that there is a 50 percent chance that he would be afflicted with Huntington disease; and, if he were positive for Huntington disease, then each of his future possible children would be faced with that same risk. This scenario produces the sort of internal conflict we are talking about. Almost everyone can imagine that the "future possible spouse" in this scenario is either herself, or a sister, or a daughter, or a best friend. It just "seems wrong" that a woman could be denied such important information for purposes of making the commitment we associate with marriage. And it "seems wrong" that those future possible children would be put at risk as well. But, as a liberal democratic society with strong commitments to the value of individual rights would we want to compromise coercively the privacy and autonomy rights of the individual at risk? This is the point at which that internal conflict is very acutely experienced. Most participants will not embrace easily or readily either of the prima facie options. The collective thought is that there must be some possible alternative that achieves some measure of reasonable balance or compromise among these conflicting social values and social interests. Individuals quickly realize at this point that rigid ideological commitments are neither relevant nor helpful. Then a cooperative social inquiry, very much of the sort that John Dewey (1929) would envision, can begin.

There are ways of guiding this discussion that can enrich and deepen the quality of the deliberative effort without steering the conversation to some predetermined conclusion. Philosophers have an important social role to play in accomplishing this if participants in the deliberative effort lack a sufficiently rich background of information. Again, in our actual community dialogues we introduced alternative examples to the Huntington disease case as a way of providing a range of possibilities. We asked participants how they would react to our original scenario if we were talking about the *BRCA1* gene and a woman who knew she was positive for a genetic variant that increased significantly her lifetime risk of breast cancer. And, to bring this discussion closer to the focus of this chapter, we asked in a hypothetical mode about some complex genetic test that would inform an individual that his bipolar disorder had a strong genetic link, which could have obvious consequences for future possible children.

This brings us to our second norm for assessing the moral and political integrity of these deliberative efforts, which can be captured in the motto "science matters." Put in question form, we ask whether dialogue participants have been given the capacity *to use available scientific knowledge honestly* to inform their ethics and policy judgments, recognizing always the fallibility of such scientific knowledge, as well as the different degrees of confidence that might be attached to one or another scientific claim. This is where expertise has an important role to play in contributing to the value and integrity of these democratic deliberative efforts (Garland, 1999). Good ethics and policy must be informed by sound science (which is still fallible science). And good ethics and policy can be severely subverted by science badly presented in the media, sometimes initiated by scientists themselves seeking to exaggerate the significance of their research (Lee, 2003).

As noted already, it is relatively rarely that science is ultimately determinative of our ethical or policy judgments. What our science does most often is speak strongly against possible ethical or policy judgments we might consider in the abstract, in effect saying those judgments ought to be put off the table, but leaving on the table many other possible ethical or policy judgments that remain compatible with our best science. Again, by way of quick illustration, there are scientifically important differences between Huntington disease and breast cancer associated with the *BRCA1* gene (which likely represents no more than 10% of breast cancer in women). Huntington disease is virtually 100 percent penetrant and we have at present no medical capacity to cure or even forestall disease progression. By way of contrast, there are several hundred variants of the *BRCA1* gene, and it is described as a "susceptibility gene" because having one of these variants will increase the lifetime risk of breast cancer for an affected individual by 45 to 85 percent. Further, there are medical interventions that can alter the feared fatal course of breast cancer. These facts would seem to have a significant bearing on possible policy judgments we might endorse, especially if one of our major concerns is the question of what sort of social responsibility we ought to embrace with respect to the genetic health of future possible children, that is, children who have not yet been conceived but whose circumstances of conception could be modified in various ways by various social policy options.

Again, returning to the focus of this chapter, it is ethically and politically relevant that, as a matter of science, there are multiple possible genotypes associated with each of the behavioral disorders we are considering. Further, there are numerous, complex, poorly understood environmental factors, as well as numerous epigenetic possibilities associated with the actual expression of these behavioral disorders (Ridley, 2003; Ehrlich and Feldman, 2003; Hamer, 2002; Kitcher, 1996). This is why only 65 percent of identical twins will both exhibit schizophrenia if one is affected with schizophrenia. Likewise, 43 percent of individuals with two copies of the short version of the *5-HTT* gene were likely to experience serious depression in response to stressful life events, as opposed to 100 percent. What this suggests is considerable policy caution with respect to testing for these genotypes, especially if we were to imagine some degree of mandatory testing, especially if such testing itself had serious potential consequences for individuals tested (as well as relatives of those individuals). If genetic testing were as personally inconsequential but therapeutically effective as drawing blood for a cholesterol count, there would be no need for rational democratic deliberation about policy options. But, as our discussion has shown, these tests have considerable uncertainty attached to them with respect to clinical utility (now and for the foreseeable future) as well as considerable risks of adverse personal consequences. Our only point for now is that good ethical and policy judgments must be rooted in good science presented in a comprehensible way to the public. Such science may be determinative in excluding some policy options, but rarely will science alone dictate a single best policy option, or whether any policy option at all ought to be pursued.

Some may be inclined to argue that the science behind behavioral genetics is just too complex for public understanding and public deliberation. But it is not obvious to me that this is a necessary truth. Many researchers may not have the capacity to communicate both clearly and accurately their scientific work and its relationship to various social problems, but there are science writers who have demonstrated the capacity to do this in a fair-minded way that would enhance rather than subvert the integrity of these democratic deliberative efforts (Baker, 2004; Ridley, 2003).

This brings us to my third norm for assessing the quality and integrity of these public deliberations. Are dialogue participants in the habit of *giving reasons* for their point of view in relation to one or another option under discussion? This is absolutely essential to appreciating what is distinctive about this deliberative process. This is intended to be *rational* democratic deliberation. Some critics have suggested disdainfully that this emphasis represents an academic or philosophic bias, that what we are attempting to advocate as a social ideal is the academic seminar. However, I would contend that this criticism is unfair. The process of reason giving is an ordinary and essential part of our lives, both as members of a moral community and as members of a political community. While practices of reason giving are manifold and complex, the critical importance of the practice is that it permits us to relate to one another in a distinctively human way, as rational beings capable of cooperating freely with one another to create and advance common goals, as opposed to having to be coerced by formal authority into participating in specific social practices. There is nothing especially esoteric or "merely academic" about such a practice.

The fourth norm is closely related to the third. Have dialogue participants been able to distinguish *specific value judgments that belong in the domain of public reason* from others that have a legitimate role only in their personal lives or in much narrower social groups? Again, this has something of an esoteric ring to it. Citing Rawls's work in this regard, as I did earlier, would likely reinforce that belief. Most members of our society would struggle to understand the central points of Rawls's *Political Liberalism*. However, Rawls's central concerns in that volume are not that distant or that intrinsically unintelligible to most citizens of our society, as my earlier examples about Hindus and vegetarians and beef prohibitions were intended to illustrate. Most of our citizens are familiar with the phrase "separation of church and state," and have at least a rough appreciation of the importance of that political commitment. We argue about the edges of that commitment, but the core is something that is very widely endorsed as central to the liberal nature of our society. We are not at all inclined to embrace the theocratic society of the Taliban. Consequently, when we must work together to shape public policy about a social problem suffused with these conflicting values (as illustrated above), and we want to achieve agreement that is sufficiently rational and reasonable to assure stability, we realize that we must be careful about the kinds of reasons we can invoke to elicit the free agreement of other citizens. I will concede to my putative critic that as a matter of fact we have only a limited number of social and political practices that exemplify this norm; and consequently, that considerable political education and political practice development will be necessary to make more common and feasible this deliberative model. But, given what is happening in genetics and most other fields of medicine, where we see raised with increasing frequency novel ethical and policy issues that are potentially very controversial, that ought to serve as a motivator for developing our democratic deliberative capacities.

The remaining norms for assessing the integrity of these democratic deliberative efforts may be presented more succinctly, with less in the way of explanation and comment. Our fifth norm is this: Are dialogue participants recognizing the *numerous values* that have a bearing on the particular problem under discussion? This norm makes explicit what Rawls would refer to as the fact of value pluralism (Rawls, 1993, chapter IV). In our personal lives we may choose to give supremacy to one value with respect to which we organize our lives. But in our lives as liberal citizens this is a political impossibility. The flip side of this norm (and related to the public reason norm) is that we might mistakenly dismiss from the deliberative conversation a value seen as attached to a specific religious worldview. I have in mind something like "respect for human life," which might be embedded in a rich religious perspective represented by a "sanctity of life ethic." That value can be abstracted from the religious belief system in which it may be embedded for some. To the extent that is possible it is a legitimate member of the numerous values that need to be considered in our deliberative conversations.

Sixth, do dialogue participants see the deliberative process as a whole as *fair and impartial,* not designed in a way aimed at manipulating participants to endorse some predetermined outcome? All will recognize that this will be a challenging norm to satisfy in practice, but there are all sorts of ways of coming close to meeting this challenge. Failure to satisfy this challenge sufficiently clearly undermines the legitimacy of any policy choices that might emerge from the deliberative process. In our actual community dialogues under the ELSI grants we deliberately recruited participants associated with Right to Life and with various disability organizations and with religious groups. Our thought was that failure to include these voices would almost certainly undercut entirely the legitimacy of our deliberative model.

Our next three norms can be bundled together. Seventh, do dialogue participants feel comfortable because they are genuinely *speaking to one another as equals?* Eighth, do dialogue participants consistently *show respect* to one another, avoiding behaviors that others would often regard as being signals of disrespect? Ninth, is there evidence in the dialogue process that *mutual understanding* is being achieved, that individuals are truly engaged in a common task and not just serially expressing opinions? These are all process norms, but no less important for that reason. In the deliberative process we are all there "as citizens," as equal members of this society. Social standing, wealth, levels of formal education, and so on are all irrelevant so far as democratic deliberation is concerned. Likewise, being respectful is critical to the success of the deliberative process. By definition, the process has been initiated because there are some deeply controversial issues that need to be addressed. Participants will disagree with one another, but that disagreement can be expressed in ways that are fundamentally respectful of the other. If such mutual respect can be maintained, then the likelihood of achieving mutual understanding is improved, which in turn will provide the footing for the difficult compromises and balancings of competing values that will be needed in some chosen policy option.

Our next three norms may again be bundled together. Tenth, have dialogue participants been able *to identify and express some shared values* that are relevant to the issue being discussed? Eleventh, have dialogue participants been able to identify and assess both *assumptions and consequences* associated with their point of view? Twelfth, have dialogue participants been able to identify what they regard as *public interests or common interests* that ought to be used as reference points for assessing any public policies related to genetics and emerging genetic technologies? These three norms are associated with practical things that must occur to move the conversation forward. They are very much internal norms associated with specific democratic deliberations. There is a recognition that the conversation began with a diversity of points of view, but that virtually all within the conversation are experiencing the internal conflict described above. In addition, there is a shared (albeit diffuse) sense that some sort of policy response is necessary to address the problem, that it would not be good to just allow the problem to simmer unaddressed. Further, there are multiple policy options that might be articulated but some common reference points are needed to assess those options. Hence, one of the mediating goals of the conversation is to identify or construct or reconstruct some shared values that would assist with policy assessment. Likewise, judging the degree to which there is a shared appreciation of the likely consequences of different policy options is important. And again, what justifies the public nature of the conversation is the initial judgment that there are public interests that are at stake that somehow need to be protected or adjudicated. To accomplish that it may be necessary to refine and further specify the nature of those public interests. This will include a critical assessment of those public interests. Thus, in an earlier part of the chapter, I raised a question suggesting it might be desirable to genetically test all children for one or another genotype in the future that might be associated with an increased disposition to depression or to alcohol dependence. It was suggested that this might be for therapeutic purposes, which has a benign and noble ring to it. However, therapeutic intent is no guarantee that there will not be intolerable consequences for individuals. This is the sort of general cautionary note that needs to be part of these deliberative conversations.

Finally, there are three more norms that we can discuss as a cluster. Thirteenth, is there evidence from the dialogue process that there has been successful *mutual civic education,* that individuals have learned what they judge to be important things from one another for making better judgments in matters of public policy related to emerging genetic knowledge and technologies? Mutual civic education is not just about scientific matters. More important, it is about the gradual evolution of new or more complex shared value perspectives, the sorts of commitments that build more stable reference points (what Rawls would call "considered value judgments") for addressing what will surely be a steady flow of other social policy problems related to these new technologies. That will have the effect of softening the intensity of future value conflicts related to these technologies as social capacities are created for addressing the problems raised. Again, what we gradually seek to achieve as each problem reaches the social agenda is what Rawls would refer to as a "social reflective equilibrium" (Rawls, 1993, chapter III, esp. 95–99; Daniels, 1996).

Our fourteenth norm is this: Is there evidence from the dialogue process that participants have a better understanding of the *complexity of the issues* they have been discussing and the *inherent uncertainty* that must characterize such discussions? Given the potentially far-reaching effects that many social policies can have once accepted, it may be a bit unnerving to think about all the uncertainties that are inherently part of these deliberative efforts. Such uncertainty could yield timidity, an unwillingness to face at all the policy response that may be called for by a particular genetically related social problem. But timidity can have its own costs; it can hardly be seen as a morally or politically "safe" response. Better, I would argue, that the deliberative process develop within our citizens a capacity to deal fairly and intelligently with these inherent uncertainties, with regard to the relevant scientific knowledge as well as the consequences of putting novel policies into practice.

Finally, our fifteenth norm is: Do dialogue participants see themselves as expressing *greater toleration* for choices related to genetics that others might make that they might not make for themselves? This is really a critical hallmark of a liberal society. Public policy can serve many very broad social purposes. It may be used to *prohibit* certain options, such as cloning or physician-assisted suicide. That represents a restriction of personal liberty that might be justified if certain uses of that liberty threatened substantial harm to important public interests. Public policy might also be used to *prioritize,* to regulate and balance conflicts among important public values and public interests. And public policy might also be used to *protect and promote* certain space for the exercise of individual liberty, even when that liberty is used in ways that others might find offensive or contrary to their visions of what it means to live a good life in a decent society. Developing a public capacity to understand the political importance of mutual tolerance in those controversial areas is a very important task for democratic deliberation in a liberal society, most especially when those controversial areas are linked to very intimate aspects of our lives as persons, as is clearly true with regard to most matters of genetics, behavioral traits, and reproductive decision making.

Conclusions

Two questions were at the core of this chapter. The first is the question of *why* we need a *public* conversation about behavioral genetics. The short answer is that there are at least perceived social problems involving public interests that are raised by emerging knowledge in the field of behavioral genetics. At least some in the field suggest that work in the field will importantly affect our general understanding of ourselves as human beings. Others have suggested that such research may affect particular social practices, like the sentencing of criminals. We have no way of knowing now what measure of truth may be attached to those predictions. It may prove to be the case that emerging knowledge in behavioral genetics may alter these understandings much less than some predict. But even that will require these rational democratic deliberative efforts to ratify and stabilize our understanding of the social implications of this knowledge.

Our second core question was about *how* we should go about creating this broad public conversation *as a rational conversation*. Our most critical conclusion is that we need to do two things in particular. First, we need to create within the minds of each member of a broad segment of the public an internal conflict so far as the conflicting values are concerned that are associated with some policy problem linked to something in behavioral genetics. This creates the necessary condition for a cooperative social problem-solving response as opposed to a fractious and socially corrosive ideological struggle. Second, we need to build our social capacity to be skillful in crafting and giving public reasons as the primary mechanism through which the deliberative process progresses. And we need to build our social capacity for understanding the public implications of complex science. These are difficult social challenges, but they are not utopian. Alternative social problem-solving approaches are far less worthy, given the ideals that define a liberal democratic society.

Finally, what I have presented here is a general and idealized model of what rational democratic deliberation ought to look like. Considerable empirical work is needed to develop practical working versions of this model in specific policy arenas. The two largest challenges would be the following. Designers must anticipate ways in which the deliberative process could be subverted or perverted and then put in place corrective mechanisms (Sunstein, 2001, 13–47). This would likely be an ongoing effort, analogous in many respects to the challenges of campaign finance reform. The other challenge is to develop effective linkages to deliberative policymaking bodies, such as state legislatures or Congress. Rational democratic deliberation would be reduced to an academic exercise if it were entirely disjoined from long-established policymaking processes and institutions. Of course, the results of the deliberative process could be perverted if those results were processed though "business as usual" policymaking bodies. Consequently, our ultimate hope is that broad practices of rational democratic deliberation would have a transformative effect on the often less-than-rational, less-than-deliberative policymaking practices that define the work of legislative bodies today.

NOTES

1. Collins and colleagues (2001) note that even single-gene disorders have turned out to be more genetically complex than was at first believed. He cites the example of sickle cell disease. It has been discovered that fetal hemoglobin genes can control the expression of adult hemoglobin genes. Those fetal genes usually turn off a few months after birth. But sometimes they remain in the "on" position, the result being a less severe form of sickle cell disease for those more fortunate individuals.

2. Over the past 15 years a substantive literature has emerged around the topic of deliberative democracy. The seminal article that provoked much of this discussion was by Cohen (1989). This movement is largely a reaction to (1) the demeaning of politics when politics is thought of as no more than self-centered interest group competition; or (2) the professionalization of politics, which diminishes what are supposed to be the democratic wellsprings of our political life; or (3) the trivialization of democratic engagement and value commitment reflected in the heavy use of largely mindless and ephemeral opinion polling to shape public policy. Deliberative democracy is intended to offer an alternative vision of what our political life ought to look like. The goal is to satisfy the Rawlsian ideal of a political system that represents a fair system of social cooperation. Cohen writes, "When properly conducted, then, democratic politics involves *public de-*

liberation focused on the common good, requires some form of *manifest equality* among citizens, and *shapes the identity and interests* of citizens in ways that contribute to the formation of a public conception of common good" (1989, 19). Among the more important books that have shaped this discussion would be Rawls (1993), Gutmann and Thompson (1996), Dryzek (2000), Bohman and Rehg (1997), Bohman (1996), Richardson (2002),Young (2000), and Goodin (2003).

3. *Note:* It may be necessary at times to have public deliberation in order to achieve public recognition and understanding that a particular option being considered must be put off the table because it violates one of these constitutional principles of political morality. In other words, we ought not assume that these constitutional principles of political morality are perfectly self-evident, especially with regard to concrete application in complex circumstances. This is essentially why in the domain of law the institution of the Supreme Court is necessary to make final and authoritative judgments when it is alleged that a particular law or policy violates the Constitution of the United States in some way. This also calls attention to the fact that our constitutional principles do in fact undergo interpretive evolution in response to changing social, political, economic, and technological features of our world.

REFERENCES

Abate, T. (2003). "State's Little Known History of Shameful Science; California's Role in Nazis' Goal of 'Purification.'" *San Francisco Chronicle* (March 10).
Baker, C. (2004). *Behavioral Genetics: An Introduction to How Genes and Environments Interact through Development to Shape Differences in Mood, Personality, and Intelligence.* Washington, D.C.: AAAS Publication Services.
Barrett, T. B., et al. (2003). "Evidence That a Single Nucleotide Polymorphism in the Promoter of the G Protein Receptor Kinase 3 Gene is Associated with Bipolar Disorder." *Molecular Psychiatry* 8(May): 546–57.
Beckwith, J., and J. Alper. (2002.) "Genetics of Human Personality: Social and Ethical Implications." In J. Benjamin, R. Ebstein, and R. Belmaker, eds. *Molecular Genetics and Human Personality.* Washington, D.C.: American Psychiatric Publishing: 315–31.
Bickenbach, J. E. (1998). "Disability and Life-ending Decisions." In M. Battin, R. Rhodes, and A. Silvers, eds. *Physician Assisted Suicide: Expanding the Debate.* New York: Routledge: 123–32.
Blakeslee, S. (2003). "A Pregnant Mother's Diet May Turn the Genes Around." *New York Times* (October 7).
Bohman, J. (1996). *Public Deliberation: Pluralism, Complexity, and Democracy.* Cambridge, Mass.: MIT.
Bohman, J., and W. Rehg, eds. (1997). *Deliberative Democracy: Essays on Reason and Politics.* Cambridge, Mass.: MIT.
Buchanan, A., D. Brock, N. Daniels, et al. (2000). *From Chance to Choice: Genetics and Justice.* New York: Cambridge University Press.
Caspi, A., et al. (2003). "Influence of Life Stress on Depression: Moderation by a Polymorphism in the 5-HTT Gene." *Science* 301: 386–89.

Citrin, T., and L. Fleck. (2001). "Communities of Color and Genetics Policy Project: Policy Reports and Recommendations." Supported by a grant from NIH, National Human Genome Research Institute, Ethical Legal and Social Implications Program (1999–2001).

Clark, C. (2003). "University of California-San Diego Will Lead Effort to Fathom Schizophrenia; Genes at Root of Traits to be Studied." *San-Diego Union Tribune* (June 3).

CNN.com. (2003). "Study: Sexual Identity Hard-wired by Genetics." October 20, reporting work of Dr. Eric Vilain, UCLA School of Medicine, published in the October issue of *Molecular Brain Research*.

Cohen, J. (1989). "Deliberation and Democratic Legitimacy." In A. Hamlin and P. Pettit, eds. *The Good Polity.* Oxford: Blackwell: 7–34.

Collins, F., L. Weiss, and K. Hudson. (2001). "Heredity and Humanity." *New Republic* 224: 27–30.

Daniels, N. (1996). *Justice and Justification: Reflective Equilibrium in Theory and Practice.* Cambridge: Cambridge University Press.

Dennis, C. (2003). "Epigenetics and Disease: Altered States." *Nature* 421: 686–88.

Dewey, J. (1929). *Experience and Nature.* New York: Dover.

Dryzek, D. (2000). *Deliberative Democracy and Beyond: Liberals, Critics, Contestations.* Oxford: Oxford University Press.

Duster, T. (1990). *Backdoor to Eugenics.* New York: Routledge.

Ehrlich, P., and M. Feldman. (2003). "Genes and Cultures: What Creates Our Behavioral Phenome?" *Current Anthropology* 44(February): 87–95.

Fleck, L. (2002). "Just Caring: Do Future Possible Children Have a Just Claim to a Sufficiently Healthy Genome?" In R. Rhodes, M. Battin, and A. Silvers, eds. *Medicine and Social Justice: Essays on the Distribution of Health Care.* New York: Oxford University Press: 446–57.

Fleck, L. (1996, 1997). *Genome Technology and Reproduction: Values and Public Policy, Fall 1996 Dialogue Report; Genome Technology and Reproduction: Values and Public Policy, Spring 1997 Dialogue Report.* Funded by the Ethical, Legal, and Social Implications Program, National Human Genome Research Institute, NIH (1995–98).

Florencio, P. (2000). "Genetics, Parenting, and Children's Rights in the Twenty-first Century." *McGill Law Journal* 45(May): 527–57.

Garland, M. (1999). "Experts and the Public: A Needed Partnership for Genetic Policy." *Public Understanding and Science* 8: 241–54.

Goodin, R. (2003). *Reflective Democracy.* Oxford: Oxford University Press.

Gutmann, A., and D. Thompson. (1996). *Democracy and Disagreement: Why Moral Conflict Cannot Be Avoided in Politics, and What Should Be Done about It.* Cambridge, Mass.: Harvard University Press.

Hamer, D., S. Hu, V. Magnusun, et al. (1993). "A Linkage between DNA Markers on the X Chromosome and Male Sexual Orientation." *Science* 261(5119): 321–27.

Hamer, D. (2002). "Rethinking Behavior Genetics." *Science* 298: 71–72.

Herman A., J. Philbeck, N. Vasilopoulos, et al. (2003). "Serotonin Transporter Promoter Polymorphism and Differences in Alcohol Consumption Behavior in a College Student Population." *Alcohol and Alcoholism* 38(September): 446–49.

Jamison, K. R. (1995). *An Unquiet Mind: A Memoir of Moods and Madness.* New York: Vintage.

Kevles, D. (1985). *In the Name of Eugenics: Genetics and the Uses of Human Heredity.* Berkeley: University of California Press.

Kitcher, P. (1996). *The Lives to Come: The Genetic Revolution and Human Possibilities.* New York: Simon and Schuster.

Lee, J. (2003). "Public Understanding of Science: Mind the Gap." *Physiology News* 51: 1–5.

Lemonick, M. (2003). "The Search for a Murder Gene." *Time Magazine* (January 12).

Nuffield Council on Bioethics. (2002). "Genetics and Human Behavior: The Ethical Context." London: Nuffield Council on Bioethics.

Parens, E., ed. (1998). *Enhancing Human Traits: Ethical and Social Implications.* Washington, D.C.: Georgetown University Press.

Rakowski, E. (2002). "Who Should Pay for Bad Genes?" *California Law Review* 90: 1345–1414.

Rawls, J. (1993). *Political Liberalism.* New York: Columbia University Press

Richardson, H. S. (2002). *Democratic Autonomy: Public Reasoning about the Ends of Policy.* Oxford: Oxford University Press.

Ridley, M. (2003). *Nature via Nurture: Genes, Experience, and What Makes Us Human.* New York: HarperCollins.

Schoen, J. (2003). "Confronting North Carolina's Eugenics Legacy." *Herald-Sun* (February 23).

Silvers, A. (1998). "Protecting the Innocents from Physician Assisted Suicide." In M. Battin, R. Rhodes, and A. Silvers, eds. *Physician Assisted Suicide: Expanding the Debate.* New York: Routledge: 133–48.

Smith, W. J. (1997). *Forced Exit: The Slippery Slope from Assisted Suicide to Legalized Murder.* New York: Times Books.

Sunstein, C. (2001). *Designing Democracy: What Constitutions Do.* Oxford: Oxford University Press.

Vedantam, S. (2003). "Variation in One Gene Linked to Depression; Contrast Emerges in Response to Stress." *Washington Post* (July 18).

Walzer, M. (1983). *Spheres of Justice: A Defense of Pluralism and Equality.* New York: Basic.

Wasserman, D. (2001). "Genetic Predispositions to Violent and Antisocial Behavior: Responsibility, Character, and Identity." In D. Wasserman and R. Wachbroit, eds. *Genetics and Criminal Behavior.* Cambridge: Cambridge University Press: 303–27.

Wong, J. E., and F. Lieh-Mak. (2001). "Genetic Discrimination and Mental Illness: A Case Report." *Journal of Medical Ethics* 27: 393–97.

Young, I. M. (2000). *Inclusion and Democracy.* Oxford: Oxford University Press.

CHAPTER THIRTEEN

Laypeople and Behavioral Genetics

Celeste Condit, Ph.D., Roxanne Parrott, Ph.D.,
and Tina Harris, Ph.D.

A substantial number of scientific studies have recently been devoted to link-ing genes with particular behavioral tendencies such as alcoholism, aggression, or sexual preference. In response to these efforts, several scholars have enu-merated a large list of potential negative social impacts of such research. In the midst of this scholarly tug-of-war, however, there have been relatively few at-tempts to explore the ways in which laypeople might actually be incorporat-ing behavioral genetics into their worldviews, or to assess the cultural resources laypeople might bring to bear to limit the negative potentials of this new re-search. This chapter reports on the discussions of laypeople about genetics, to contribute to our understanding of lay resources for responding to behavioral genetics research. These discussions indicate that laypeople already assign a substantial role to both genes and environment in human behaviors, varying this assignment among different behaviors. In spite of their perception that genes play a significant role in human behaviors, the majority of laypeople do not apply deterministic frameworks when incorporating genetics into their views of human behavior. Instead, they employ several different models of the relationships among genes, environment, and free will in a fashion that typically holds individuals responsible for overcoming their genetic predispositions. These lay accounts can be faulted on grounds of accuracy or social desirability, but they do not support the idea that the incorporation of genetics research into lay understandings will promote genetic determinism and the social ills that go with it.

To illuminate the contrast between critical concerns about behavioral genetics and lay opinions, and to frame the choices we made in analyzing our data, this chapter begins with a brief review of the common critiques of behavioral genetics, followed by a description of the method of our study, our findings, and a discussion of the implications.

The Social Critique

As has been explained at length in Part 1 of this volume, behavioral geneticists investigate how genetic differences between individuals influence phenotypic differences between them (Clark and Grunstein, 2002; Flint, 2000; Hamer and Copeland, 1998; McGuffin et al., 2001; Pfaff et al., 2000; Plomin et al., 1997; Rowe 1994, 64). This research program has inspired substantial criticism.

Critics of genetic determinism have identified a range of potential negative consequences that might flow from scientific validation and social propagation of the "results" of the behavioral genetics research program. They suggest that this research may cause the "dismantling of the welfare state" (Nelkin, 1999), heightened racism (Andrews, 1999; Lewontin et al., 1984; Nelkin, 1999), and social inequalities of many forms (Lewontin et al., 1984; Nelkin, 1999; Rothstein, 1999). They worry that behavioral genetics will disrupt the criminal justice system by eliminating concepts of personal responsibility, or that it will encourage surveillance, mandatory detention, or forced training or medication of those who are diagnosed as "predisposed" to violence (Andrews, 1999; Wasserman and Wachbroit, 2001). Given existing social patterns, this would likely mean increased discrimination against minorities. Critics have also suggested that the findings of behavioral genetics might be used to "blame the victims" of alcoholism or drug abuse, instead of establishing social structures that effectively prevent addiction or rehabilitate addicts. At the least, the critics suggest that behavioral genetics research will heighten stigma for people who are predisposed to patterns of behavior such as alcoholism or schizophrenia, without providing them any aid or assistance (Turney and Turner,

2000). Critics also worry that attributing sexual preference to genetic factors might result in abortions of fetuses that are tested and shown to be "at risk," without enhancing any legal protections for those who are shown to be born with a homosexual disposition (Brookey, 2001).

While there is a fairly diverse range of critical responses to behavioral genetics, a large number of critics identify at least two core beliefs that may lead to the potentially broad range of its negative outcomes. First, they suggest that behavioral genetics is inherently deterministic (Lewontin et al., 1984; Andrews, 1999). Consequently, it may tend to legitimate the status quo because it suggests that the social order is as it must and should be. Most critics, however, are not explicit about what counts as genetic determinism. It is therefore unclear whether the undesirable consequences of genetic determinism arise only from statements and research asserting an absolute role for genes, from those suggesting a large role for genes, or from all research assigning any role for genes at all. For some critics, it appears that any attention to genes is tantamount to determinism. Dorothy Nelkin and Susan Lindee would appear to use such a definition when they provide as an example of discourse that discusses "addictive behavior in *absolute* genetic or biological terms," a quotation from a self-help book that states that "Obsessive Compulsive Disorder is *partially* genetically transmitted" (Nelkin and Lindee, 1995, 93; our emphases). Peter Conrad, another experienced sociologist, likewise provides as examples of a "genes-cause-alcoholism" frame in news media stories a broad range of statements. Some lie at the more deterministic end of the scale, such as "the myth that alcoholism is always psychologically caused is giving way to a realization that it is, in large measure, biologically determined" (Conrad and Weinberg, 1966, 10). Many of his examples, however, assume more moderate levels of genetic influence, and use qualifying terms such as *tendency, susceptibility, prone,* or *one factor.* One of his examples states: "some children of alcoholics inherit certain physiological traits that may indicate a tendency toward alcoholism" (12). What precisely counts as genetic determinism, or excessive mention of genetics, thus appears to be variable, or at least unclear. Wherever the lines are drawn, however, critics tend to agree that heightened emphasis or overemphasis on the role of genes in behavior supports undesirable beliefs that current social conditions are natural and unchangeable.

A second common critique is grounded in the belief that behavioral genetics draws attention to the individual rather than to the social, and thus discourages social solutions to social problems. While behavioral geneticists sometimes deny that the products of genes are "immutable" or that individual inequality is tantamount to group inequality (Plomin et al., 1997, 84–85), the fact that behavioral genetics–style arguments have been used historically for racist, classist, and sexist agendas, and that there are still active advocates who use them for such purposes (Comings, 1996; Herrnstein and Murray, 1994), gives substantial force to the concerns these critics raise.

The critics' concerns, however, are worries about the future, and most predictions of human futures are difficult to ground. Moreover, much of the predictive power of these worries is mediated by assumptions about how the results of behavioral genetics will be taken up into the social meaning structures that govern our shared laws and our attitudes and actions toward one another. Dorothy Nelkin identified many instances in which behavioral genetics has been used in precisely the negative senses about which the critics worry in mass media discussions of genetics. However, these instances do not necessarily define the social trend. Understanding social trends requires not only a balanced assessment of the relative frequency and placement of deterministic interpretations of genetics in the mass media, but also a sense of the degree to which these published attitudes are reflected in the attitudes of the lay public who watch the media, but who do not necessarily always agree with it.

Many social critics of genetics appear to assume that the lay public simply absorbs and adopts whatever values and attitudes the mass media offer to it. Indeed, Lori Andrews asserts that the public too often accepts behavioral genetics research "without question" (1999, 119). This perspective is called the "magic bullet" theory of communication, and it has been widely discredited by research in communication studies (Tompkins, 1982, 224). Instead, clear evidence indicates that members of the lay public interpret the messages they receive from the mass media using their preexisting beliefs and attitudes, as well as new experiences outside the media's frame of reference (Morley, 1980; Radway, 1984). Sometimes members of the public agree with the messages they hear, and sometimes they disagree. Very often, people selectively perceive materials in accord with their prior attitudes, and seek out media that confirm their prior beliefs. There are certainly limits on the abilities of lay members of the public to counterinterpret media products, but those abilities are enhanced by the existence of prior belief sets (Condit, 1989). Thus, one important input for predicting how the results of behavioral genetics might impact our culture is an understanding of how laypeople already think about the relationships among genes and human behavior.

Method

To assess whether and how laypeople incorporate the ideas of genetics into their thinking about human behavior, we used focus group research. Focus group methods involve gathering people to talk together about a particular topic (Morgan, 1993; Stewart and Shamdasani, 1990). Moderators use questions and prompts that are designed to elicit extended talk about a targeted topic area, without providing narrow frames that suggest particular vocabularies or answers. The strength of good focus group research is that it allows researchers to hear how laypeople frame issues in their own words and priorities. In contrast, closed question surveys provide a specific and limited set of options from which to choose and frame the issues in a singular vocabulary that may not represent the research participants' preferred choices or vocabulary. Focus groups are thus superior to closed answer surveys in this respect. Focus groups also are advantageous compared to interviews in some ways. Focus groups allow interaction among laypeople, rather than simple responses to an interviewer. The dynamics of discussions among several participants may produce more open and varied discussion than replies in an interview (especially where interviewers use an objectivist protocol that does not enable them to "discuss" the issue with the participants). With good questions and moderators, therefore, focus group methodology may elicit sustained, varied talk about an issue that reflects perspectives of the participants that are more strongly influenced by their discussion with other laypeople, rather than by the researchers' preconceptions.

For this research project, we utilized transcripts of 17 focus groups that were conducted to assess lay understandings of genetics in general. In order to enhance the likelihood that participants would feel free to express opinions on contentious issues that might bear on racial or gender differences, each group in the study was homogeneous for race and gender, as socially defined in their community and by the participants. Our groups included 4 with white men, 4 with white women, 5 with black women, and 4 with black men. Participants were recruited from a town associated with a large land grant university in the southeastern United States in the winter and spring of 2000 through telephone solicitation via random digit dialing (n = 24), community sponsor recruitment (n = 40), and a snowball technique (n = 19) in which individuals recruited to participate were invited to bring an acquaintance (which could include friends or family members). Individuals who had received genetic testing or counseling, or who indicated in screening questions that they "know all there is to know" or "know a great deal" about human genetics were eliminated from further consideration for participation as a method of defining the "lay" as compared to a more knowledgeable or experienced and expert public.

Participants (N = 82) in the 17 focus groups included 39 women (including 19 blacks) and 43 men (including 23 whites). The average age of participants was 28.55 years (SD = 6.19). Their income included 16 percent who made less than $10,000, 24 percent in the $10,000 to $25,000 range, 29 percent making $25,000 to $40,000, 10 percent in the $40,000 to $55,000 range, and 16 percent making $55,000 or more. Nearly half of the participants had some college, with 49.4 percent indicating that they had completed a college course in biology. Another 38.6 percent reported that they had taken a biology class in high school. Our group was thus somewhat more educated than the national average, although they were relatively typical of a college town. The participants included a broad range of economic classes and purposeful demographic overrepresentation of African Americans, to ensure ample opportunity for the representation of one regionally important minority voice.

After general introductions, the focus group leader, who was matched for race with the participants, introduced a series of open-ended questions about the group's understanding of genetics. We culled all these responses to all questions for any reference to human behaviors. The resulting subset of data was analyzed by recording what particular behaviors were linked to genes and what models of the relationship between genes, environment, and behavior were applied by the discussants. Behaviors were categorized in five types including personality, actions, mental conditions, addictions, and "other." These categories arose from an interaction between items and item-types identified in the academic literature and the specific behaviors listed by participants. The models were constructed from statements by participants. In the report below, male participants are those with odd numbers, and females have even numbers. Participants numbered from 1 to 50 are African American, and those from 50 to 100 are European American.

One bias in the findings reported below needs to be highlighted in advance of their presentation. The quotations used to illustrate various positions below are heavily loaded toward those behaviors that are socially stigmatized (especially alcoholism and homosexuality). Our participants talked about less stigmatized behaviors (such as a personal tendency to "speak one's mind" or self-esteem), but these topics did not elicit extended disagreement or discussion, and so in such cases the underlying structure of their attitudes is not articulated in as clear a fashion. We will address the implications of the resulting overrepresentation of stigmatized behaviors in the conclusions, but it should be kept in mind when reading the following findings.

Findings

Many Different Traits are Linked to Genes by Different People

As Table 13.1 indicates, participants in every group linked a wide variety of behaviors to genes. Some categories of behavior were linked to genes by persons of every race and gender. All groups had some members identifying personality, sexuality, and alcoholism as related to a person's genes. However, some categories of behavior were linked to genes solely by persons of particular races. Thus, some African Americans in both women's and men's groups linked self-esteem to genetics, while some European Americans in both women's and men's groups linked "everything" to genes. Some categories of behavior were listed in some, but not all groups (mental illnesses), whereas some behaviors are listed only by one group ("retardation," "gambling," "alcohol tolerance"). Wording from the focus groups is used in reporting the particular behaviors linked to genes in Table 13.1 in order to avoid imposing researcher biases on the lay perspectives (except that we have changed *Down's syndrome* to *Down syndrome* in respect for the preferences of the associated support groups). However, several behaviors within categories probably repeat across groups, in spite of differences in phrasing. For example, "mood" is a term used by European American men, whereas "emotions" is used by European American women, and these may be essentially the same characteristic.

This wide variety of behaviors linked to genes nonetheless shows substantial variability by individuals within the groups. Thus, participant 32 indicated that "I think they [genes] play a very big role. Who we are and our personality and stuff like that," whereas participant 12 said, "I don't think genetics play a lot of role in personality. Maybe I'm wrong but I don't think so." However, it is not simply that some people attribute a large role to genes and some a small role. Rather, participants see genes as playing a larger or smaller role in particular traits. Thus, participant 18 indicated that genes play a large role in shaping human beings in general, saying that "it plays a great deal because

Table 13.1. *"Behaviors" Treated by Participants as Having a Genetic Component*

	Personality	Actions	Mental Disorders	Addictions	Other
African American women	Personality Self-esteem Personal strength	Mannerisms	Mental illness Schizophrenia ADD Down syndrome	Alcoholism Smoking	Homo- Sexuality
European American women	Personality Coping skills Reactions Disposition Emotional stuff	Behaviors Conversational patterns Body language How act	Mental health	Alcoholism	Everything Sexual orientation
African American men	Personality Attitude Sensititivy Spirituality Personal strength Passivity Reactions Mood swings Predisposition to anger Self-esteem Being loving Will to live	Crime Violence How you're going to act	Down syndrome Retardation	Alcoholism Addictive personality Overeating	Homo- sexuality Alcohol tolerance
European American men	Personality Handling stress Greed Religion Bad mood Greed "Vulnerable" to victim- hood	Behaviors Crime Violence How you behave The way you act Sex offender	Autism	Alcoholism Drug abuse Gambling	Everything Sexuality

294 Celeste Condit, Roxanne Parrott, and Tina Harris

your genes determine who you are," but she thought that homosexuality was not genetic, because "if we are going to argue that it's genetic then it's like saying that God doesn't know what He's doing . . . and we know it's not in God's plan to have homosexual relations." In direct contrast, participant 14 emphasized environment over genes in general discussions, saying that "again, it can just be the environment in which the kid is raised," but with regard to homosexuality she said that "I don't think it is always the point that you have a choice, especially when it happens early on." These individuals differed, therefore, not just in a global assessment of the role of genes in behavior, but rather in their assessment of the relative importance of genes in producing particular behaviors.

Some participants even indicated that the role of genes versus environment varied by individual case. Thus, participant 1 shared with 14 the idea that homosexuality might result from different factors in different cases, suggesting that "some males are just born with a certain amount of female genes. And some people . . . some guys turn gay. It's a mental thing you know. They can't compete. You know you have some guys who turn gay because they can't compete with the guys. So it's half and half to me." Individuals thus appeared to negotiate their sense of the role of genes in producing behaviors with regard to their particular attitudes about particular characteristics, and even to allow for different degrees of influence from different characteristics in different individuals.

In spite of this fairly wide variety of attitudes, and their trait-dependence, most participants attributed some substantial role to genes in behavior. Even most of those who emphasized environment assigned a fairly significant role to genes in shaping behavior. For example, participant 54 said that "I actually think genetics is pointed to too much I think as far as how people are. I mean I'm more of an environmentalist. I think the environment has a lot to do with it. If I had to do like percentages I would probably say like 30 percent genetics and 70 percent environmental factors." Her view does not appear to be atypical of the participants. One of the tasks we asked group members to undertake was to assign percentages to genetic versus environmental influences by filling in pie charts for specific human features. Because our research agenda at the time was focused on ascertaining the extent to which participants incorporated genetic accounts into their understandings, we did not encourage or create a viable way for them to indicate a percentage for gene-environment interactions. We also did not ask them specifically to rate "behavior," but we did ask them to rate mental abilities and talents. The former is included by several

Table 13.2. Estimates of Genetic Influence on Human Characteristics

	Mean %	Highest Assigned %	Lowest Assigned %
Height	71	100	12.5
Weight	41	NA	NA
Cancer <40	54	100	10
Talents	26	82	5
Mental abilities	40	87	0

behavior geneticists in their studies and the latter by a few. On average, participants assigned 40 percent of mental abilities to genes, but the range went from a low of zero percent to a high of 87 percent and they assigned 26 percent of one's talents to genetics, with a low of 5 percent and a high of 82 percent. The attribution of mental ability is strikingly similar to attributions of weight, though lower than height and cancer. (The mean for cancer was 54%, with a range from 10 to 100%, whereas the mean for height was 71%, with a range from 12.5 to 100% [Parrott et al., 2003]; see Table 13.2.)

These estimates are certainly within the range of heritabilities that behavioral geneticists invoke, if somewhat at the low end of the range. However, there was also a class of "discretionary" behaviors that most respondents indicated were clearly dominated by environment. Thus, for example, participant 66 indicated that "if you live in South Georgia, you're probably not going to be skiing very much." Similarly, participant 25 noted that "if you take a black kid and he is raised in a white household I think he's pretty much going to listen to country music or rock and roll or heavy metal or whatever as opposed to rap or whatever we listen to." Behavioral geneticists, of course, have not claimed to address or account for such situated or cultural components of behavior. In this respect, our participants thus seemed to consider a more comprehensive scope in their considerations of behavior than do the experts. Overall, though there was some variability in their accounts, the lay perspective seemed to assign a substantial role to both genes and environment in human behaviors, but to vary this assignment among different behaviors.

Varying Models of Genes and Behavior

Because most participants included both genes and environment as causal forces in their worldview, few articulated positions that might be called either singularly "genetically determinist" or "socially determinist." They also integrated a very strong dose of the idea that individuals exercised personal will and that this also accounted for human behaviors. As a consequence of their acceptance of the multiple causal inputs into human behavior, they needed to talk about responsibility for these behaviors through informal models of the relationships among genes and environment, or genes, environment, and personal will. Four different components of such informal models appeared in more than one group and with enough detail for us to describe their assumptions and features. Some of these informal models are relatively complete in themselves, and some constitute merely components of broader models of the causal forces that shape human behavior, which could be combined with other components to form more complete models. Different individuals combined these different modular components with regard to different traits in different ways. For simplicity of diction, and because informal reasoning does not always function in well-elaborated models, we refer to both the more limited components and the fuller accounts as informal "models."

Equal Genetic Capacities Means the Environment Determines

One of the most emphatically expressed views of the relationship between genes, environment, and personal will held that genes influence human behaviors, but that such influence does not produce overwhelming differences among individuals. On this view, because individuals were basically the same in their genetically produced capacities, the environment played the determining role in differential outcomes for individuals. This position was most emphatically produced by participant 8, who argued,

> with having the basic needs and personal needs and those things taken care of first where they can get to the point where they can use their intellectual ability, you know to the fullest extent. That the genes may be there . . . that they're highly capable, but because they haven't had the basic needs and . . . you know the sense of loving and belonging all of those things are missing . . . they can't perform well academically. So I think in a sense environment.

This participant held this view even with regard to severe mental retardation. In the face of a challenge in this regard by other participants she replied, "You don't believe you could take a child that's had that kind of head start in life and maybe put them with a family that is nurturing and maybe all of those other things . . . You don't think that person can over come that?" This participant did not deny that genes were necessary to produce certain human out-comes. As she says, "the genes were there," but simply not able to act because of an inadequate environment. While she pushed the position much farther than any of the other participants, this was a position held with less absolutism by some other participants. Thus, another participant made a distinction be-tween those who are normal and those who are not normal, but indicated, "'Cause if you have, I don't want to say good genes or bad genes . . . but you know if you have normal genes then the rest of these things have more influ-ence" (participant 2).

On this view, genes are important to human behavioral capacities, but the genetic differences between individuals are not decisive, except perhaps in some very extreme cases. All but a few of the people who articulated this view would recognize that extreme genetic malfunctions could destroy human ca-pacities. But within this model, in most cases genes don't vary enough to over-come the greater differences in environment. This position is at odds with the research program of many behavioral geneticists, but as we will note in our dis-cussion below, these participants were arguably taking into account greater variability in both populations and environmental variations than has been included in the majority of the surveys in behavioral genetics research. While several people held this position, it was not a position expressed by the ma-jority, or even a substantial plurality.

The Environment Catalyzes Different Predispositions

A somewhat more common view of the relationship between environment and genetics recognized differences in genetic potentials among at least some individuals, but held that these potentials were only activated when environ-mental conditions catalyzed them. Thus, participant 54 suggested that "men-tal health is a big deal for me and environment plays a very big role in that. Genetics definitely predisposes you to a lot of mental illnesses as well as to other illness but environment is usually the catalyst." As this example suggests, this model of the relationship between environment and genes was applied with particular frequency to mental health as a "behavioral trait." The model was compatible with other traits, however, as indicated by participant 51's gen-eralized statement that "sometimes the effect of these genes are triggered by some environment stressor that you may want to avoid."

Although the catalytic model did not assume equal genetic capacities, it was similar to the equal capacities model in that it placed environment as the active agent and genes as the passive agent. This is opposite of the thrust of much of the behavioral genetics program, which has developed stories of "niche picking" to describe the ways in which a person's genes actively select those environments that allow the genes to manifest themselves most comfortably. Thus, a behavioral geneticist might argue that a person whose genes predisposed her to alcoholism would select peers and environments where alcohol consumption was encouraged (Plomin et al., 1997, 256). In contrast, these lay stories portray the environment as an active agent that functions to enable the genetic predisposition, which is dormant until activation. The role of individual will, understood as something independent from the genetic predisposition itself, is not explicitly stated in this model, which is compatible either with environmental determinism or with a sense of personal will. The catalytic model is, for example, compatible with the most popular model of the sources of behaviors articulated by our participants, the idea that genetic predispositions can be thwarted.

Malleable Genetic Predispositions

Probably the most common model in these discussions of human behaviors held that undesired genetic predispositions can be overridden. From this perspective, either individuals or social groups are capable of consciously thwarting the predispositions generated by genes. Participant 38 articulated the idea that individuals have a responsibility to override their predispositions when she stated that

> even though you might receive a gene for high tolerances . . . alcohol gene. Or anybody in your family has an alcoholic gene and was more likely to be an alcoholic, but you have to make the choice to be an alcoholic. Or if you receive any kind of trait like I know my dad is stubborn and I am stubborn like him too but that . . . that means I can change my mind not to be stubborn all the time.

Some participants also added to this sense of individual control the idea that social groups can play a role in overriding undesirable predispositions. Participant 58 expressed this combined view, saying:

> There are a lot of people who probably would never have measured very high on IQ test, even maybe a good one. But because of a nurturing environment and maybe good teachers and good work habits and a certain drive to succeed or a certain caring about a certain cause have achieved great things.

This view of genetic legacies as malleable was expressed with particular frequency in regard to alcoholism, but whether it was applied to homosexuality or personal conversational style, the presumed ability to override a negative predisposition generally was taken as a responsibility to override that predisposition. Mechanisms for overriding such negative predispositions included changing one's personal actions or controlling one's environment (e.g., to avoid alcoholism). Thus, for example, though she appears to mix social learning and genetics as causal elements, participant 20's discussion of her personal traits illustrates this view:

> I think it's genetic in that aspect . . . Y'all might disagree with me, but my mom was a very high strong, high willed domineering woman and I learned to be that way and I be forward with people and don't really know that I'm doing it but I see it in my mom. You know she's really direct, she don't care what you think just let the truth. And I see that in me and I kind of hate myself for doing that sometimes because people can't really take me. That's why I have to choose my friend wisely.

This excerpt highlights the ways in which lay individuals using this model might portray environment or genes as either active or passive, and still hold the individual personally accountable for personal behavior, because they held personal will to be capable of trumping the other predispositions. This is the way in which the lay accounts may differ most strongly from either the genetically determinist accounts of behavioral genetics or the socially determinist accounts of many of the critics of genetics. A related lay model held that all individuals, not just those with negative predispositions, were responsible for their behaviors. This informal model held that you had to "play the hand you're dealt."

You've Gotta Play the Hand You're Dealt

One of the most common sentiments about genes and human behavior articulated by the participants was a resignedly pragmatic one we call the maximizing model. This view held that genetic predispositions might well be unfairly distributed among people, and that one might not be able to compensate for that unfairness, but one nonetheless had a responsibility to make the best of what you were given. This model was expressed by participant 62, who responded that "I think it is kind of like the hand you are dealt. Just what you start with but then you know what you do with that." Though this model is compatible with perceptions that different individuals had different levels of genetic "gifts" it is also compatible with a relatively nonhierarchical perspective on genetic abilities. Participant 60 seems to have been focusing on the diversity of different possibilities individuals have available to them rather than using a dichotomous advantage/disadvantage model when she declared, "I don't think that everything is mapped out for you. I think you are given so much and then you use your abilities to go and take your abilities to do something with it . . . Do with it what you will." This maximization model was applied to people with talents as well as those with deficits. As participant 31 noted, "You're not just born with a basketball in your hand. You have to work on it." Thus, "playing the hand you're dealt" required work on whatever talent set you might have.

Pregenetic Views of Nature and Nurture

As the comments above indicate, most of our participants had a view of the relationship between genes, environment, and behaviors that was in gross outline similar to the view of molecular genetics. That is, like the molecular geneticists, the laypeople understood genes and environment as basically separate, if interacting, entities. Many of our participants appeared to accept a view of the process of natural selection, though some of the participants articulated relatively Lamarckian accounts and perspectives that did not distinguish between nature and nurture with regard to heredity.

Lamarckian perspectives hold that the actions of an individual or the impact of the environment on that individual are passed directly to offspring. On this view, parents who lift weights will have children with stronger muscles. These perspectives were relatively common among scientists at the end of the nineteenth and beginning of the twentieth centuries, but the theory died out as several experiments demonstrated the failure of the theory in obvious cases, such as the fact that rats whose tails were chopped off did not bear tail-less offspring (though the abandonment of the theory was not without controversy and counterexperiments). Pro-Lamarckianism appeared in popular media in the United States until the late 1930s. When the Soviet Union became associated with Lamarckian perspectives through Lysenkoism, however, the American media rapidly turned against the theory because it came to represent communist orthodoxy (Condit, 1999, 69–70). Some of our participants, however, expressed Lamarckian perspectives. Participant 24 gave the fullest articulation to this perspective when she said, "Sometimes the genetics may not take place until a later date in a family . . . when that person chose [to smoke] that became a part of their genetic makeup . . . and then that is passed on to the next generation . . . Where there may be a little bit more genetic as opposed to a choice." This captures the rough practical truth that it may be harder to avoid becoming addicted to smoking in a family with a history of smoking than in a family that does not have such a history. Which is to say that in daily life, it often doesn't matter much whether an inherited predisposition is genetic or familial-environmental.

Before the era of molecular genetics, "heredity" was not aligned with "genetics" as opposed to "environment" as it is in current parlance. Even among the discourse of the classical eugenicists, "heredity" included both one's genes and the family environment through which one inherited one's culture as well as one's material "inheritance." One of the key impacts of molecular genetics on lay discourse was the drawing of a relatively rigid separation between physiological "inheritance" and familial-environmental "inheritance" (Condit, 1999). In many realms of daily life, however, this separation is of no particular relevance. As participant 25's comments indicate, in many cases it doesn't matter whether what your family passes on to you arrives in your genes or your enculturation: "Because if you grew up in a household that shows a lot of love and affection that's pretty much going to take effect for you as opposed to people being cold-hearted . . . So it's hard to say whether it's genetic or something learned." Whether your parents are "cold hearted" by nature or simply by training, the effects on you are likely to be the same. The perseverance of these two models in lay discourse suggests that a key factor in the uptake of behavioral genetics may well be whether it makes any useful difference in daily life to think about the source of inherited behavior in terms of genetics as opposed to environment.

Conclusions and Implications

This research indicates that many, probably even most, laypeople in the United States already incorporate the idea that genes play a role in human behavior into their ways of understanding their world. If we understand as genetic determinism a belief that the role played by genes exerts a causal force that is not subject to other effective influences, then the lay public has made this integration of genetics research without becoming genetic determinists.

They manage belief in the influence of genes without resorting to genetic determinism by employing a variety of models that integrate the contributions of multiple factors—including genes, environments, and personal will—in different relationships to one another. The equal genetic capacities model holds that while genetics determine human capacities, differences among individuals are nonexistent or not pragmatically significant, except perhaps in cases of serious abnormality. The catalytic model holds that genes and environment both contribute to differences, but that the environment is the active agent because it must be manipulated to produce the genetic effect. The malleable genetic predispositions model suggests that differences in genetic predispositions exist, but it holds individuals responsible for overcoming these predispositions by using their other talents and abilities. Finally, the maximization model admits to genetically based differences and accepts inequality, but holds that individuals should maximize whatever potentials they have. The last three of these models together appear to constitute a dominant lay perspective.

The gene-inclusive models all accept a substantial influence from genes on human behavior, but they do not thereby conclude either that human behavior is uncontrollable or that genes are the primary fulcrum for changes in human behavior. Instead, they emphasize "personal will" and the other talents and capacities that individuals may have as counterweights to genetic influences. These views may be judged negatively on the grounds that they are empirically incorrect, excessively optimistic, or even down-right disadvantageous to social justice in many ways, but they provide a robust source of resistance to genetic determinism. Thus, even in the face of significant acceptance of the role of genes in human behaviors, lay attitudes do not simply abandon concepts of personal responsibility and familial care and support. Instead, the genes are accepted as a real force, perhaps even a potent biasing factor in life outcomes, but one that can and should be worked against.

While a quantitative study with a representative sample will be necessary to establish more precisely what percentage of the population has integrated the basic premises of behavioral genetics with more traditional notions of will and family responsibility, it would be extremely difficult to pin down what percentage of the population uses each particular model, because the different models can be applied by the same individual to different behavioral traits and even to the same trait in different cases. Nonetheless, there would probably be utility in broadening this study to additional groups to search for more models and to establish more clearly whether there are particular patterns by which large numbers of people associate particular models with particular behavioral traits (such as aggression as opposed to alcoholism or cognitive abilities).

In addition to revealing a strong set of preexisting attitudes about behavior and genes, this study gives reason to suggest that in some ways the lay models offer more comprehensive and more sophisticated accounts of the role of genes in human behavior than one sometimes still sees in some behavioral genetics publications. It is worth enumerating the virtues of these lay accounts. First, laypeople seem to be keenly aware that different types of traits carry different levels of influence. As their discussion of model 1 (equal capacities) indicates, most laypeople appear to be able to distinguish between the different magnitude of effects of what scientists would probably call "single-gene" disorders that create serious abnormalities, as opposed to the range of normal polymorphisms, which produce a much smaller range of differences.

Laypeople may simply conclude that "for all practical purposes" most people's genetic endowment is roughly equivalent (and employ the equivalence model). If this is true, laypeople may be unconcerned about the statistically significant results offered by behavioral genetics if those statistically significant differences do not translate into meaningful differences in lay practice. Thus, a behavioral geneticist might be impressed by the fact that 62 percent of the variance in a "relaxed" communicator style is accounted for by biological heredity, but a lay person might find the ability to account for this variance unimpressive, given that, for example, the relatively small difference between the means and standard deviations for this variable is practically less meaningful than the larger variation in the means and standard deviations for a variable such as "contentiousness," in which genetics seems to account for a much smaller part of the variance (12%: relaxed: DZ: mean 2.87; SD 0.91; MZ: mean 2.95; SD 0.90; contentious: DZ: mean 3.10; SD 1.02; MZ: mean 2.98; SD 0.93 [Hovarth, 1995, 402]). Contentiousness may be of more concern in a pragmatic sense and it certainly appears to be more variable, so that the lack of importance of genes in this more variable and perhaps more important feature may overshadow the high heritability of other features such as openness in communicator style.

Lay understandings of the role of genes in behavior also recognize that individual cases may vary. While the best behavioral geneticists emphasize the idea that heritability only indicates how much genetic variation helps to explain phenotypic variation within a given population and a given environment at a given time (e.g., Plomin et al., 1997, 83), this is not the banner headline of the research program. Instead, probably because they tend to define environment as "family" environment and because they rely on twin and adoption studies that do not usually cross cultural lines, a large group of behavioral geneticists focus their discourse on the lack of role played by (family) environment. However, our respondents, who include substantial representatives of minority groups, who regularly face the realities of cultural differences, are attentive to the fact that large cultural differences (i.e., social environment) may have a significant impact on individual outcomes (King, 1988; Phillips, 1995). They are thus able to take a "case by case" approach, which indicates that in some instances a strong environmental influence overrides a weaker genetic input, whereas in other instances that genetic input is manifested. Scientists, of course, are also disciplinarily dissuaded from a case-by-case approach by the imperative to generalize.

Another difference caused by the nature of academic discourse as opposed to lay discourse is that laypeople take into account a wider range of behaviors than do these scientists. Behavioral science has generally only been interested in behaviors that can be studied "regardless of context, culture, or time" (Hovarth, 1995, 405). Thus, behavioral genetics has usually focused on stable, individual patterns. But much significant human behavioral difference operates at the cultural level (working 9 to 5 or with the seasons? leaving one's birth family at marriage or moving into the family compound? farming or hunting and gathering?), and such variation has significant impacts on individual human lives. Our lay participants had not been "disciplined" to ignore culture and its role on behavior. If it is to provide a comprehensive account of human behavior, behavioral genetics needs to maintain focus on individual differences and work actively to incorporate cultural variation and population variation in its studies, including accounts of the wide range of human behaviors that are not traitlike, and ways in which social motivations may lead to a focus on particular traits as problems (see chapter 6).

We need, of course, to attend to the limitations of our own study as well. One of these limitations is the assumption that the majority attitudes of the lay public are significant in policy outcomes. We are concerned that, in fact, lay attitudes may be disregarded in social policy. It may be that the attitudes of social elites and the mass media ultimately control policy outcomes, and these attitudes might indeed be genetically determinist, even if the attitudes of the lay public are not.

A second limitation of our study arises because, as we noted in the methods section, focus group methodology is dependent upon what lay participants will talk about without excessive direction. This is in many ways a great strength of the method, but in this case, it also reflects a potential bias. Because our participants discuss stigmatized behaviors in more depth than nonstigmatized behaviors, we articulate their mental models of behavior and genetics based on their models of stigmatized behaviors. The first risk here is that this misrepresents the underlying models of behavior, environment, and genetics that laypeople employ because laypeople might employ very different models for stigmatized and nonstigmatized behavior. We have several examples of nonstigmatized behaviors that fit within the models we have described, so we believe that we are not making such a misrepresentation. But substantial additional research using different methods is needed to confirm that the range of models applied in heavily stigmatized behavior is similar to the range of models applied to less stigmatized behavior. Second, we worry that the focus on stigmatized behavior reinforces the stigmatization. By re-presenting stigmatizing comments and by re-presenting statements that assign individual responsibility for overcoming such behaviors, we might contribute to the process of social stigmatization. Consequently, we need also to highlight the ways in which the existing lay perspectives on stigmatized behaviors are problematic.

We were especially struck by the fact that in the gene/environment/free will formulations offered by our lay participants, "environment" rarely seemed to incorporate the pervasive social structures that influence our lives. Environment was more likely to mean family (as with the behavioral geneticists) or culture. This absence of attention to social structures was problematic because most of our participants agreed not only that the predispositions of genes could be overcome, but also that individuals had a *responsibility* for overcoming them. Thus, families and individuals on their own were assigned as the agents for overcoming genetic inequities, even in the face of rigid social structures that might augment the inequities. Assuming that cultures are too diffuse to act as directive agents of change, and assuming that social structures are potential sources of directed change, and clearly of input to human behaviors as well (e.g., taxes, zoning, restrictions on public intoxication, dress, "decency," etc.), the lay models of the arsenal for overcoming the power of genes and/or faulty early environments seem to be seriously underpowered.

In part, many of our participants believe that a "higher power" provides another resource for augmenting personal will. Several of our participants invoked prayer and faith as sources of support available to the individual for overcoming negative personal predispositions or more generally guiding one's life course. However, the "higher power" itself was conceived either as a supplement to personal will or as autonomous and insurmountable. It was not portrayed as a force that might be engaged at the social level of action (for a more detailed discussion of the role of religion and genetics, see Harris et al., 2004). Thus, viewing God as a resource for overcoming genetic predispositions did not relieve the responsibility assigned to individuals to solve their own problems, even in the face of social structures that worked against their efforts.

Finally, we would suggest that the contrast between the lay discourse about genetics and the critics' discourse about behavioral genetics also provides some insight. We think that the flexibility of the lay accounts makes clear that the assumption of some critics that conceding any amount of genetic role in human behavior is tantamount to positing the dominance of genes over environment (Kerr et al., 1998, 188) is simply untrue. Thus, the community of social critics may need to begin to discuss more carefully the parameters of what counts as "genetic determinism." Second, we think that the community of social critics may need to direct their efforts beyond merely cataloguing the worst imaginable outcomes of the behavioral genetics program. While warning of the worst-case possibilities, as several critics have done to date, is surely a useful social function, we would suggest that a next step would be to try to identify which social reactions to the behavioral genetics program are most likely, given the existing lay understandings of the role of genes in behavior and the strengths and weaknesses in lay resources for dealing with additional information about genetics. This will require a more fine-grained analysis of the many potential problems with behavioral genetics worldviews than have been enumerated to date, and it may even bring to light problems that have not appeared to be so obvious.

At the least, we hope that this chapter makes clear that the lay public, although unfamiliar with the details of molecular genetics and the methodologies of twin studies, has existing schemas for reflecting on the role of genes in human behavior. Through observations of the people and families around them, as well as through critical filtering of mass mediated reports on behavior genetics, they have developed a set of accounts of human behavior that factor in a wide range of variables and conditions as causal inputs. While the popular account is surely less quantitatively precise (or at least explicit) than that of the scientific experts in the area, the lay accounts are in some ways more comprehensive and complex. This does not make current lay accounts "ideal," nor does it mean that we must accept them as permanent or inviolable. However, we believe that this chapter demonstrates that understanding how the lay public has processed genetic research to date may enable better assessment of the social impact of genetic research in the future.

REFERENCES

Andrews, L. B. (1999). "Predicting and Punishing Antisocial Acts: How the Criminal Justice System Might Use Behavioral Genetics." In R. A. Carson and M. A. Rothstein, eds. *Behavioral Genetics: The Clash of Culture and Biology.* Baltimore and London: Johns Hopkins University Press: 116–55.

Beatty, M. J., J. C. McCroskey, and A. D. Heisel. (1998). "Communication Apprehension as Temperamental Expression: A Communibiological Paradigm." *Communication Monographs* 65: 197–219.

Berrettini, W. H. (2000). "The Search for Susceptibility Genes in Bipolar Disorder." In D. W. Pfaff, W. H. Berrettini, T. H. Joh, et al., eds. *Genetic Influences on Neural and Behavioral Functions.* Boca Raton, Fla.: CRC: 31–46.

Brookey, R. A. (2001). "Bio-rhetoric, Background Beliefs and the Biology of Homosexuality." *Argumentation and Advocacy* 37(Spring): 171–83.

Clark, W. R., and M. Grunstein. (2000). *Are We Hardwired? The Role of Genes in Human Behavior.* New York and Oxford: Oxford University Press.

Comings, D. E. (1996). *The Gene Bomb: Does Higher Education and Advanced Technology Accelerate the Selection of Genes for Learning Disorders, Addictive and Disruptive Behaviors?* Duarte, Calif.: Hope.

Condit, C. M. (1989). "The Rhetorical Limits of Polysemy." *Critical Studies in Mass Communication* 6: 103–22.

Condit, C. M. (1999). *The Meanings of the Gene.* Madison: University of Wisconsin Press.

Conrad, P., and D. Weinberg. (1966). "Has the Gene for Alcoholism Been Discovered Three Times since 1980? A News Media Analysis." *Perspectives on Social Problems* 8: 3–25.

Flint, J. (2000). "Genetic Influences on Emotionality." In D. W. Pfaff, W. H. Berrettini, T. H. Joh, and S. C. Maxson, eds. *Genetic Influences on Neural and Behavioral Functions.* Boca Raton, Fla.: CRC: 431–58.

Hamer, D., and P. Copeland. (1998). *Living With Our Genes: Why They Matter More Than You Think.* New York: Doubleday.

Harris, T., R. Parrot, and K. Dorgan. (2004). "Talking about Human Genetics within Religious Frameworks." *Health Communication* 16(1): 105–16.

Herrnstein, R. J., and C. Murray. (1994). *The Bell Curve: Intelligence and Class Structure in American Life.* New York: The Free Press.

Hovarth, C. W. (1995). "Biological Origins of Communicator Style." *Communication Quarterly* 43: 394–407.

Kerr, A., S. Cunningham-Burley, and A. Amos. (1998). "Eugenics and the New Genetics in Britain: Examining Contemporary Professionals' Account." *Science, Technology, and Human Values* 23(Spring): 175–98.

King, D. K. (1988). "Multiple Jeopardy, Multiple Consciousness: The Content of a Black Feminist Ideology." *Journal of Women in Culture and Society* 14(11): 42–72.

Lewontin, R. C., S. Rose, and L. J. Kamin. (1984). *Not in Our Genes: Biology, Ideology and Human Nature*. New York: Pantheon.

McGuffin, P., B. Riley, and R. Plomin. (2001). "Toward Behavioral Genetics." *Science* 291: 1232–33.

Morgan, D. L., ed. (1993). *Successful Focus Groups: Advancing the State of the Art*. Newbury Park: Sage.

Morely, D. (1980). *The "Nationwide" Audience: Structure and Decoding*. London: British Film Institute.

Nelkin, D. (1999). "Behavioral Genetics and Dismantling the Welfare State." In R. A. Carson and M. A. Rothstein, eds. *Behavioral Genetics: The Clash of Culture and Biology*. Baltimore and London: Johns Hopkins University Press: 156–71.

Nelkin, D., and M. S. Lindee. (1995). *The DNA Mystique: The Gene as a Cultural Icon*. New York: W. H. Freeman.

Parrott R., K. Silk, and C. Condit. (2003). "Diversity in Lay Perceptions of the Sources of Human Traits: Genes, Environments, and Personal Behaviors." *Social Science and Medicine* 56: 1099–1109.

Pfaff, D. W., W. H. Berrettini, T. H. Joh, et al., eds. (2000). *Genetic Influences on Neural and Behavioral Functions*. Boca Raton, Fla.: CRC.

Phillips, L. (1995). "Who's Schooling Who? Black Women and the Bringing of Everyday into Academe, or Why We Started the Womanist." *Signs: Journal of Women in Culture and Society* 20:1007–18.

Plomin, R., J. C. DeFries, G. E. McClearn, et al. (1997). *Behavioral Genetics*. 3rd ed. New York: W. H. Freeman.

Radway, J. (1984). *Reading the Romance: Woman, Patriarchy, and Popular Literature*. Chapel Hill: University of North Carolina Press.

Rothstein, M. A. (1999). "Behavioral Genetic Determinism: Its Effects on Culture and Law." In R. A. Carson and M. A. Rothstein, eds. *Behavioral Genetics: The Clash of Culture and Biology*. Baltimore and London: Johns Hopkins University Press: 89–115.

Rowe, D. C. (1994). *The Limits of Family Influence: Genes, Experience, and Behavior*. New York: Guilford.

Rowe, D. C., and K. C. Jacobsen. (1999). "In the Mainstream: Research in Behavioral Genetics." In R. A. Carson and M. A. Rothstein, eds. *Behavioral Genetics: The Clash of Culture and Biology*. Baltimore and London: Johns Hopkins University Press: 12–34.

Stewart, D. W., and P. N. Shamdasani. (1990). *Focus Groups: Theory and Practice*. Newbury Park: Sage.

Tompkins, P. K. (1982). *Communication as Action: An Introduction to Rhetoric and Communication*. Belmont, Calif.: Wadsworth.

Turkheimer, E. (2000). "Three Laws of Behavior Genetics and What They Mean." *Current Directions in Psychological Science* 9: 160–64

Turney, J., and J. Turner. (2000). "Predictive Medicine, Genetics and Schizophrenia." *New Genetics and Society* 19: 1–22.

Wasserman, D., and R. Wachbroit, eds. (2001). *Genetics and Criminal Behavior*. Cambridge: Cambridge University Press.

CHAPTER FOURTEEN

Behavioral Genetics and the Media

Rick Weiss, M.A.

It's July 15, 1993. Torrential rains have left much of the Midwest underwater and President Clinton has just returned from a visit to the ravaged area. But reporters following the president aren't asking about the weather. Reporters live and die by deadlines, and back in January Clinton had set today as a deadline for himself. He had promised that by today he would finally decide whether to override the advice of his military leaders and reverse a 50-year-old ban on gays in the military.

The tension of that day capped a year in which gay and homosexual rights had repeatedly been prominent in the news. From Anchorage to St. Petersburg, several U.S. communities had passed local statutes either outlawing discrimination on the basis of sexual orientation or, as in the case of the Oregon farming town of Cornelius, explicitly banning the extension of civil rights to gays. In March, hundreds of thousands of gay rights activists had converged on Washington, D.C., to retake homosexuality as a natural right—as a trait as basic as race or sex. Two weeks later a furor had erupted when the Army discharged a Gulf War veteran and winner of the 6th Army's 1992 Soldier of the Year award for declaring his homosexuality at that march.

The world of culture, too, was ablaze with gay issues. Tony Kushner's epic play about AIDS in the Reagan era, *Angels in America,* was a Broadway hit. And Jonathan Tolins's new play, *The Twilight of the Golds,* was captivating audiences with its futuristic tale of a liberal Jewish couple deciding whether to abort a pregnancy after a prenatal test had predicted that the boy was likely to grow up gay.

This was the steamy political and cultural climate into which Clinton prepared to announce his now famous "don't ask, don't tell" policy. And this was the climate that news editors had been steeped in for months when, that afternoon, a 770-word wire-service story got beamed to newsroom computers around the country. "Researchers have identified a gene pattern linked to male homosexuality, adding powerful new evidence to the scientific theory that the tendency to be gay can be inherited," began the story by Paul Recer of the Associated Press (Recer, 1993). Thus began one of the bigger waves of media coverage of behavioral genetics in the past decade—and one of the bigger tests of American journalism's ability to navigate the rocky terrain of that nascent and controversy-prone branch of science.

Recer's lede was strong but also carefully worded, reflecting lessons learned in the late 1980s when "genes for" alcoholism, manic depression, and schizophrenia had been introduced with great fanfare only to slink away months later when follow-up studies could not back them up. Perhaps chastened by those experiences, Recer said nothing at the top of his story to suggest that a causative gene had actually been found, or that any single gene might by itself have the capacity to determine a person's sexual preference. Yet three paragraphs after that eminently responsible opening, the words *gay* and *gene* pop up as an irrepressible pair. "Evidence of a gay gene," the story says. Suddenly, with those words, the story slips into an old pattern. And readers on the brink of getting educated about the true nature of polygenic traits are instead invited to come to the conclusion that the Gold family is not so futuristic after all.

It's tempting to say that the coverage surrounding that 1993 study was better than the coverage that came before it and less sophisticated than the coverage that followed in years to come. And certainly to some extent that is true. Early stories in the 1980s often failed to make the distinction between the discovery of an actual gene and the mere discovery of a stretch of DNA or genetic "markers" associated with a behavioral trait. And early stories often mistakenly implied that certain genes were linked to certain ailments, rather than noting that in fact virtually everyone inherits every gene in the human genome and that only certain versions of those genes, or alleles, are problematic. Both of those errors seem less common today.

Yet problems clearly persist, including the one perpetrated by Recer in his 1993 report: many stories are plagued by that elusive "gene for," providing in one paragraph all the appropriate warnings against overinterpreting the data and then, in the next paragraph—apparently unable to resist—using language that only strengthens those misinterpretations. It's as though we writers believe we can claim legal immunity as long as we scatter enough caveats throughout our stories. Unfortunately, phrases such as "gay gene" are likely to stick with readers more than the staid warnings found elsewhere in a story. Which means that, in behavioral genetics at least, news reports may need to be nearly perfect if they are to avoid doing more harm than good. And unfortunately, as described below, that's going to be an increasingly difficult standard to achieve given some worrisome trends in journalism that are making it more difficult than ever for reporters to include the details such reporting requires.

This chapter does not try to quantify the accuracy of news coverage of behavior genetics or document objective trends. Rather, what follows is a set of examples and impressions from someone who has participated in the lurching journalistic effort to cover the field during the past decade or so—with prime emphasis on newspaper coverage, with which I am most familiar. And in the fine journalistic tradition of billboarding the main points up high in a story so a copy editor can cut from the end with impunity, let's just say right up front that mistakes have been made. Some stories have oversimplified the links between genes and behaviors and others have overstated the certainty of new findings. At the same time, even some of the first reports of links between genes and behaviors included many of the caveats one would hope to find in such stories (although some should have appeared higher in the stories than they did). And happily, lessons seem to have been learned—not only with regard to the scientific content of articles but also with regard to their placement and play. Nowadays it's not easy to get a story about a putative behavioral gene on the front page, and rightly so.

In many respects, of course, the challenges inherent in covering behavioral genetics—and the failings that have ensued—are no different than those seen in other fields of science. Scientific truth has a long history of being maimed in the process of being extruded through the die of science journalism. Every branch of science has been abused, and all types of scientists have been burned at one time or another as their findings flew from the lab bench to the lino-type machine.

Some of these problems are inevitable. The art of science and the art of jour-nalism may share important principles, among them the standard of inde-pendent verification. (Just as scientists know that an "n of 1" tells little about the larger universe, editors don't waste a lot of ink on single-source stories.) But journalistic truth and scientific truth are not the same things, and a first rough draft of history cannot pretend to be a peer-reviewed journal article.

But while every branch of science takes its chances when it dares to com-mit news, each has its own Achilles heel when it comes to precisely how or why the media is likely to misrepresent its findings. Behavioral science has at least three.

First, it involves molecular genetics, a relatively new science the basic tenets of which remain unfamiliar to many reporters and the public. It's been two and a half decades since Cambridge, Massachusetts, townsfolk got uppity about recombinant research going on at local laboratories, launching the mod-ern era of genetics news coverage (McElheny, 1975; McWethy, 1975). Today, countless column inches later, a large core of Americans remains unsure about what DNA really is, or whether a gene is bigger or smaller than a cell. Just a few years ago, a majority of people surveyed in Britain agreed with the statement that the main difference between genetically engineered tomatoes and con-ventional tomatoes was that the former have genes while the latter do not (An-gell, personal communication). Oh, well.

Second, behavioral genetics takes place in a world of higher-level mathe-matics and statistics that few reporters or readers really grasp. Given the real-ity that even simple behaviors emerge from the interactions of many genes, the search for statistically meaningful correlations between individual genes and complex behaviors demands sophisticated computations. Without some mathematical and statistical grounding, it's easy for reporters and the public to get fooled by flawed evidence of linkage or causality. At times it seems as though we'd all inherited the gene for gullibility.

Third, behavioral genetics can lead to conclusions that are personally trou-bling and politically explosive. The discovery of links between genes and be-havior can seem to challenge deeply held beliefs about free will, predestiny, blame, shame, personal responsibility, heroism, altruism, laziness, greed, and criminal justice. It can seem to challenge bedrock notions of democracy and egalitarianism. Given all that, writers can be excused for sometimes tying themselves in knots as they try to report on new findings in the field. And readers may be excused if they are sometimes too quick to accept findings that jibe with their own prejudices, social theories, or religious beliefs—or for being too dismissive of findings that contradict those beliefs.

So how has journalism handled the challenge? The modern era of reporting on behavioral genetics arguably began on February 26, 1987. That was the day an issue of *Nature* came out with a genetic study of manic-depressive illness in a cohort of Amish people in Lancaster County, Pennsylvania (Egeland et al., 1987). It was a tricky story to write because, unlike other studies from that era linking newly discovered genes to diseases, this study did not identify any single gene. Rather, it found a link between manic depression and a region of chromosome 11.

Here is how Malcolm Ritter of the Associated Press first reported the finding: "Scientists for the first time have linked some cases of manic-depressive illness to a defective gene, a breakthrough they say could improve the understanding of schizophrenia and other psychiatric disorders" (Ritter, 1987). One can almost hear the whistles and see the red flags. Most important, and most obvious: that sure sounds like scientists have found a gene. Not until the last sentence of this 572-word story do we learn that, in fact, no gene has been identified. And in retrospect, at least, the leap to those "other psychiatric disorders" seems a bit premature.

To his credit, though, Ritter noted in his lede that the link is only to "some" cases of manic-depressive illness—an implicit acknowledgment of two other articles in that same week's issue of *Nature*—articles that found no link between that particular genetic locus and depressive illness in two other cohorts (Hodgkinson et al., 1987; Detera-Wadleigh et al., 1987). Little could Ritter have known that in the years to come such contradictions among behavioral genetics studies would become the rule.

Like the AP, the *Washington Post* overstated the nature of the new findings in a front- page story: "Researchers have located a gene that triggers a form of depression, establishing biological proof of the theory that it is an inheritable, genetically based disease," wrote Philip J. Hilts (Hilts, 1987). Only in the fourth paragraph from the last in this 21-paragraph story did readers get a hint—and only a hint—that in fact, no gene had yet been found. Moreover, the terms *inheritable* and *genetically based* never got defined, leaving readers unclear about the possible role of other factors.

But if blame is to be doled out for these overly deterministic takes on manic depression, at least some must be laid on scientists and mental health experts, many of whom were heady at the time with the promise then being posed by the new genetics. "If there was anyone who doubted still the biological nature of mental illness, this is a critical demonstration of that fact," National Institute of Mental Health clinical director Rex Cowdry is quoted as saying in Hilts's article (Hilts, 1987). One would like to think that today such a quote could not pass without the addition of some defining nuances about the meaning of "biological nature."

Erring somewhat differently, Thomas H. Maugh II of the *Los Angeles Times* led this way: "The first strong proof that psychiatric illnesses can be inherited has emerged from a decade-long study, and the discovery could be a major advance in the detection and treatment of mental illness, scientists are reporting today" (Maugh, 1987).

Of course, it's the predisposition and not the illness that's inherited, and epidemiological studies had already offered plenty of "strong proof" that manic depression and other mental illnesses had a heritable component. Helping the situation, the *Los Angeles Times* ran that page 1 story to the tune of 979 words, a generous allotment that allowed Maugh to make important clarifying points farther down. Importantly, for example, he paraphrased a scientist saying, "not everyone who has the gene will develop the illness, and . . . environmental factors are also important" (Maugh was quoting biologist and study author David E. Housman of MIT). Later he had the same scientist warning that "manic-depressive illness is so widespread in the general population that more than one gene may be associated with a predisposition to it." Those caveats would later become commonplace in behavioral genetics stories. And even way back then in 1987, Maugh raised with some prescience a key social implication of the research that would later arise with the "gay gene" study and others, noting that the discovery "may remove some of the stigma from mental illness."

A month later, United Press International botched an interpretation of a follow-up study, reporting wrongly that a team had "traced the gene that causes" manic-depressive illness in a different group of families when in fact the researchers had simply identified a link to the X chromosome (Young, 1987). That report also mischaracterized the previous month's findings involving the Amish, saying scientists had in that case "reported discovery of the gene that causes manic depression in Pennsylvania Amish families."

Over time, however, most reporters learned the difference between actually finding a gene associated with a disease and simply finding a chromosomal region associated with that trait—a lesson that was in evidence by November 1988, when news broke about a putative gene linked to schizophrenia (Sherrington et al., 1988). "Researchers have found evidence that a single gene can help trigger schizophrenia, and have estimated its approximate location," wrote AP's Ritter (Ritter, 1988a), who deserves kudos for his use of the conditional word *evidence* and his instant acknowledgment that no exact genetic location had been mapped. A rewrite by Ritter the following day softened the lede even more, saying: "A study has found evidence of a hereditary link to schizophrenia" (Ritter, 1988b).

In an uncharacteristic but workable punt, the *New York Times* fell back on the scientists' own words to describe what, exactly, had been found in that schizophrenia study. "An international research team has announced that it has found 'the first concrete evidence for a genetic basis to schizophrenia,' one of the most devastating and widespread varieties of mental illness," wrote Harold M. Schmeck Jr. on page 1 (Schmeck, 1988). A few sentences later, Schmeck added other important details, saying the study "finds a link between schizophrenia and an abnormally functioning gene or cluster of genes on a part of chromosome 5, one of the 46 human chromosomes that contain the complete archive of heredity for every person. The gene itself is still unidentified, but the discovery of its approximate location may help scientists identify the specific gene that is abnormal in these cases."

And importantly, as part of an explanation for why other studies had found no link between the locus and the disease in other schizophrenics, Schmeck made the point that such studies are complicated by the squishiness of the diagnostic criteria for schizophrenia: "schizophrenia is really a catch-all term for a biologically heterogeneous group of diseases that produce much the same symptoms," Schmeck wrote.

Interestingly, Maugh of the *Los Angeles Times* led with the same quote used by Schmeck, but by substituting some of his own words in that sentence he inflicted an unfortunate change upon its meaning (Maugh, 1988). "An international team of researchers today reported 'the first concrete evidence' that schizophrenia can be caused by a genetic defect," Maugh wrote, adding the worrisome word *caused,* with all its implications that environmental influences may be irrelevant.

About a year and a half later, in April 1990, behavioral genetics was again in the news, this time with a report in the *Journal of the American Medical As-*

sociation finding a link between a particular gene variant and alcoholism (Blum et al., 1990). This time, the *New York Times,* which played the news on the front page, was among those outlets that withheld until relatively low in the story some of the standard caveats one might wish to see: "A gene that puts people at risk of becoming alcoholics has been identified for the first time, scientists report in a study being published today," wrote Lawrence K. Altman, who apparently trusted the findings enough to avoid the conditional construction of "appears to put people at risk" or "may put people at risk" (Altman, 1990). That lede was followed by no fewer than eight paragraphs of additional details that generally presumed the validity of the results before the story turned to some warnings, arguably a tad too late: "Scientists generally accept the notion that alcoholism is based on complex genetic, cultural and social factors . . . The researchers said no single gene, including this one, caused all forms of alcoholism . . . Social and cultural factors may set off the affliction for many alcoholics who are not genetically predisposed to the disease."

Most reporters took a more cautious approach. And why not? By now the field of behavioral genetics, young as it was, was already getting a reputation for unreliability. Those previous studies identifying genetic links with schizophrenia and manic depression had already been undermined in follow-up studies (Detera-Wadleigh et al., 1989; Berrettini et al., 1990). And while those negative studies got less coverage than the initial findings—a problem that has long plagued science journalism—reporters were starting to worry that they had been a bit too willing to buy into the earlier work.

The *Washington Post*'s Malcolm Gladwell led his page 3 story (Gladwell, 1990) with at least three warning flags: "Scientists say they have found, for the first time, a genetic abnormality strongly linked to alcoholism, a discovery that—if confirmed and extended—could lead to more effective understanding and treatment of one of mankind's most debilitating diseases." Note the use of the word *say* in the first clause, the words *strongly linked to,* and the mention of a need for further confirmation.

Similarly, Brenda Coleman of the Associated Press opened her story this way: "Researchers say they have pinpointed for the first time a gene that may make people prone to alcoholism, adding weight to the argument that alcoholism is a disease and not a moral weakness" (Coleman, 1990). The very next sentence made the additional points that the study, while provocative, was preliminary and that it would be wrong to conclude that an "alcohol gene" had been discovered. Coleman also made it clear that the risk of alcoholism in the study was linked not just to a gene, but to a particular version, or allele, of that gene.

USA Today's Tim Friend also went with a cautious lede—indeed, one so riddled with caveats that it's almost surprising it made it onto the front page: "A specific gene associated with alcoholism appears to have been located for the first time, new research suggests" (Friend, 1990). Note the words *associated with* instead of *that may cause,* the words *appears to be* instead of *has been,* and the popular warning phrase "new research suggests." Not only that, the first few words of the next sentence are: "The discovery must be confirmed." That's four elements of conditionality in the first sentence and a half.

Several of the stories written about the alcoholism link brought into focus a common problem in behavioral genetics reporting: how to balance the twin desires to absolve people of blame for their illnesses and to not take from people the belief that they still have some control over their lives. The *USA Today* story, for example, was one of many that day that focused on the study's implication that alcoholism is more properly a matter of medicine, not morality. The new research, Friend wrote, supported the idea that "alcoholism is hereditary rather than a 'moral weakness.'" Yet much later in the story, the point is made that people who inherit the gene (actually the allele, of course) "are not destined to develop alcoholism because environment and behavior also play a role." The reference to environment is a welcome one. Yet the mention of behavior as an additional influencing factor is curious. What does it mean? Is that a reference to free will? And if so, does that suggest that alcoholism is in fact, at least in part, a "moral failing" after all?

It was around this time that the unreliability of behavioral genetics findings was becoming as big a story as the latest findings themselves, with several reporters doing wrap-up stories tracking the rise and fall of various candidate genes. As *Newsday*'s Robert Cooke wrote in an October 1990 story about the emerging pattern of overturned behavioral genetics findings: "A critical lesson from the race to uncover important genes is that it pays to keep an eraser handy" (Cooke, 1990).

The uncertainties inherent in behavioral genetics research became unavoidable news in October 1991 when the *Journal of the American Medical Association* came out with a pair of contradictory studies in the same issue, one confirming the 1990 link between alcoholism and a particular dopamine receptor gene allele and the other finding no such association (Cloninger, 1991; Gelernter et al., 1991).

The *Washington Post* story carried the sober headline: "Genetic Studies Yield Opposite Results; Connection between DNA 'Marker' and Alcoholism Remains Unclear" (Brown, 1991). "The murky realm of science in which genes are searched for possible effects on complex human behaviors has yielded two contradictory studies about the risks for alcoholism laid out back-to-back in the same scientific journal," wrote the *Post*'s David Brown. "One study found a strong relationship between alcoholism and possible defects in a particular gene active in the brain. The other found no relationship whatsoever," Brown wrote.

Yet not everyone was willing to live with that uncertainty. Under a one-sided headline that read "Study Supports Genetic Link to Alcoholism," the *Los Angeles Times* led its story that day with three full paragraphs about the gene-confirming study (Scott, 1991). Only halfway through the fourth paragraph is there even a mention of the contradictory research published in the same issue of the journal. Perhaps it is just a coincidence that the initial 1990 study and the confirmatory 1991 study both were led by Californians while the dissenting research came out of Yale.

Then, in 1993, came the most explosive behavioral genetics story yet: Dean Hamer's now famous study suggesting that a single chromosomal region might predispose men to being gay (Hamer et al., 1993). My favorite report from that Thursday morning's batch of newspapers was the one on the front page of the *New York Times* (though, in the interest of full disclosure, it was written by my wife): "Ushering the politically explosive study of the origins of sexual orientation into a new and perhaps more scientifically rigorous phase, researchers report that they have linked male homosexuality to a small region of one human chromosome," Natalie Angier wrote (Angier, 1993).

The *perhaps* in that lede was bold, almost cheeky. And the second paragraph is quick with the caveats: "The results have yet to be confirmed by other laboratories, and the chromosomal region implicated, if it holds up under further scrutiny, is almost surely just a single chapter in the intricate story of sexual orientation and behavior." And while the findings "indicate that sexual orientation often is at least partly inborn, rather than being solely a matter of choice," Angier's story continues, "researchers warn against over-interpreting the work, or in taking it to mean anything as simplistic as that the 'gay gene' had been found."

The *Washington Post*'s Boyce Rensberger also struck the right balance (Rensberger, 1993). "Scientists at the National Institutes of Health have discovered evidence that some gay men have inherited one or more genes that predisposed them to be homosexual," the story opened, with all the conditionality one could hope for. The story continued: "The findings—which must be confirmed by a repeat study—do not prove there is a 'gay gene' that invariably causes homosexuality or that all gay men have it. But they strongly suggest there are genes that increase the likelihood that males will turn out to be homosexual and that such genes played a role in influencing the sexual orientation of a significant—though still unknown—percentage of homosexual men." The next sentence also made it clear that what was really at issue was a version of the gene in question, not the gene itself. On the other hand, it wasn't until eight long paragraphs into that story that Rensberger explicitly notified readers that, in fact, no individual gene had yet been identified but rather a chromosomal region.

USA Today, doing what it does best, seemed to say it all in just a few words: "A predisposition to homosexuality appears to be written into the very genes of some men," Kim Painter wrote with elegant simplicity (Painter, 1993). Painter was also one of several writers quick to make the provocative point that the gene locus in question was on the X chromosome, which boys get from their mothers. Some, including the *San Francisco Chronicle*'s Charles Petit, couldn't resist putting that fact in the very first sentence: "A government genetic research team reported strong new evidence linking a gene or set of genes to homosexuality in men, and it said the trait was passed down by their mothers," Petit wrote (Petit, 1993).

Alas, some newspapers fell back on the by-then discredited "gene for" construction. The *Dallas Morning News* said scientists had found the location of "a possible gene or set of genes for homosexuality" (Beil, 1993). And even the next sentence, which warns that no "gay gene" has been found, seems to hint that there may be one out there to find: "The scientists . . . say they haven't pinpointed a gay gene. But they have narrowed down the location to a small stretch of the X chromosome, which in men is always inherited from their mothers."

Television was even faster and looser with the terminology. The *MacNeil/Lehrer NewsHour* that Thursday night led with a teaser that invited viewers to stay tuned for a major report "on the search for the homosexual gene" (MacNeil/Lehrer, 1993). After devoting some time to the Midwestern floods, the show announced the new findings and jumped right to an interview with the parents of three grown sons, two of them heterosexual and one gay. The parents recalled a Christmas when the boys were still quite young, when the two who eventually turned out to be heterosexual were playing with the war toys they'd asked for and the one who turned out gay was playing with the toys he had asked for: a baby doll and kitchen set. The presumption seems to be that not only does a gene encode homosexuality but also the gene somehow determines one's taste for culturally determined sex-role-appropriate playthings. On *Nightline* that same night, Ted Koppel announced: "A new study identifies the very genes that may be a key to male homosexuality" (ABC News, *Nightline*, 1993). A few seconds later, Koppel made the additional mistake of using the "D-word," saying the new study "shows that male homosexuality may be genetically determined."

Did Hamer's work deserve to be on the front pages of so many of the nation's newspapers and at the top of the evening news on television? Even ignoring what we know now—that Hamer's findings have failed to be independently replicated—one could argue that, given the poor track record of the previous years' findings in behavioral genetics, editors should have been more cautious in their coverage. But I'd argue that the story was played correctly. After all, a lot goes into the decision of which seven or eight stories should make it onto the front page, and scientific reliability is just one of them for science stories.

Indeed, some criteria for choosing front-page stories are quite the opposite of those used by scientists. Counterintuitiveness, for example, is a selling point in the news business. Everyone knows that it's news when a man bites a dog, but not the reverse. By contrast, scientists are skeptical of findings that don't fit existing models, and tend to demand extra proof before giving those findings much display. Most important, however, homosexuality and gay rights had loomed large in the news for months before Hamer's study went to press. And for better or worse, news judgment tends to be very inertial, with topics already deemed newsworthy more likely to get followed while others have to fight for their debut. Given the context of the previous months' events, even preliminary evidence of a genetic component to homosexuality—with all its implications for genetic discrimination and molecular "correction"—was virtually assured of getting the play it got.

The more pressing question is not whether such stories belong on the front page (the process of selecting A1 stories will always be quirky) but whether reporters, in the future, will be able to continue to improve their coverage given some worrisome trends in journalism—and science journalism in particular.

Perhaps prime among them is that of the Incredible Shrinking News Hole. In news-speak, the news hole is the amount of page space available for news, as opposed to space for advertisements, photographs, or other purposes. Some newspapers have historically had larger news holes than others. The *Los Angeles Times* is famous, and in some circles infamous, for the generous lengths of its feature stories. At the other end of the spectrum, *USA Today* has invented what amounts to journalistic haiku. And television and radio news spots are almost comically short when it comes to the number of words or ideas actually communicated in a typical 30-second or even one-minute science piece.

The news business is a business, of course, and the news is not the part of that business that directly brings in revenue. From the point of view of my fellow *Washington Post* workers who sell ads, the news is but a sales vehicle—essentially a lure—to get people to plop down 35 cents for a package of ads. Most publications would not go so far as to share the philosophy I once saw espoused in an editor's office at the *National Geographic* magazine: "Words," a little sign in that office declared, "are the walls upon which we hang our pictures." Still, news holes are increasingly seen as financial liabilities, and on average they are growing smaller at many newspapers. And while longer stories do not always do a better job of explaining science than shorter stories, smaller allocations of space make it less likely that a complex concept will get properly fleshed out and its nuances reliably explicated and balanced.

One might guess that the recent move toward more and more news on the Internet might act as an antidote to the space crunch. Newspapers and other news organizations are placing an ever-growing emphasis on their Web sites, in part to reach an audience far more geographically dispersed than can be achieved with actual home delivery of newsprint. Given the essentially infinite capacity for information on the Web, it seems logical that news-outlet Web sites could serve as "overflow" areas for all the details and fine print that may not make it into the paper or onto that 45-second newscast. But in general, news stories on the Internet tend to be, if anything, even more abbreviated than those that appear in print editions. This is a manifestation of two phenomena, both of which undermine news organizations' ability to educate the public about science.

First, in keeping with the longstanding emphasis on "scooping" the competition, news Web sites are mostly used as outlets for breaking news—that is, as a means of being the first to report that something happened. First reports of breaking news are typically short, if for no other reason than little is known.

It's not reasonable to expect the jumpy editors at News.com to spend their time editing a 100-inch thumb-sucker on the uncertain roles of various genes on various behaviors. The second reason news Web sites are not making up for shrinking print news holes is that, according to Webmeisters who have studied such stuff, people reading their news on the Web do not want to read long, detailed documents on their computers. Web readers are in a hurry, have short attention spans, and want the Cliff's Notes version of whatever they are looking at. If anything, they want to devote *less* time to a story than they would devote to the newsprint version.

Exacerbating the problem of the Incredible Shrinking News Hole for those who are trying to publish good science journalism is the problem of the Increasingly Shameless Marketing of Science. More and more science is trying to fit into less and less space. And just as a candidate for office can sometimes get elected not because of a superior grasp of the issues but because of a flashier campaign, so some stories make it into the news more on the basis of salesmanship than science. That means that even as reporters struggle for the space to explain the latest findings, they are also having to filter out a growing amount of overhyped material washing over the transom.

Many readers in the general public are not aware of how scientific discoveries get pitched to the media, much less how much more aggressively they are pitched today than they were, say, 10 years ago. Most of the major scientific journals release summaries of upcoming issues to reporters in advance, including full-text versions of key papers and contact information to ease the job of interviewing the relevant scientists. But they don't stop there. Many journal editors send these along to the media accompanied by introductory comments that are, in essence, little sales pitches to encourage reporters to follow up on the stories. Scientific journals, no less than scientific personages, have an interest in seeing their names in the newspaper. It is no coincidence that most of the major weekly journals come out on their own days of the week— the *Proceedings of the National Academy of Sciences* on Monday, the *Journal of the American Medical Association* on Tuesday, *Nature* (and, in a rare conflict, the *New England Journal of Medicine*) on Wednesday, *Science* on Thursday, and the *Lancet* on Friday—assuring a minimum of competition for that shrinking daily news hole.

The language in these weekly "poop sheets" (a newsroom term with roots in the phrase "What's the poop?" but which also carries with it an increasingly appropriate implication of a need for hip boots) at times borders on hyperventilation. There seems to be a fear among science journal editors that science writers may not appreciate a huge breakthrough when they see one. The downside, of course, is that preliminary findings—especially in young fields like behavioral genetics—are likely to get touted as being more certain or more meaningful than they are.

Scientists themselves seem similarly drawn to selling, or overselling, their work. One scientist, speaking to a colleague of mine at the *New York Times* a few years ago, went so far as to admit that, as far as he was concerned, the second most important recognition of his scientific worth, other than winning a Nobel Prize, would be to have his work featured on the front page of the *Times*. So it is that universities and other research institutions unleash a weekly torrent of news releases, advisories, backgrounders, and assorted poop sheets of their own, touting the work of their faculty members, no matter how unformed or unreplicated the findings. Some of these professionals go even further. They call and e-mail to cajole reporters, sometimes cleverly noting as an aside that, by the way, the other big newspaper in town is working up a story on this. "Just trying to be helpful," they say. "Wouldn't want you to look like you missed a story."

Geneticists in particular seem to have learned the fine art of making their work accessible by giving cute names to the genes or gene-altered creatures to which they have devoted their lives. When scientists at Princeton a few years back made a gene-altered mouse with an enhanced ability to remember and learn, they called the rodent the "Doogie mouse," after the precocious television medical doctor Doogie Hauser, M.D. (Tang et al., 1999). Only an editor with a tin ear for news could pass that story up. Only later did it come out, to far less fanfare, that the "genius gene" also played a role in pain signal transmission—and that Doogie and his other seemingly medical school-bound mice were living their lives in chronic pain (Wei et al., 2001). So much for that ticket to gene-based smart pills. And so much for the prolonged honeymoon that behavioral genetics enjoyed during the first decade or so of its modern existence. In recent years very few "discoveries" of behavioral genes have cleared the bar of newsworthiness as gun-shy editors demand some assurance that the findings will not disappear like so many others. Those stories that do see the light of day typically run small, inside, and are heavily laden with caveats.

Given the difficulties posed by the field of behavioral genetics generally, and the forces within journalism that today are making it difficult for reporters to fully interpret and explicate the latest findings, perhaps a few basic rules for such coverage are in order. I suggest the following catechism as a start, to be repeated daily by all reporters covering this problematic field:

1. I believe that behaviors are complex traits, representing the concatenation of multiple genetic and environmental influences. Never again shall I write the words "a gene for" or the words "the [your trait here] gene."
2. I recognize that the separation between genes and environment is to a degree contrived, with the actions of each constantly influencing the other, muddying the boundary between the two. Never again, lacking evidence of true autosomal dominance and close to 100 percent penetrance, shall I write that a gene "causes" a disease-behavioral or otherwise.
3. I appreciate that the techniques used by behavior geneticists are often imprecise and easily misinterpreted, in part because of the way behaviors or phenotypes are categorized or diagnosed in the first place.
4. I know that the discovery of a gene that merely contributes to a behavior says nothing about the moral or social acceptability of that behavior, and so does not logically insist upon any particular public policy response to that behavior.
5. Yea, though the mathematics used by behavior geneticists are often beyond me and seem too difficult to explain, I will find myself a reliable source to bounce those stats off of before going to print.

I also recommend that reporters covering behavioral genetics use two unassuming but powerful questions that are favorites of investigative reporters but which are so simple they often go unasked: "What do you mean?" (as in, "What do you mean that manic depression is heritable?") and "How do you know that?"

In the years to come, behavioral genetics is sure to pose ever more findings to be interpreted and transmitted by the media. And just as other hot topics in recent years—including reproductive biology, gene therapy, and stem cell research—have required science reporters to get educated about much more than the science itself, the coming revolution in behavioral genetics will demand that science reporters become knowledgeable about much more than behavior and genetics. We will need to talk to experts and read up on such diverse subjects as the history of notions of intelligence; the theories of personal responsibility and criminal justice; and the philosophies of free will and predestiny. That's a big assignment. But not too much to ask as we chase what is, really, the only story ever worth writing: the story of who we are as humans, and what makes us tick.

REFERENCES

ABC News. (1993). *Nightline,* July 15, "The Genetic Link to Male Homosexuality."
Altman, L. K. (1990). "Scientists See a Link between Alcoholism and a Specific Gene." *New York Times* (April 18): A1, column 1.
Angell, P. (former director of corporate communications for Monsanto). Personal communication.
Angier, N. (1993). "Report Suggests Homosexuality Is Linked to Genes." *New York Times* (July 16): A1, column 2.
Beil, C. (1993). "Study Links Genetics to Homosexuality; Scientists See Possibility of Other Causes, Need for More Research." *Dallas Morning News* (July 16): 1A.
Berrettini, W. H., L. R. Goldin, J. Gelernter, et al. (1990). "X-Chromosome Markers and Manic-Depressive Illness: Rejection of Linkage to Xq28 in Nine Bipolar Pedigrees." *Archives of General Psychiatry* 7(4): 366–73.
Blum, K., E. P. Noble, P. J. Sheridan, et al. (1990). "Allelic Association of Human Dopamine D2 Receptor Gene in Alcoholism." *Journal of the American Medical Association* 63(15): 2055–60.
Brown, D. (1991). "Genetic Studies Yield Opposite Results; Connection between DNA 'Marker' and Alcoholism Remains Unclear." *Washington Post* (October 2): A3.
Cloninger, C. R. (1991). "D2 Dopamine Receptor Gene Is Associated But Not Linked with Alcoholism." *Journal of the American Medical Association* 266(13): 1833–34.
Coleman, B. C. (1990). "Researchers Say They Have Identified Gene Linked to Alcoholism." Associated Press, April 17, Tuesday a.m. cycle.
Cooke, R. (1990). "Now You See 'Em, Now You Don't; Scientists Trying to Identify Single Genes among the 100,000 in Human Chromosomes Often Seem to Have One Cornered, Then Lose It." *Newsday* (New York) (October 23): 6.
Detera-Wadleigh, S. D., W. H. Berrettini, L. R. Goldin, et al. (1987). "Close Linkage of c-Harvey-ras-1 and the Insulin Gene to Affective Disorder Is Ruled Out in Three North American Pedigrees." *Nature* 325(6107): 806–8.
Detera-Wadleigh, S. D., L. R. Goldin, R. Sherrington, et al. (1989). "Exclusion of Linkage to 5q11–13 in Families with Schizophrenia and Other Psychiatric Disorders." *Nature* 340(6232): 391–93.
Egeland, J. A., D. S. Gerhard, D. L. Pauls, et al. (1987). "Bipolar Affective Disorders Linked to DNA Markers on Chromosome 11." *Nature* 325(6107): 783–87.
Friend, T. (1990). "Heredity, Alcoholism Link Seen." *USA Today* (April 18): 1A.
Gelernter, J., S. O'Malley, N. Risch, et al. (1991). "No Association between an Allele at the D2 Dopamine Receptor Gene (DRD2) and Alcoholism." *Journal of the American Medical Association* 266(13): 1801–7.
Gladwell, M. (1990). "Genetic Tie to Alcoholism Is Reportedly Discovered; Aberrant Gene Is Found in Most Cases Studied." *Washington Post* (April 18): A3.

Hamer, D. H., S. Hu, V. L. Magnuson, et al. (1993). "Linkage between DNA Markers on the X Chromosome and Male Sexual Orientation." *Science* 261(5119): 321–27.

Hilts, P. J. (1987). "Manic-Depression Gene Found; Hereditary Nature of Disease Established." *Washington Post* (February 26): A1.

Hodgkinson S., R. Sherrington, H. Gurling, et al. (1987). "Molecular Genetic Evidence for Heterogeneity in Manic Depression." *Nature* 325(6107): 805–6.

MacNeil/Lehrer *NewsHour* (1993) July 15, Thursday, Transcript 4711, "Sexual Chemistry."

Maugh, T. H., II. (1987). "Genetic Marker Found; Psychiatric Illnesses Can Be Inherited, Study Shows." *Los Angeles Times* (February 26): 1, column 1.

Maugh, T. H., II. (1988). "Study Ties Schizophrenia to Genetic Flaw." *Los Angeles Times* (November 10): A44, column 1.

McElheny, V. K. (1975). *New York Times* (January 22, February 28); *Newsweek* (March 10).

McWethy, J. (1975). "A Move to Protect Mankind." *U.S. News and World Report* (April 7): 66.

Painter, K. (1993). "Is There a Gay Gene? Key Evidence: More Maternal Kin Are Gay." *USA Today* (July 16): 1A.

Petit, C. (1993). "New Evidence of 'Gay Gene' in Some Men; Study Says Hereditary Trait Is Passed Along by Mothers." *San Francisco Chronicle* (July 16): A1.

Recer, P. (1993). "Researchers Find Genetic Link to Homosexuality." Associated Press, July 15, Thursday a.m. cycle, Washington Dateline.

Rensberger, B. (1993). "Study Links Genes to Homosexuality; NIH Finds Gay Men Share Chromosomal Characteristics." *Washington Post* (July 16): A1.

Ritter, M. (1987). "Scientists Link Manic-Depressive Illness to Faulty Gene." Associated Press, February 25, Wednesday a.m. cycle.

Ritter, M. (1988a). "Gene May Help Trigger Schizophrenia, New Study Says." Associated Press, November 9, Wednesday a.m. cycle.

Ritter, M. (1988b). "Evidence of Hereditary Link to Schizophrenia Reported." Associated Press, November, Thursday p.m. cycle.

Schmeck, H. M., Jr. (1988). "Schizophrenia Study Finds Strong Signs of Hereditary Cause." *New York Times* (November 10): A1, column 1.

Scott, J. (1991). "Study Supports Genetic Link to Alcoholism; Medicine: Duarte City of Hope Researchers Say Their Findings Confirm Controversial Earlier Results. But They Suspect That the Gene Is a 'Modifying' One That, with Other Factors, Increases Risk." *Los Angeles Times* (October 2): B1, column 2.

Sherrington, R., J. Brynjolfsson, H. Petursson, et al. (1988). "Localization of a Susceptibility Locus for Schizophrenia on Chromosome 5." *Nature* 33 (6195): 164–67.

Tang, Y. P., E. Shimizu, G. R. Dube, et al. (1999). "Genetic Enhancement of Learning and Memory in Mice." *Nature* 401(6748): 63–69.

Wei, F., G. D. Wang, G. A. Kerchner, et al. (2001). "Genetic Enhancement of Inflammatory Pain by Forebrain NR2B Overexpression." *Nature Neuroscience* 4(2): 164–69.

Young, G. (1987). "Second Genetic Link to Manic Depression Found." United Press International, March 18, Wednesday a.m. cycle.

Index

Page numbers in *italics* refer to figures or tables.